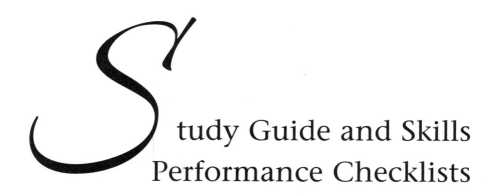

Study Guide and Skills Performance Checklists

to Accompany

Canadian Fundamentals of Nursing

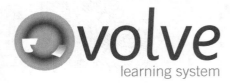

volve
learning system

Evolve provides online access to free learning resources and activities designed specifically for the textbook you are using in your class. The resources will provide you with information that enhances the material covered in the book and much more.

Visit the Web address listed below to start your learning evolution today!

http://evolve.elsevier.com/Canada/Potter/fundamental

Evolve® Student Learning Resources for Potter & Perry, Canadian Fundamentals of Nursing, 4th Edition, offer the following features:

Student Resources

- **Audio Summaries for each chapter are downloadable to an MP3 device or CD.**
- **Student Learning Activities include Hangman, Match Its, and Drag and Drop exercises.**
- **Animations feature exciting images related to various chapters in the textbook.**
- **Video Clips demonstrate important aspects of various nursing skills described in the textbook.**
- **Web links are a useful resource that allows you link to hundreds of Web sites carefully chosen to supplement the content of the textbook.**
- **Content Updates include the latest information from the authors of the textbook to help you keep abreast of recent developments in select areas of study.**

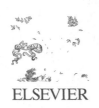

ELSEVIER

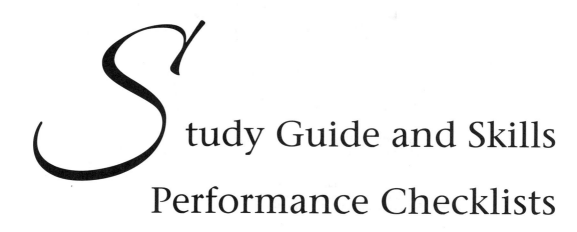

Study Guide and Skills Performance Checklists

to Accompany

POTTER/PERRY
Canadian Fundamentals of Nursing
4th edition

Geralyn Ochs, RN, MSN, BC-ACNP, ANP
Assistant Professor of Nursing
St. Louis University School of Nursing
St. Louis, Missouri

Skills Performance Checklists by
Jerilee LaMar, PhD, RN, BC
Assistant Professor of Nursing
University of Evansville
Evansville, Indiana

Linda Turchin, RN, MSN
Assistant Professor
Fairmont State University
Fairmont, West Virginia

Canadian Editors
Janet C. Ross-Kerr, RN, BScN, MS, PhD
Professor Emeritus
Faculty of Nursing
University of Alberta
Edmonton, Alberta

Marilynn J. Wood, BSN, MSN, DrPH
Professor Emeritus
Faculty of Nursing
University of Alberta
Edmonton, Alberta

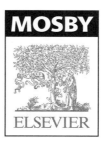

MOSBY

ELSEVIER

MOSBY
ELSEVIER

NOTICE

Knowledge and best practice in this field are constantly changing. As new research and expertise broaden our knowledge, changes in practice, treatment, and drug therapy may become necessary or appropriate. Readers are advised to check the most current information provided (i) on procedures featured or (ii) by the manufacturer of each product to be administered and to verify the recommended dose or formula, the method and duration of administration, and contraindications. It is the responsibility of the practitioner, relying on his or her own experience and knowledge of the client, to make diagnoses, to determine dosages and the best treatment for each individual client, and to take all appropriate safety precautions. To the fullest extent of the law, neither the Publisher nor the Authors assume any liability for any injury and/or damage to persons or property arising out of or related to any use of the material contained in this book.

The Publisher

Library and Archives Canada Cataloguing in Publication

Study guide and skills performance checklists to accompany Potter/Perry Canadian fundamentals of nursing, fourth edition / [edited by] Geralyn Ochs; Canadian editors, Janet C. Ross-Kerr, Marilynn J. Wood; skills performance checklists by Jerilee LaMar, Linda Turchin.

ISBN-13 978-1-8974-2219-9
ISBN-10 1-8974-2219-9

1. Nursing–Problems, exercises, etc. 2. Nursing–Handbooks, manuals, etc.
I. Kerr, Janet C., 1940- II. Wood, Marilynn J. III. Ochs, Geralyn
IV. Title.

RT41.P68 2009 Suppl.   610.73   C2009-901665-6

Vice President, Publishing: Ann Millar
Developmental Editor: Toni Chahley
Managing Developmental Editor: Martina van de Velde
Managing Production Editor: Lise Dupont
Copy Editors: Jane Clark and Holly Dickinson
Cover, Interior Design: Christine Rae, Interrobang Graphics, Inc. (cover); Amy Buxton (interior)
Typesetting and Assembly: Macmillan Publishing Solutions
Printing and Binding: Transcontinental Printing

Elsevier Canada
905 King Street West, 4th Floor
Toronto, ON, Canada M6K 3G9
Phone: 1-866-896-3331
Fax: 1-866-359-9534

Printed in Canada

2 3 4 5   14 13 12 11 10

Working together to grow
libraries in developing countries

www.elsevier.com | www.bookaid.org | www.sabre.org

ELSEVIER   BOOK AID
International   Sabre Foundation

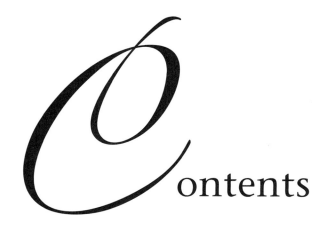

ontents

Unit I   Health and Health Care in Canada

Unit II   Foundations of Nursing Practice

Unit VII   *Scientific Basis for Nursing Practice*

Unit VIII   *Basic Physiological Needs*

$\mathcal{S}$kills Performance Checklists

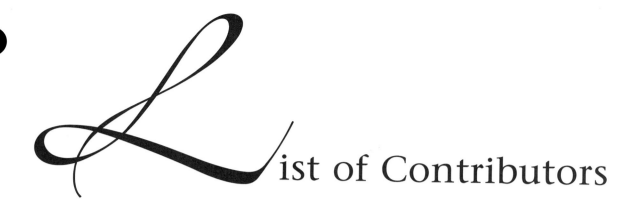

List of Contributors

Canadian Editors

Janet C. Ross-Kerr, RN, BScN, MS, PhD
Professor Emeritus, Faculty of Nursing
University of Alberta
Edmonton, Alberta

Marilynn J. Wood, BSN, MSN, DrPH
Professor Emeritus, Faculty of Nursing
University of Alberta
Edmonton, Alberta

Canadian Contributors

Barbara J. Astle, RN, PhD
University of Calgary
Calgary, Alberta

Colleen Astle, RN, MN
Nurse Practitioner, Nephrology
University of Alberta Hospital, Grey Nuns
    Hospital
Edmonton, Alberta

Sylvia S. Barton, RN, PhD
Associate Professor
University of Alberta
Edmonton, Alberta

Yvonne G. Briggs, RN, BScN, MN
Faculty, School of Nursing
Grant MacEwan College
Edmonton, Alberta

Corinne Crockett, RN, BScN, MHS(c)
Clinical Assistant, School of Nursing
UBC Okanagan
Kelowna, British Columbia

Susan M. Duncan, RN, PhD
Dean
School of Nursing
Thompson Rivers University
Kamloops, British Columbia

Kaysi Eastlick Kushner, RN, PhD
Associate Professor, Faculty of Nursing
University of Alberta
Edmonton, Alberta

Nancy A. Edgecombe, RN-NP, BN, MN, PhD
Assistant Professor, School of Nursing
Dalhousie University
Halifax, Nova Scotia

Frances Fothergill Bourbonnais, RN, BScN, MN, PhD
Full Professor
School of Nursing, Faculty of Health Sciences
University of Ottawa
Ottawa, Ontario

Jo-Ann E. T. Fox-Threlkeld, RN, BN, MSc, PhD
Professor Emeritus
McMaster University
Hamilton, Ontario

Michelle Funk, RN, BScN, MSN
Nurse Educator, School of Nursing
Thompson Rivers University
Kamloops, British Columbia

Nicole Harder, RN, BN, MPA, PhD(c)
Coordinator, Learning Laboratories
Faculty of Nursing
University of Manitoba
Winnipeg, Manitoba

Jim Hunter, RN, BSN, MSN
Program Head, Year 2
British Columbia Institute of Technology
Burnaby, British Columbia

Anne Katz, RN, PhD
Adjunct Professor
University of Manitoba
Winnipeg, Manitoba

Rosemary Kohr, RN, BA, BScN, MScN, PhD, ACNP(cert)
Advanced Practice Nurse
London Health Sciences Centre
Assistant Professor
Faculty of Health Sciences
University of Western Ontario
London, Ontario

Nicole Letourneau, RN, PhD
Canada Research Chair in Healthy Child
    Development
Peter Lougheed/CIHR New Investigator
    (honorary)
Professor, Faculty of Nursing and Research
    Fellow CRISP
University of New Brunswick
Fredericton, New Brunswick

Angela Luciani, RN, BScN, MN
Instructor, Faculty of Nursing
Nunavut Arctic College
Iqaluit, Nunavut

Melanie L. T. MacDonald, BScN, RN, MHSA, PhD(c)
Assistant Professor, School of Nursing
University of Prince Edward Island
Charlottetown, Prince Edward Island

Sally Naphan, RN, BA, BN, MA
Nursing Instructor
Nunavut Arctic College
Iqaluit, Nunavut

Judee E. Onyskiw, RN, PhD
Instructor and Research and Scholarship Advisor
School of Nursing
Faculty of Health and Community Studies
Grant MacEwan College
Edmonton, Alberta

Harry E. Peery, MS, PhD(c), RN
Brock University
St. Catharines, Ontario
University of Saskatchewan
Saskatoon, Saskatchewan
McMaster University
Hamilton, Ontario

Pammla Petrucka, RN, BSc, BScN, MN, PhD
Associate Professor
University of Saskatchewan
Regina, Saskatchewan

Cheryl Sams, RN, BScN, MSN
Professor
Seneca College
Toronto, Ontario

Michael Scarcello, RN, HBScN, MA(N)(c)
Faculty, Practical Nursing Program
Confederation College
Thunder Bay, Ontario

Lynne Thibeault, RN(EC), BScN, MEd, DNP(c)
Professor, Health Sciences, Confederation
    College
Nurse Practitioner, NorWest Community Health
    Centre
Thunder Bay, Ontario

Jill E. Vihos, RN, BScN, MN, PhD(c)
Faculty Lecturer
University of Alberta
Edmonton, Alberta

Debra Walker, RN, BA, MDE, PhD(c)
Nursing Professor, Health and Community
    Services
Confederation College
Thunder Bay, Ontario

Kathryn Weaver, RN, PhD
Associate Professor, Faculty of Nursing
University of New Brunswick
Fredericton, New Brunswick

Introduction

The *Study Guide and Skills Performance Checklists* to accompany *Canadian Fundamentals of Nursing*, Fourth Edition, has been developed to encourage independent learning among beginning nursing students. As you begin to read the textbook, you may notice a difference in style and format from other books you have used in the past. The terms you'll find in *Canadian Fundamentals of Nursing* are new and the focus of the content is probably different than you are accustomed to. You may be wondering, "How will I learn all of the material in this chapter?" The essential objective of this study guide is to assist you in this endeavour—to help you learn what you need to know and then self-test with hundreds of review questions.

This study guide follows the textbook content chapter for chapter. Whatever chapter your instructor assigns, you will use the same chapter number in this study guide. The outline format was designed to help you learn to read nursing content more effectively and with greater understanding. Each chapter of this study guide includes the following sections to assist your comprehension and recall.

The *Preliminary Reading* section is designed to teach prereading strategies. You need to become familiar with the chapter by first reading the chapter title, the key concepts and key terms, and all headings, and then by reviewing all of the photographs, drawings, tables, and boxes. This can be done rather quickly and will give you an overall sense of the content of the chapter.

The *Comprehensive Understanding* section is next and appears in outline format. This will prove to be a very valuable tool, not only as you first read the chapter, but also as you prepare for tests. This outline identifies the topics and main ideas of each chapter as an aid to concentration, comprehension, and retaining textbook information. By completing this outline, you will learn to "pull out" key information from the chapter. As you record your answers in the study guide, you will reinforce that content. Once completed, this outline will serve as a review tool when preparing for exams.

The *Review Questions* in each chapter provide a valuable means of testing and reinforcing your knowledge of the material read and the answers you recorded in the outline. Each question is multiple choice. As a further aid for independent learning, each answer requires a rationale (the reason why the option you selected is correct). After you have completed the review questions, you can check the answers at the end of the study guide.

Chapters 26 to 30 and 36 to 49 include exercises based on the care plans that appear in the textbook. These exercises allow you to practice synthesizing the nursing process and critical thinking as you, the nurse, care for clients. Taking into account one aspect of the nursing process, you will be asked to imagine you are the nurse in the case study and to think about what knowledge, experiences, standards, and attitudes might be used in caring for the client. Write your answers in the appropriate boxes and check them against the answer key.

When you finish answering the review questions and synthesis exercises, take a few minutes to check your answers against the answer keys. If you answered a question incorrectly, analyze the thoughts that led you to the wrong answer:

- Did you miss the key word or phrase?
- Did you make assumptions about something that was not actually stated in the textbook?
- Did you misunderstand the subject matter?
- Did you use an incorrect rationale when selecting your response?

Each incorrect response is an opportunity to learn. Go back to the textbook and re-read any content that is still unclear. In the long run, this will be a time-saving activity.

The *Skills Performance Checklists* section features a checklist for each of the skills presented in the text. The checklists may be used by instructors to evaluate your competence in performing the techniques. Note that you may need to adapt these skills in order to meet a client's special needs or to follow the particular policy of an institution.

The learning activities presented in this study guide will help you to complete the semester with a firm understanding of nursing concepts and processes that you will rely on throughout your professional career.

1

Health and Wellness

Preliminary Reading

Chapter 1, pp. 1–13

Comprehensive Understanding

Conceptualizations of Health

1. Compare three different conceptualizations of health.

   _____

   _____

   _____

Historical Approaches to Health in Canada

2. Historically, the three different approaches to health in Canada have been medical, behavioural, and socioenvironmental. Identify the distinguishing features of each of these approaches.

   a. Medical:

   _____

   _____

   b. Behavioural:

   _____

   _____

   c. Socioenvironmental:

   _____

   _____

3. Identify the contributions of the following Canadian documents to the understanding of health and health determinants.

   a. *Lalonde Report*:

   _____

   _____

   b. *Ottawa Charter*:

   _____

   _____

   c. *Epp Report*:

   _____

   _____

   d. *Strategies for Population Health*:

   _____

   _____

   e. *Toronto Charter*:

   _____

   _____

Determinants of Health

4. Identify major determinants of health as outlined by Health Canada, the *Ottawa Charter*, and the *Toronto Charter*.

   _____

   _____

   _____

5. Why is it important for nurses to understand the concept of health determinants?

   _____

   _____

   _____

Strategies to Influence Health Determinants

6. The concepts of *health promotion* and *disease prevention* are distinct yet interrelated. Briefly explain each one.

   a. Health promotion:

   _____
   _____

   b. Disease prevention:

   _____
   _____

7. Define the three levels of prevention and give an example of each.

   a. Primary prevention:

   _____
   _____

   b. Secondary prevention:

   _____
   _____

   c. Tertiary prevention:

   _____
   _____

Health Promotion Strategies

8. Define the five health promotion strategies contained in the *Ottawa Charter* and give examples of activities in each strategy.

   a. Strengthen community action:

   _____
   _____

   b. Build healthy public policy:

   _____
   _____

   c. Create supportive environments:

   _____
   _____

   d. Develop personal skills:

   _____
   _____

   e. Reorient health services:

   _____
   _____

Population Health Promotion Model: Putting It All Together

9. What are the four major elements of the Population Health Promotion Model?

   a. _____
   b. _____
   c. _____
   d. _____

10. Provide an example of how you might use this model in your practice.

   _____
   _____

Review Questions

Select the appropriate answer and cite the rationale for choosing that particular answer.

1. The "watershed" document that marked the shift from a lifestyle to a social approach to health was the
   a. *Lalonde Report*
   b. National Forum on Health
   c. *Toronto Charter*
   d. *Ottawa Charter*

   Answer: _____   Rationale: _____
   _____
   _____

2. The major determinants of health in a socioenvironmental view of health are
   a. Psychosocial risk factors and socioenvironmental risk conditions
   b. Physiological risk factors and behavioural risk factors
   c. Behavioural and psychosocial risk factors
   d. Behavioural and socioenvironmental risk factors

   Answer: _____   Rationale: _____
   _____
   _____

3. The main reason that intersectoral collaboration is a necessary strategy to reach the goal of "Health for All" is
   a. The determinants of health are broad
   b. Intersectoral collaboration is cost-effective
   c. Intersectoral collaboration encourages problem solving at a local level

d. Intersectoral collaboration is less likely to result in conflict

Answer: _____   Rationale: _____

_____

_____

4. Providing immunizations against measles is an example of
   a. Health promotion
   b. Primary prevention
   c. Secondary prevention
   d. Tertiary prevention

Answer: _____   Rationale: _____

_____

_____

5. Which of the following statements does *not* accurately characterize health promotion?
   a. Health promotion addresses health issues within the context of the social, economic, and political environment.
   b. Health promotion emphasizes empowerment.
   c. Health promotion strategies focus primarily on helping people develop healthy behaviours.
   d. Health promotion is political.

Answer: _____   Rationale: _____

_____

_____

6. The belief that health is primarily an individual responsibility is most congruent with which approach to health?
   a. Medical
   b. Behavioural
   c. Socioenvironmental
   d. Public health

Answer: _____   Rationale: _____

_____

_____

7. All of the following statements accurately describe the Population Health Promotion Model, *except*
   a. The model suggests that action can address the full range of health determinants
   b. The model incorporates the health promotion strategies of the *Ottawa Charter*

c. The model focuses primarily on interventions at the society level
d. The model attempts to integrate the concepts of population health and health promotion

Answer: _____   Rationale: _____

_____

_____

8. Which of the following is the most influential health determinant?
   a. Personal health practices
   b. Income and social status
   c. Health care services
   d. Physical environment

Answer: _____   Rationale: _____

_____

_____

9. A medical approach to health is to health services as a behavioural approach is to
   a. Income and social status
   b. Employment and working conditions
   c. Physical environments
   d. Personal health practices

Answer: _____   Rationale: _____

_____

_____

10. Understanding the context in which health behaviours occur most accurately reflects which approach to health?
    a. Behavioural
    b. Medical
    c. Socioenvironmental
    d. Primary prevention

Answer: _____   Rationale: _____

_____

_____

2

The Canadian Health Care System

Preliminary Reading

Chapter 2, pp. 14–27

Comprehensive Understanding

Evolution of the Canadian Health Care System

1. Canada has constructed a social safety net for the protection of its citizens. Medicare is an important part of this safety net. Briefly explain the role of the following in the development of Medicare.

   a. *British North America Act:*

   _____

   _____

   b. Great Depression:

   _____

   _____

   c. Tommy Douglas:

   _____

   _____

   d. *Medical Care Act* (1966):

   _____

   _____

   e. *Canada Health Act* (1984):

   _____

   _____

The Organization and Governance of Health Care

2. Briefly explain the following.

   a. The four areas of federal jurisdiction for health in Canada:

   _____

   _____

   _____

   _____

   b. The role of the provincial and territorial governments in the organization and delivery of health care:

   _____

   _____

   _____

   _____

   c. The five principles enshrined in the *Canada Health Act:*

   _____

   _____

   _____

   _____

   _____

Health Care Spending

3. In 2007, a Conference Board of Canada study stated that despite our significant increase in health care spending, Canada ranked _____ in a comparison of 17 industrialized countries. How did Canada compare in health spending and health status with these other countries?

   _____

   _____

Trends and Reforms in Canada's Health Care System

4. Describe the main recommendations of the Romanow and Kirby reports.

_____

_____

_____

_____

_____

Right to Health Care

5. Explain the role and influence of the *Canada Health Act* in establishing health care as a right for all Canadians.

_____

_____

_____

_____

_____

Primary Health Care

6. Explain the difference between primary care and primary health care.

_____

_____

_____

_____

_____

7. Explain the four pillars of primary health care.

a. _____

b. _____

c. _____

d. _____

8. Describe the benefits and potential drawbacks involved with increasing funding to primary health care and home care services.

_____

_____

_____

_____

_____

Settings for Health Care Delivery

9. Explain the role of each of the following institutions in delivering health care.

a. Hospitals:

_____

_____

b. Long-term care facilities:

_____

_____

c. Psychiatric facilities:

_____

_____

d. Rehabilitation centres:

_____

_____

10. Explain the role of each of the following in delivering health care in the community.

a. Public health:

_____

_____

b. Physician offices:

_____

_____

c. Community health centres and clinics:

_____

_____

d. Assisted living:

_____

_____

e. Home care:

_____

_____

f. Adult day care centres:

_____

_____

g. Community and voluntary agencies:

_____

_____

h. Occupational health:

_____

_____

i. Hospice and palliative care:

_____

_____

j. Parish nursing:

_____

_____

Levels of Care

11. List and briefly describe the five levels of health care.

a. _____

b. _____

c. _____

d. _____

e. _____

12. Explain primary care, secondary care, and tertiary care.

_____

_____

_____

_____

_____

Challenges to the Health Care System

13. Describe three cost accelerators in the Canadian health care system.

a. _____

b. _____

c. _____

Review Questions

Select the appropriate answer and cite the rationale for choosing that particular answer.

1. When the *Canada Health Act* of 1984 amalgamated the previous acts of 1957 and 1966, it added which principle to the existing four?
   a. Accessibility
   b. Comprehensiveness
   c. Portability
   d. Public administration

   Answer: _____   Rationale: _____

   _____

   _____

2. The amount of money (public and private) Canada spent on health care per capita in 2006 was approximately
   a. $1870
   b. $3839
   c. $4548
   d. $2440

   Answer: _____   Rationale: _____

   _____

   _____

3. A 16-year-old student sees a physician at a walk-in clinic to find out if she is pregnant. This service can be best described as an example of
   a. Primary care
   b. Primary health care
   c. Tertiary care
   d. Secondary care

   Answer: _____   Rationale: _____

   _____

   _____

4. The 16-year-old student attends a community program on prenatal health for teenage mothers. The program is taught by a nurse, a nutritionist, and a social worker. This service can best be described as an example of
   a. Primary care
   b. Primary health care
   c. Tertiary care
   d. Secondary care

   Answer: _____   Rationale: _____

   _____

   _____

5. Which of the following is a *false* statement?
   a. Most nurses work in institutional settings in Canada.
   b. Most nursing graduates are diploma prepared.
   c. Most nurses are over age 50.
   d. Most nurses work part-time or in other than full-time positions.

   Answer: _____   Rationale: _____

   _____

   _____

3

The Development of Nursing in Canada

Preliminary Reading

Chapter 3, pp. 28–40

Comprehensive Understanding

1. Define *nursing* (according to the International Council of Nurses [ICN]).

   _____
   _____
   _____

Early History of Nursing in Canada

The First Nurses and Hospitals in New France

2. What was the contribution of Mme Hébert to health care in the new colony?

   _____
   _____
   _____

3. List five important milestones in the development of nursing in Canada.

   a. _____
   b. _____
   _____
   _____
   c. _____
   _____
   _____
   d. _____
   _____
   _____
   e. _____
   _____
   _____

Nursing During the British Regime

4. How did British nursing compare with French nursing during the eighteenth century?

   _____
   _____
   _____

5. _____ carried by _____ and _____ spread rapidly in the British colonies. Established French-Canadian orders expanded their services, and new English-speaking orders were founded to help the sick and the poor.

Nursing Education in Canada

6. What was the main reason for establishing the first Canadian nursing schools?

   _____
   _____
   _____

7. Describe the growth of hospital nursing schools in the late nineteenth century.

   _____
   _____
   _____

The Impact of Nursing Organizations on Nursing Education

8. How did the ICN influence the development of nursing organizations worldwide?

   _____
   _____
   _____

9. How did the struggle for women's rights influence nursing?

_____

_____

_____

The First University Programs

10. When and where was the first university program in nursing established?

_____

_____

_____

From the Depression to the Post–World War II Years

11. The Great Depression brought _____ and _____ to nurses.

12. How did World War II affect health education?

_____

_____

_____

Expansion in the 1950s and 1960s

13. Describe the development of graduate programs during these years.

_____

_____

_____

Nursing Education Today

14. Where does the responsibility for monitoring standards of nursing education lie?

_____

_____

15. A master's degree in nursing is necessary for _____.

16. Nurses with doctorates can _____

_____.

Continuing and In-Service Education

17. Define *continuing education*.

_____

_____

Professional Roles and Responsibilities

18. Briefly describe the following nursing roles.

a. Advanced practice nurse:

_____

_____

b. Clinical nurse specialist:

_____

_____

c. Nurse practitioner:

_____

_____

d. Nursing educator:

_____

_____

e. Nursing administrator:

_____

_____

f. Nursing researcher:

_____

_____

Professional Nursing Organizations

19. What is the role of a professional organization? How does the Canadian Nurses Association (CNA) fulfill this role?

_____

_____

_____

Unions

20. How did the Supreme Court decision of 1973 change the situation for Canadian nursing? Within a decade, every province had both _____ and _____.

Standards of Nursing Practice

21. Nursing is a self-regulating profession and sets its own standards of practice. Standards are developed and established based on _____ and _____.

22. Briefly describe the responsibility of nurses under the Ontario standards of practice in the following areas.

a. Accountability:

_____

b. Knowledge:

_____

c. Application of knowledge:

_____

d. Ethics:

_____

e. Continuing competence:

_____

Ethical Standards of Practice

23. The Code of Ethics provides nurses with direction for ethical decision making and practice in everyday situations.

Registration and Licensure

24. In all provinces and territories, nursing practice acts regulate _____ and ___ _____ of nursing. Legislation in each province outlines nursing's scope of practice.

Certification

25. Define *certification*.

_____

_____

26. In Canada, certification is offered by the CNA.

Review Questions

Select the appropriate answer and cite the rationale for choosing that particular answer.

1. Hippocrates is considered the father of scientific medicine because
   a. He was the first to make observations of clients and develop treatments on the basis of symptoms
   b. He recognized the importance of fresh water and hygiene for public health
   c. He believed in a spiritual basis of illness
   d. He recognized the importance of nutrition in maintaining health

Answer: _____   Rationale: _____

_____

_____

2. The first visiting nurses in Canada were
   a. Led by Jeanne Mance in 1642
   b. The first three Augustinian nuns in 1639
   c. Marie Rollet Hébert and her surgeon-apothecary husband in 1617
   d. The Grey Nuns under Margaret d'Youville in 1737

Answer: _____   Rationale: _____

_____

_____

3. Which of the following is *not* attributed to Florence Nightingale?
   a. Dramatically reduced morbidity and mortality rates among the wounded
   b. Developed nursing as a profession independent from medicine
   c. Introduced nursing to the British army during the Crimean War
   d. Made nursing an acceptable field of work for middle- and upper class women outside the home

Answer: _____   Rationale: _____

_____

_____

4. The first integrated basic undergraduate degree program in nursing in Canada was developed at
   a. St. Francis Xavier University
   b. University of Toronto
   c. University of Alberta
   d. University of British Columbia

Answer: _____   Rationale: _____

_____

_____

5. Which of the following specialty groups was the first to offer certification under the program sponsored by the CNA?
   a. Neuroscience nurses
   b. Occupational health nurses
   c. Enterostomal nurses
   d. Perioperative nurses

Answer: _____   Rationale: _____

_____

_____

4

Community Health Nursing Practice

Preliminary Reading

Chapter 4, pp. 41–52

Comprehensive Understanding

1. Community health nursing care focuses on
   _____
   _____
   _____

Promoting the Health of Populations and Community Groups

2. Distinguish between a *population* and a *community* and give an example of each.
   _____
   _____
   _____

3. Compare the characteristics of a *healthy population* and a *healthy community*.
   _____
   _____
   _____

Community Health Nursing Practice

4. Describe the scope of community health nursing practice.
   _____
   _____
   _____

5. Briefly explain the nursing focus in primary health care.
   _____
   _____
   _____

6. Briefly explain the nursing focus on empowerment in community health nursing guided by primary health care.
   _____
   _____
   _____

7. Describe each of the components identified in the Canadian Community Health Nursing Practice Model.
   a. Values and beliefs:
      _____
      _____

   b. Community health nursing process:
      _____
      _____

   c. Standards of practice:
      _____
      _____

   d. Sociopolitical environment:
      _____
      _____

8. Briefly describe the contributions of public health and population health to public health nursing.

_____

_____

9. Give an example of each of the strategies identified in the framework for public health programs.

   a. Promote individual and family action:

   _____

   _____

   b. Provide direct care:

   _____

   _____

   c. Influence the environment:

   _____

   _____

   d. Build partnerships:

   _____

   _____

10. A strong theoretical foundation for home health nursing is provided by

   _____

   _____

11. Briefly describe key distinctions between public health nursing and home health nursing.

   a. Public health nursing:

   _____

   _____

   b. Home health nursing:

   _____

   _____

The Changing Focus of Community Health Nursing Practice

Vulnerable Populations

12. Vulnerable populations of clients are those who are

   _____

   _____

13. Explain how a nurse approaches diversity to provide culturally sensitive, competent, and safe care.

_____

_____

_____

_____

14. List some of the reasons why vulnerable populations typically experience poorer health outcomes.

_____

_____

_____

15. Briefly describe the following vulnerable groups and identify the circumstances that contribute to their vulnerability.

   a. Poor and homeless people:

   _____

   _____

   b. People in precarious circumstances:

   _____

   _____

   c. People with chronic conditions and disabilities:

   _____

   _____

   d. People who engage in stigmatizing risk behaviours:

   _____

   _____

Competencies, Roles, and Activities in Community Health Nursing

16. A nurse in a community health practice must have a variety of skills and knowledge to assist individuals and families within the community, as well as communities broadly. Briefly explain the competencies the nurse needs in the following roles.

   a. Communicator:

   _____

   _____

   b. Facilitator:

   _____

   _____

c. Collaborator:

_____

_____

d. Coordinator:

_____

_____

e. Consultant:

_____

_____

f. Educator:

_____

_____

g. Direct care or service provider:

_____

_____

h. Community developer:

_____

_____

i. Social marketer:

_____

_____

j. Policy formulator:

_____

_____

k. Researcher:

_____

_____

Community Assessment

17. The community is viewed as having three components. Briefly explain each one.

a. Locale or structure:

_____

_____

b. Social systems:

_____

_____

c. People:

_____

_____

18. Briefly describe each of the following strategies to assess the locale or structure of a community.

a. Windshield or walking survey:

_____

_____

b. Observation of activities:

_____

_____

c. Key informant interviews:

_____

_____

d. Population data review:

_____

_____

e. Focus group interviews:

_____

_____

Promoting Clients' Health

19. The challenge is how to promote and protect the client's health, whether within the context of the community or with the community as the focus. The most important theme to consider, in order to be an effective community health nurse, is to

_____

_____

_____

_____

20. Identify some factors that nurses must consider in community nursing practice.

_____

_____

_____

_____

Review Questions

Select the appropriate answer and cite the rationale for choosing that particular answer.

1. Which of the following would *not* typically be considered an example of primary health care?

a. Lunch-time nutrition and activity program in an inner-city school run by nurses, nutritionists, social workers, and teachers

b. A rehabilitation program in a hospital provided by physiotherapists, physicians, nurses, and social workers for clients and families recovering from a stroke
c. Activities provided by child care workers in a day care centre at a corporation
d. A well-baby clinic conducted by nurses and nutritionists for new mothers at a neighbourhood health centre

Answer: _____   Rationale: _____
_____
_____

2. Among the communication skills needed to provide nursing care to community clients is the ability to
   a. Clarify client values and care expectations
   b. Follow medical prescriptions in many settings
   c. Manage generational interfamilial conflict
   d. Speak the client's language or dialects

Answer: _____   Rationale: _____
_____

3. Which of the following is *not* a known risk factor for abuse in families?
   a. Immigration to Canada within the past five years
   b. Mental health problems
   c. Substance abuse
   d. Socioeconomic stressors

Answer: _____   Rationale: _____
_____
_____

4. When the community health nurse refers clients to appropriate resources and monitors and coordinates the extent and adequacy of services to meet family health care needs, the nurse is functioning in the role of
   a. Collaborator
   b. Educator
   c. Consultant
   d. Coordinator

Answer: _____   Rationale: _____
_____
_____

5. Which of the following is *not* identified as a challenge in community health nursing?
   a. Increased task orientation, specialization, and working in silos
   b. Staying current on health information
   c. Limited demand for acute care in the community
   d. Conflict between prescribed programs and community partnership activities

Answer: _____   Rationale: _____
_____
_____

5

Caring for the Cancer Survivor

Preliminary Reading

Chapter 5, pp. 53–62

Comprehensive Understanding

The Effects of Cancer on Quality of Life

1. A cancer survivor is at risk for a wide range of treatment-related problems. Briefly explain the following.

   a. Second cancer:

   _____

   _____

   b. Late effects of chemotherapy:

   _____

   _____

   c. Neuropathy:

   _____

   _____

   _____

   d. Fatigue:

   _____

   _____

   _____

   e. Cognitive changes:

   _____

   _____

   _____

2. Identify the persistent symptoms that may occur after either a lumpectomy or a mastectomy.

   _____

   _____

   _____

3. Explain the following psychosocial effects of cancer.

   a. Distress:

   _____

   _____

   b. Post-traumatic stress disorder:

   _____

   _____

   c. Disrupted interpersonal relationships:

   _____

   _____

4. Identify the social impact that cancer causes across the lifespan.

   a. Adolescents and young adults:

   _____

   _____

   b. Adults (30 to 59 years):

   _____

   _____

   c. Older adults:

   _____

   _____

5. Cancer survivors most at risk for spiritual distress are those with

   a. _____

   b. _____

   c. _____

   d. _____

   e. _____

Cancer and Families

6. Identify some of the reasons that caring for a client with cancer causes family distress.

_____

_____

_____

Implications for Nursing

7. List the type of questions that you may use to assess the cancer survivor.

_____

_____

_____

8. The nurse's responsibilities with client education for the client who initially receives a diagnosis of cancer are

_____

_____

_____

Components of Survivorship Care

9. The four essential components of survivorship care are

a. _____

b. _____

c. _____

d. _____

Review Questions

Select the appropriate answer and cite the rationale for choosing that particular answer.

1. Many cancer survivors report attention problems, loss of memory, and difficulty recognizing and solving problems. This is an example of impaired
   a. Social well-being
   b. Physical well-being

   c. Spiritual well-being
   d. Psychological well-being

   Answer: _____   Rationale: _____

   _____

   _____

2. All of the following are the numerous social concerns that older adults are faced with as a result of cancer *except*
   a. Retirement
   b. Fixed income
   c. Isolation from social supports
   d. Ample medical insurance coverage

   Answer: _____   Rationale: _____

   _____

   _____

3. The essential components of survivorship are all of the following *except*
   a. Surveillance for cancer spread
   b. Care for the client by oncologists only
   c. Intervention for consequences of cancer
   d. Prevention and detection of new cancers and recurrent cancer

   Answer: _____   Rationale: _____

   _____

   _____

6

Theoretical Foundations of Nursing Practice

Preliminary Readings

Chapter 6, pp. 63–73

Comprehensive Understanding

1. Define the terms *theory* and *nursing theory* and explain why knowledge of nursing theory can help nurses become better practitioners.

_____

_____

_____

Early Nursing Practice and the Emergence of Theory

2. Briefly describe how developments in science and technology affected the development of nursing as a science.

_____

_____

_____

3. Explain the relationship between the development of nursing theory and the challenge of building curriculum for nursing education.

_____

_____

_____

_____

_____

4. Describe the purpose of nursing theory.

_____

_____

_____

Nursing Process

5. Describe the four basic steps of the nursing process.

a. Assessment:

_____

_____

b. Planning:

_____

_____

c. Intervention:

_____

_____

d. Evaluation:

_____

_____

6. The relationship between clinical judgement and nursing process is

_____

_____

_____

Conceptual Frameworks

7. Briefly describe how systematic thinking using conceptual nursing models differs from linear reasoning processes.

_____

_____

_____

Metaparadigm Concepts

8. Explain the importance of each metaparadigm concept for the clinical reasoning process in nursing.

   a. Person:

   _____

   _____

   b. Environment:

   _____

   _____

   c. Health:

   _____

   _____

   d. Nursing:

   _____

   _____

9. For each metaparadigm concept, identify at least two possible ways it might be defined for the purpose of guiding nursing practice.

   a. Person:

   _____

   _____

   b. Environment:

   _____

   _____

   c. Health:

   _____

   _____

   d. Nursing:

   _____

   _____

Philosophy of Nursing Science

10. Kuhn's ideas about paradigms helped nurses understand the scientific basis of nursing not simply as theoretical propositions but as

    _____

11. Chaos theory provided nurses with a new way to think about

    _____

Ways of Knowing in Nursing Practice

12. List four forms of knowledge identified by Carper that have contributed to excellent nursing practice.

    a. _____

    b. _____

    c. _____

    d. _____

Paradigm Debates Within Nursing

13. The two distinct paradigms that have been associated with debates surrounding nursing's theoretical development are

    _____

    _____

Nursing Diagnosis

14. Identify advantages and disadvantages of adopting a fixed list of diagnostic categories for nursing care.

    a. Advantages:

    _____

    _____

    _____

    b. Disadvantages:

    _____

    _____

    _____

Major Theoretical Models

15. Identify one characteristic of each of the following categories of theoretical models.

    a. Practice-based theories:

    _____

    b. Needs theories:

    _____

    c. Interactionist theories:

    _____

    d. Systems theories:

    _____

    e. Simultaneity theories:

    _____

16. Name one theory or theorist as an example for each of these categories.

    a. _____

    b. _____

    c. _____

    d. _____

    e. _____

Review Questions

Select the appropriate answer and cite the rationale for choosing that particular answer.

1. Which of the following is *not* an intended outcome of a grand theory?
   a. To provide guidance for specific nursing interventions
   b. To provide a framework for broad ideas about nursing
   c. To provide a structural framework within which smaller range theories can be developed
   d. To stimulating critical thinking about nursing ideas

Answer: _____   Rationale: _____
_____
_____

2. Which of the following is *not* an intended outcome of a prescriptive theory?
   a. To provide insight into general and broad phenomena
   b. To be action oriented
   c. To test validity
   d. To predict the consequence of a specific intervention

Answer: _____   Rationale: _____
_____
_____

3. Which nursing theorist's model conceptualizes the person as an adaptive system?
   a. Virginia Henderson
   b. Rosemary Parse
   c. Hildegard Peplau
   d. Sister Callista Roy

Answer: _____   Rationale: _____
_____
_____

4. Which nursing theorist's model conceptualizes the person as an irreducible energy field, coextensive with the universe?
   a. Adam's interactionist theory
   b. Orem's self-care theory
   c. Rogers's simultaneity theory
   d. Watson's transpersonal theory

Answer: _____   Rationale: _____
_____
_____

5. Which of the following levels of abstraction is *not* part of Liaschenko's ideas about nursing knowledge?
   a. Knowing the case
   b. Knowing the client
   c. Knowing the disease
   d. Knowing the person

Answer: _____   Rationale: _____
_____
_____

7

Research As a Basis for Practice

Preliminary Reading

Chapter 7, pp. 74–88

Comprehensive Understanding

Why Evidence?

1. Define *evidence-informed practice*.

   _____

   _____

   _____

2. Briefly describe the relationship between research and practice.

   _____

   _____

   _____

3. What are the sources of evidence used to inform practice?

   _____

   _____

   _____

Researching the Evidence

Ask the Clinical Question

4. Describe a PICO question.

   _____

   _____

   _____

   _____

Critique the Evidence

5. How is research evidence assessed for applicability in practice?

   _____

   _____

   _____

6. The typical research article has the following parts. Briefly explain each section.

   a. Introduction:

   _____

   b. Methods:

   _____

   c. Results:

   _____

   d. Discussion (Clinical Implications):

   _____

   e. References:

   _____

Collect the Best Evidence

7. Describe where and how to find research studies in nursing.

   _____

   _____

   _____

Evidence-Informed Practice and Research

8. Differentiate *research-based practice* from *evidence-informed practice*.

   _____

   _____

   _____

Knowledge Development in Nursing

9. Briefly describe Carper's four patterns of knowing in nursing.

   _____

   _____

   _____

   _____

The Development of Research in Nursing

10. Nursing research involves

    _____

    _____

    _____

11. Identify the priorities for nursing research as identified by the Canadian Association of Schools of Nursing.

    _____

    _____

    _____

12. Briefly describe the relationship between research and theory.

    _____

    _____

    _____

The History of Nursing Research in Canada

13. Briefly explain the significance of each of the following.

    a. Florence Nightingale:

       _____

       _____

       _____

    b. Development of master's and doctoral programs in nursing

       _____

       _____

       _____

    c. Establishment of nursing research journals

       _____

       _____

       _____

Nursing Research

The Scientific Paradigm

14. The scientific paradigm gave rise to *the scientific method*, a _____ means of acquiring and testing knowledge, by which researchers try to _____, _____, and _____ or _____ nursing phenomena.

15. The dominant paradigm for most of the nineteenth and twentieth centuries has been _____.

16. *Positivism* emphasizes _____ and _____ experience, rather than speculation, and focuses on the search for _____ and _____ relationships to explain phenomena.

17. Wood and Ross-Kerr described the research process as beginning with a researchable question, reviewing the literature to determine what is already known about the topic of the question, and then designing a study to answer the question. A goal of scientific research is to understand phenomena so that the knowledge can be applied generally, not just to isolated cases. Researchers conduct studies that contribute to the testing or development of theories, thereby advancing knowledge that can be applied in practice.

The Qualitative (Interpretive) Paradigm

18. _____ is an alternative to positivism and promotes the idea that many truths exist depending on the perceptions of people in the situation. This philosophy leads to _____, which strives to understand the situation from the perspective of the participant, not the researcher.

Research Designs

19. The two broad approaches to research are _____ and _____.

Scientific Nursing Research

20. Briefly describe the three requirements of a true experiment.

    _____

    _____

    _____

21. A quasi-experiment is one in which groups are formed and the conditions are controlled, but

   _____
   _____
   _____

22. Surveys are designed to

   _____
   _____

23. Exploratory descriptive designs provide in-depth descriptions of populations or variables not previously studied.

Qualitative Nursing Research

24. Qualitative studies stem from questions that cannot be quantified and measured.

25. Define the following designs that are used with qualitative research.

   a. Ethnography:

      _____

   b. Phenomenology:

      _____

   c. Grounded theory:

      _____

Conducting Nursing Research

26. Who should conduct nursing research?

   _____
   _____

Ethical Issues in Research

27. Describe the purpose and responsibilities of a research ethics board.

   _____
   _____
   _____

28. Informed consent means that research subjects

   _____
   _____
   _____

29. Briefly describe the eight guiding ethical principles for research in Canada.

   a. _____
   b. _____

   c. _____
   d.
   e. _____
   f. _____
   g. _____
   h. _____

Applying Research Findings to Nursing Practice

30. To use findings in clinical practice, nurses must _____
   _____,
   and _____
   _____.

Review Questions

Select the appropriate answer and cite the rationale for choosing that particular answer.

1. The researcher's refusal to disclose the names of subjects is
   a. Respect for privacy and confidentiality
   b. Minimizing harm
   c. Informed consent
   d. Balancing harms and benefits

   Answer: _____ Rationale: _____
   _____
   _____

2. The purpose of a research ethics board is to
   a. Ensure that federal funds are equitably appropriated
   b. Conduct research benefiting the public
   c. Determine the risk status of clients in research projects
   d. Ensure that ethical principles are being upheld

   Answer: _____ Rationale: _____
   _____
   _____

3. Research studies can most easily be identified by
   a. Looking for the word "research" in the title of the report
   b. Looking for the study only in research journals

c. Examining the contents of the report
d. Reading the abstract and conclusion of the report

Answer: _____   Rationale: _____
_____
_____

4. Which statement concerning research articles is accurate?
   a. Nursing textbooks are primary sources of information.
   b. Primary sources are those written by one of the researchers in the study.
   c. The fact that a report is a primary source guarantees its accuracy.
   d. Secondary sources are the best source of information about the research study.

Answer: _____   Rationale: _____
_____
_____

5. A research article includes all of the following *except*
   a. A summary of literature used to identify the research problem
   b. The researcher's interpretation of the study results
   c. A summary of other research studies with the same results
   d. A description of methods used to conduct the study

Answer: _____   Rationale: _____
_____
_____

8

Nursing Values and Ethics

Preliminary Reading

Chapter 8, pp. 89–101

Comprehensive Understanding

1. A value is a

   _____

   _____

2. Ethics is the study of

   _____

   _____

Values

3. Values formation is

   _____

   _____

4. Value conflict occurs when

   _____

   _____

5. Values clarification is

   _____

   _____

6. Identify three values clarification questions.

   a. _____

   b. _____

   c. _____

Ethics

7. Define *ethics* or *morality*.

   _____

   _____

   _____

   _____

Professional Nursing and Ethics

8. A *code of ethics* serves

   _____

   _____

9. Identify and briefly describe the seven values that must be upheld by Canadian nurses according to the Canadian Nurses Association.

   a. _____

   b. _____

   c. _____

   d. _____

   e. _____

   f. _____

   g. _____

10. Define the following terms and explain how they apply to the role of the nurse.

    a. *Responsibility*:

    _____

    _____

    b. *Accountability*:

    _____

    _____

    c. *Advocacy*:

    _____

    _____

Ethical Theory

11. Define the following terms and explain how they apply to the role of the nurse.

a. *Deontology*:

_____

_____

b. *Utilitarianism*:

_____

_____

c. *Bioethics*:

_____

_____

d. *Autonomy*:

_____

_____

e. *Beneficence*:

_____

_____

f. *Nonmaleficence*:

_____

_____

g. *Justice*:

_____

_____

h. *Social justice*:

_____

_____

i. *Feminist ethics*:

_____

_____

j. *Relational ethics*:

_____

_____

k. *Environment*:

_____

_____

l. *Embodiment*:

_____

_____

m. *Mutuality*:

_____

_____

n. *Engagement*:

_____

_____

How to Process an Ethical Dilemma

12. An ethical dilemma is

_____

_____

13. Briefly describe each of the seven steps in the processing of an ethical dilemma.

a. Step 1:

_____

_____

b. Step 2:

_____

_____

c. Step 3:

_____

_____

d. Step 4:

_____

_____

e. Step 5:

_____

_____

f. Step 6:

_____

_____

g. Step 7:

_____

_____

Ethical Issues in Nursing Practice

Client Care Issues

14. Explain the following client care issues and how they apply to nursing.

a. Informed consent:

_____

_____

b. Futile care:

_____

_____

c. Advance directives:

_____

_____

d. Withdrawal of food and hydration:

_____

_____

Review Questions

Select the appropriate answer and cite the rationale for choosing that particular answer.

1. Nursing codes of ethics fulfill which of the following purposes?
   a. They help nurses and the public understand professional nursing conduct.
   b. They outline actions to be implemented in specific nursing care situations.
   c. They define the scope of nursing practice on a national level.
   d. They define the roles of the nurse, the client, other health care professionals, and society.

Answer: _____ Rationale: _____

_____

_____

2. Identify the statement below that is *not* accurate regarding advance directives.
   a. Advance directives offer direction of care goals to health care professionals.
   b. Two broad categories exist within an advance directive: proxy and interactive.
   c. The instructive directive is commonly called a durable power of attorney.
   d. Proxy directives permit clients to name a surrogate decision maker on their behalf.

Answer: _____ Rationale: _____

_____

_____

3. With regard to ethical situations in client care, the most important nursing responsibility is to
   a. Remain neutral in clinical decisions
   b. Realize that the professional health care team collectively must be responsible for deciding ethical questions
   c. Be accountable for the morality of one's own actions
   d. Act only when absolutely certain that the action is ethically correct

Answer: _____ Rationale: _____

_____

_____

4. You are working with the parents of a seriously ill newborn. Surgery has been proposed for the infant, but the chances of success are unclear. In helping the parents resolve this ethical conflict, you know that the next step is
   a. Exploring reasonable courses of action
   b. Collecting all available information about the situation
   c. Clarifying values related to the cause of the dilemma
   d. Identifying people who can solve the difficulty

Answer: _____ Rationale: _____

_____

_____

5. The goal of informed consent is to protect the client's right to
   a. Autonomy
   b. Beneficence
   c. Ethic of care
   d. Advocacy

Answer: _____ Rationale: _____

_____

_____

9

Legal Implications in Nursing Practice

Preliminary Reading

Chapter 9, pp. 102–113

Comprehensive Understanding

Legal Limits of Nursing

1. The legal guidelines that nurses must follow are derived from the following. Briefly explain each one.

   a. Statute law:

   _____

   _____

   b. Nursing practice acts:

   _____

   _____

   c. Standards of care:

   _____

   _____

   d. Common law:

   _____

   _____

2. Define the following terms.

   a. *Criminal law*:

   _____

   _____

   b. *Civil law*:

   _____

   _____

3. Standards of care are the legal guidelines for nursing practice and are defined by the

   _____

   _____

   _____

4. Nursing practice acts establish

   _____

   _____

5. In a negligence lawsuit, these standards are used to determine

   _____

   _____

Legal Liability Issues in Nursing Practice

6. Define *tort*.

   _____

Intentional Torts

7. Define the following.

   a. Assault:

   _____

   b. Battery:

   _____

c. Invasion of privacy:

_____

d. False imprisonment:

_____

Unintentional Torts

Negligence

8. Define *negligence*.

_____

9. Briefly explain how a nurse can avoid being liable for negligence.

_____
_____
_____

Criminal Liability

10. Describe the difference between the tort of negligence and criminal negligence charges.

_____
_____
_____
_____

Consent

11. The following factors must be verified for consent to be legally valid.
   a. _____
   b. _____
   c. _____

12. A signed consent form is required for all routine treatment, hazardous procedures, some treatment programs such as chemotherapy, and research involving clients.

13. *Informed consent* is a person's agreement to

_____
_____

14. The following factors provide adequate information for the client to form a decision and are required to have met the standard of *informed consent*.
   a. _____
   b. _____
   c. _____
   d. _____

15. The nurse's signature witnessing the consent means

_____
_____
_____

Nursing Students and Legal Liability

16. If a client is harmed as a direct result of a nursing student's actions or lack of action, who is liable?

_____
_____
_____

17. When students are employed as nursing assistants or nurses' aides when not attending classes, which tasks should they not perform?

_____
_____
_____

Abandonment, Assignment, and Contract Issues

Short Staffing

18. Briefly explain the process that a nurse needs to follow when a staffing assignment is unreasonable.

_____
_____
_____

Floating

19. Identify what the nurse's responsibility is when he or she "floats" to another nursing unit.

_____
_____
_____

Physicians' Orders

20. The physician is responsible for directing the medical treatment.

21. What is the nurse's responsibility with physicians' orders?

_____
_____
_____

22. One of the most frequently litigated issues is whether the nurse

_____
_____

23. If a verbal order is necessary, it should be written out and _____ by the physician within _____ hours.

Legal Issues in Nursing Practice

Abortion

24. Summarize the legal rights of women in Canada relative to abortion in Canada.

_____

_____

_____

_____

Drug Regulations and Nurses

25. Describe the two federal acts that control the manufacture, distribution, and sale of food, drugs, and therapeutic devices in Canada.

  a. _____

  b. _____

Communicable Diseases

26. If nurses become aware of communicable diseases in their jurisdiction, what must they do?

_____

27. What must a nurse do whenever confidential health care information is requested by a third party?

_____

Death and Dying

28. Explain the legal definition of _death_ that is used as standard medical practice across Canada.

_____

_____

_____

29. Define the following terms and explain their legal status in Canada.

  a. _Euthanasia_:

_____

_____

  b. _Assisted suicide_:

_____

_____

  c. _Withdrawing or withholding treatment_:

_____

_____

Advance Directives and Health Care Surrogates

30. Describe the function of an advance directive for health care.

_____

_____

_____

31. Differentiate an advance directive from a living will.

_____

_____

_____

32. If the existence of an advance directive for health care is known, the instructions must be followed.

33. Describe the two forms that an advance directive assumes.

  a. _____

  b. _____

Organ Donation

34. Every province and territory has human tissue legislation that provides for both _____ and _____ _____ of tissues and organs.

Mental Health Issues

35. What is true about the rights of clients admitted to a psychiatric unit on a voluntary basis?

_____

36. What special consideration must be kept in mind for a client who has a history and medical records that indicate suicidal tendencies?

_____

37. Documentation of precautions against suicide is essential.

Public Health Issues

38. Briefly explain the purpose of public health legislation.

_____

_____

_____

39. Describe nurses' obligation when child abuse or neglect is witnessed or suspected.

_____

_____

_____

Risk Management

40. Risk management is

    _____

    _____

41. The steps involved in risk management include

    a. _____

    b. _____

    c. _____

    d. _____

42. The purpose of a tool used by risk managers is the

    _____

    _____

43. Risk management includes documentation. It should be

    a. _____

    b. _____

    c. _____

Review Questions

Select the appropriate answer and cite the rationale for choosing that particular answer.

1. Nursing practice acts are an example of
   a. Statute law
   b. Common law
   c. Public law
   d. Criminal law

   Answer: _____   Rationale: _____

   _____

   _____

2. An example of an *unintentional tort* is
   a. Assault
   b. Battery
   c. Invasion of privacy
   d. Negligence

   Answer: _____   Rationale: _____

   _____

   _____

3. What should you do if you doubt a client's capacity to give informed consent?
   a. Do not be concerned if the consent is already signed
   b. Notify the physician and document your concerns
   c. Send the client for the procedure and discuss it afterward
   d. Ask a family member to give consent

   Answer: _____   Rationale: _____

   _____

   _____

4. When a client is harmed as a result of a nursing student's actions or lack of action, the liability is generally held by
   a. The student
   b. The student's instructor or preceptor
   c. The hospital or health care facility
   d. All of the above

   Answer: _____   Rationale: _____

   _____

   _____

5. A confused client falling out of bed because side rails were not used is an example of which type of liability?
   a. False imprisonment
   b. Assault
   c. Battery
   d. Negligence

   Answer: _____   Rationale: _____

   _____

   _____

6. When you stop to help in an emergency at the scene of an accident, if the injured party files suit and your employing institution's insurance does not cover you, you would probably be covered by
   a. Your automobile insurance
   b. Your homeowner insurance
   c. The Patient Care Partnership, which may grant immunity from suit if the injured party consents
   d. The Good Samaritan laws, which grant immunity from suit if there is no gross negligence

   Answer: _____   Rationale: _____

   _____

   _____

7. Treating a client without the person's consent is considered
   a. Battery
   b. Negligence
   c. Implied consent
   d. Expressed consent

   Answer: _____   Rationale: _____
   _____
   _____

9. You restrain a client without the client's permission and without a physician's order. You may be guilty of
   a. Assault
   b. False imprisonment
   c. Invasion of privacy
   d. Neglect

   Answer: _____   Rationale: _____
   _____
   _____

8. Even though the nurse may obtain the client's signature on a form, obtaining informed consent is the responsibility of the
   a. Client
   b. Physician
   c. Student nurse
   d. Supervising nurse

   Answer: _____   Rationale: _____
   _____
   _____

10. You are obligated to follow a physician's order unless
   a. The order is a verbal order
   b. The physician's order is illegible
   c. The order has not been transcribed
   d. The order is in error, violates hospital policy, or would be detrimental to the client

   Answer: _____   Rationale: _____
   _____
   _____

10

Culture and Ethnicity

Preliminary Reading

Chapter 10, pp. 114–131

Comprehensive Understanding

Understanding Cultural Concepts

1. To provide culturally competent care, you must understand cultural concepts. Briefly explain each of the following.

   a. Culture:

   _____

   _____

   b. Subculture:

   _____

   _____

   c. Ethnicity:

   _____

   _____

   d. Race:

   _____

   _____

   e. Enculturation:

   _____

   _____

   f. Acculturation:

   _____

   _____

   g. Assimilation:

   _____

   _____

   h. Multiculturalism:

   _____

   _____

   i. Cultural pluralism

   _____

   _____

   j. Cultural relativism

   _____

   _____

Cultural Conflicts

2. Define the following terms.

   a. *Ethnocentrism*:

   _____

   b. *Discrimination*:

   _____

   c. *Cultural imposition*:

   _____

   d. *Stereotypes*:

   _____

Cultural Awareness

3. Define *cultural awareness*.

   _____

   _____

4. Briefly describe two strategies a nurse can use to achieve cultural self-awareness.

   _____

   _____

   _____

Historical Development of the Nursing Approach to Culture

5. Define *transcultural nursing*.

   _____

   _____

6. Define *culturally congruent care*.

   _____

   _____

7. Define *culturally competent care*.

   _____

   _____

8. Cultural competence has five interlocking components. Briefly explain each one.

   a. _____

   b. _____

   c. _____

   d. _____

   e. _____

9. Define *cultural safety*.

   _____

   _____

Cultural Context of Health and Caring

10. Culture is the context in which groups interpret and define their experiences relevant to life transitions.

11. Culture is the framework used in defining social phenomena.

12. Briefly explain the difference between Western and non-Western cultures.

    _____

    _____

    _____

Cultural Healing Modalities and Healers

13. Foster identified two distinct categories of cross-cultural healers. Explain each one.

    a. Naturalistic practitioners:

       _____

       _____

    b. Personalistic practitioners:

       _____

       _____

Cultural Assessment

14. The goal of a *cultural assessment* is

    _____

    _____

15. Briefly explain how using a cultural assessment model or tool as a guide with a client can assist with providing culturally competent care.

    _____

    _____

    _____

    _____

16. Briefly describe the challenges of using one specific cultural assessment model or tool with every client.

    _____

    _____

    _____

    _____

Review Questions

Select the appropriate answer and cite the rationale for choosing that particular answer.

1. When providing care to clients with diverse cultural backgrounds, it is imperative for you to recognize that
   a. Cultural consideration must be put aside if basic needs are in jeopardy
   b. Generalizations about the behaviour of a particular group may be inaccurate
   c. Current health standards should determine the acceptability of cultural practices
   d. Similar reactions to stress will occur when individuals have the same cultural background

   Answer: _____   Rationale: _____

   _____

   _____

2. To be effective in meeting various ethnic needs, you should
   a. Treat all clients alike
   b. Be aware of clients' cultural differences
   c. Act as if you are comfortable with the client's behaviour
   d. Avoid asking questions about the client's cultural background

   Answer: _____   Rationale: _____

   _____

   _____

3. To provide culturally competent nursing care, you should
   a. Identify the client's values, attitudes, beliefs, and practices
   b. Make decisions based solely on your own assessment of the client
   c. Not be overly concerned with using knowledge from conceptual or theoretical models
   d. Acknowledge that a client's response to his or her health is similar among various ethnic groups

Answer: _____   Rationale: _____
_____
_____

4. To respect a client's personal space you
   a. Avoid the use of touch
   b. Explain nursing care and procedures
   c. Keep the curtains pulled around the client's bed
   d. Stand 2.5 metres away from the bed, if possible

Answer: _____   Rationale: _____
_____
_____

5. Which of the following is *not* included in providing culturally competent care to a client?
   a. Being sensitive and open to a client's cultural beliefs
   b. Providing opportunities for a client to discuss his or her view with you
   c. Ensuring that a client's traditional health care practice is handled separately from current health approaches
   d. Working collaboratively with a client in making health care decisions

Answer: _____   Rationale: _____
_____
_____

11

Nursing Leadership, Management, and Collaborative Practice

Preliminary Reading

Chapter 11, pp. 132–145

Comprehensive Understanding

Management and Leadership Roles for Nurses

1. Building a nursing team and developing a quality work environment begin with the leadership of the nurse executive.

2. Describe the leadership attributes of a Nurse Executive.

   _____

   _____

Nursing Care Delivery Models, Collaborative Practice, and Nursing Teams

3. Care delivery must be effective in helping nurses achieve desirable outcomes for their clients.

4. Briefly explain the following delivery systems.

   a. Functional nursing:

   _____

   _____

   _____

   b. Team nursing:

   _____

   _____

   _____

   c. Collaborative practice:

   _____

   _____

   _____

   d. Primary nursing:

   _____

   _____

   _____

   e. Case management:

   _____

   _____

   _____

Decentralized Decision Making

5. Briefly explain the following management structures.

   a. Centralized management:

   _____

   _____

   _____

   b. Decentralized management:

   _____

   _____

   _____

   c. Matrix:

   _____

   _____

   _____

6. Identify the responsibilities of a nurse manager in a decentralized management structure.

_____

_____

_____

7. The following are key elements in establishing decentralized decision making. Briefly explain each one.

a. Responsibility:

_____

_____

b. Autonomy:

_____

_____

c. Authority:

_____

_____

d. Accountability:

_____

_____

8. The nurse manager nurtures and supports staff involvement through the following approaches. Briefly explain each.

a. Nursing practice or professional shared governance councils:

_____

_____

b. Interprofessional collaboration:

_____

_____

c. Staff communication:

_____

_____

d. Learning organization:

_____

_____

9. Give an example of how a student nurse may be involved as a member of a learning organization in a practice setting.

_____

_____

Leadership Skills for Nursing Students

10. Summarize each of the following leadership and management competencies a student nurse may develop for entry into registered nurse practice.

a. Accountability and responsibility:

_____

_____

b. Use of best practice guidelines:

_____

_____

c. Prioritizing:

_____

_____

d. Nursing team development:

_____

_____

e. Advocacy:

_____

_____

f. Time management:

_____

_____

g. Evaluation:

_____

_____

11. Give an example of how a student nurse may be involved in nursing team development.

_____

_____

_____

12. Define *delegation*.

_____

_____

_____

13. Identify the five rights of delegation.

a. _____

b. _____

c. _____

d. _____

e. _____

14. Identify the purposes of delegation.

_____
_____
_____

15. Summarize the requirements for appropriate delegation.

a. _____
b. _____
c. _____
d. _____
e. _____

Quality Care and Client Safety

16. Define *quality improvement.*

_____
_____

Quality in Nursing Practice

17. Define each of the elements of quality nursing practice.

a. Professional standards:

_____
_____

b. Care and best practice guidelines:

_____
_____

c. Nurse-sensitive outcomes:

_____
_____

18. Give an example of a *nurse-sensitive outcome.*

_____
_____

19. Define *culture of safety for client care.*

_____
_____
_____

20. Discuss how nurses and other health care professionals can contribute to a culture of safe practice.

_____
_____
_____

21. Discuss the role of a transformational leader in health care.

_____
_____

Review Questions

Select the appropriate answer and cite the rationale for choosing that particular answer.

1. Primary nursing refers to
   a. Nurses who work with physicians in primary care
   b. Nurses who hold management positions
   c. Placing registered nurses in a continuous, direct care role with clients in health care organizations
   d. Nursing carried out in primary health care

   Answer: _____   Rationale: _____

   _____
   _____

2. A student nurse practising in a collaborative practice model would demonstrate all of the following *except*
   a. Understanding the client and family perspective
   b. Recognizing other team members for their contribution
   c. Assuming primary responsibility for planning, implementation, follow-up, and evaluation
   d. Developing listening skills and being aware of personal motivation

   Answer: _____   Rationale: _____

   _____
   _____

3. Decentralized management is best described as
   a. Care decisions being made by a manager in another location
   b. Situations in which there is a lack of coordination of care

c. Situations in which staff overrule the decisions made by managers
d. Situations in which decision making occurs at the staff level

Answer: _____   Rationale: _____
_____
_____

4. Autonomy is best described as
   a. The duties and activities that an individual is employed to perform
   b. The right to act in areas where an individual has been given and accepts responsibility
   c. The freedom to decide and act
   d. Being answerable for one's actions

Answer: _____   Rationale: _____
_____
_____

5. Which of the following is *not* a purpose for delegation?
   a. Improves efficiency
   b. Provides job enrichment
   c. Transfers accountability for client care
   d. Improves utilization of health care professionals

Answer: _____   Rationale: _____
_____
_____

12

Critical Thinking in Nursing Practice

Preliminary Reading

Chapter 12, pp. 146–157

Comprehensive Understanding

1. Critical decision making separates professional nurses from technical or ancillary personnel.

Critical Thinking Defined

2. Define *critical thinking*.

   _____
   _____
   _____

3. Describe the process of critical thinking in nursing.

   _____
   _____
   _____

4. To think critically, you must be able to

   a. _____
   b. _____
   c. _____
   d. _____
   e. _____

5. Identify the core critical thinking skills that apply to nursing.

   a. _____
   b. _____
   c. _____
   d. _____
   e. _____
   f. _____

6. Learning to think critically helps a nurse to care for clients as their advocate and to assist them in making better informed choices about their care.

Levels of Critical Thinking in Nursing

7. Three levels of critical thinking in nursing have been identified. Briefly describe each.

   a. Basic:

   _____
   _____

   b. Complex:

   _____
   _____

   c. Commitment:

   _____
   _____

Critical Thinking Competencies

8. Critical thinking competencies are the cognitive processes a nurse uses to make judgements.

General Critical Thinking Competencies

Scientific Method

9. Define *scientific method*.

   _____
   _____
   _____

10. List the steps of the scientific method.

   a. _____

   b. _____

   c. _____

   d. _____

   e. _____

Problem Solving

11. Define *problem solving*.

   _____

   _____

12. Solving a problem in one situation allows you to apply the knowledge to future client situations.

Decision Making

13. Define *decision making*.

   _____

   _____

14. Explain the process that an individual needs to go through to make a decision.

   _____

   _____

   _____

Specific Critical Thinking Competencies in Clinical Situations

Diagnostic Reasoning and Inference

15. Explain the process of diagnostic reasoning.

   _____

   _____

   _____

Clinical Decision Making

16. The clinical decision-making process requires

   _____

   _____

17. List the criteria for decision making.

   a. _____

   b. _____

   c. _____

18. After determining a client's priorities, a nurse selects therapies most likely to solve each problem.

19. Cite some examples of how nurses make decisions about their clients.

   _____

   _____

   _____

Nursing Process As a Critical Thinking Competency

20. The nursing process is a systematic and comprehensive approach for nursing care. List the five steps of the nursing process.

   a. _____

   b. _____

   c. _____

   d. _____

   e. _____

Developing Critical Thinking Skills

21. Define *reflection*.

   _____

   _____

22. Provide some examples of how a nurse can use reflection.

   _____

   _____

   _____

23. Identify a common approach to reflection that the student nurse may use.

   _____

   _____

24. To become a critical thinker, a nurse must be able to use language precisely and clearly. It is important not only to communicate clearly with clients and families but also to be able to communicate findings clearly to other health care professionals.

A Critical Thinking Model for Clinical Decision Making

25. Summarize the critical thinking model and list its five components.

   _____

   _____

   _____

   _____

   _____

Specific Knowledge Base

26. Identify what constitutes a nurse's knowledge base.

   _____

   _____

Experience

27. Identify the ways in which critical thinking is developed through experience.

_____

_____

_____

Critical Thinking Synthesis

28. Define *critical thinking*.

_____

_____

_____

29. The nursing process is the traditional critical thinking competency that allows nurses to make clinical judgements and take actions based on reason.

30. Briefly explain how the nursing process and the critical thinking model work together.

_____

_____

_____

Review Questions

Select the appropriate answer and cite the rationale for choosing that particular answer.

1. Clinical decision making requires you to
   a. Improve a client's health
   b. Establish and weigh criteria in deciding the best choice of therapy for a client
   c. Follow the physician's orders for client care
   d. Standardize care for the client

Answer: _____   Rationale: _____

_____

_____

2. Which of the following is *not* one of the five steps of the nursing process?
   a. Planning
   b. Evaluation
   c. Hypothesis testing
   d. Assessment

Answer: _____   Rationale: _____

_____

_____

3. Gathering, verifying, and communicating data about the client to establish a database is an example of which component of the nursing process?
   a. Assessment
   b. Planning
   c. Evaluation
   d. Nursing diagnosis
   e. Implementation

Answer: _____   Rationale: _____

_____

_____

4. Completing nursing actions necessary for accomplishing a care plan is an example of which component of the nursing process?
   a. Assessment
   b. Planning
   c. Evaluation
   d. Nursing diagnosis
   e. Implementation

Answer: _____   Rationale: _____

_____

_____

13

Nursing Assessment and Diagnosis

Preliminary Reading

Chapter 13, pp. 158–177

Comprehensive Understanding

1. The nursing process is used to _____, _____, and _____ human responses to _____ and _____.

Critical Thinking Approach to Assessment

2. Nursing assessment is the systematic process of _____, _____, and _____.

3. Identify the purpose of the assessment.

   _____

   _____

4. As you initiate the assessment component for a specific client, you are also synthesizing critical knowledge, experience, standards, and attitudes simultaneously.

5. Accurate assessment makes it possible to develop appropriate nursing diagnoses and to devise appropriate goals and strategies.

Data Collection

6. Identify some nonverbal behaviours that you may observe during an assessment.

   _____

   _____

   _____

7. A comprehensive nursing health history includes

   _____

   _____

8. It is important for the nurse's assessment to first consider the _____.

9. Assessment data must be _____, _____, and _____.

10. The collection of inaccurate, incomplete, or inappropriate data leads to incorrect identification of the client's health care needs and subsequent inaccurate, incomplete, or inappropriate nursing diagnoses.

11. Whichever approach is used, you must cluster cues of information and identify emerging patterns and potential problems.

Types of Data

12. Define each of the following.

    a. Subjective data:

       _____

       _____

    b. Objective data:

       _____

       _____

Sources of Data

13. Each source provides information about the client's level of wellness, anticipated prognosis, risk factors, health practices and goals, and patterns of health and illness.

Client

14. Identify the types of information a client can provide.

    a. _____

    b. _____

    c. _____

    d. _____

    e. _____

Family and Significant Others

15. Families can be an important secondary source of information about the client's health status. Give an example.

    _____

    _____

    _____

Health Care Team

16. Identify the ways that health care team members identify data.

    a. _____

    b. _____

    c. _____

Medical Records

17. By reviewing medical records, you can _____ _____, _____, and _____.

18. Identify records that may contain pertinent health care information.

    _____

    _____

Literature

19. Reviewing nursing, medical, and pharmacological literature about an illness helps the nurse complete the database.

Nurse's Experience

20. A nurse's ability to make an assessment will improve as he or she uses _____, applies _____, and focuses _____.

Methods of Data Collection

Interview

21. During an interview, nurses have the opportunity to

    a. _____

    b. _____

    c. _____

    d. _____

    e. _____

22. Describe the phases of the interview.

    a. _____

    b. _____

    c. _____

23. The nurse uses various types of interview techniques. Describe some of the information obtained in an interview.

    _____

    _____

    _____

Nursing Health History

24. The nursing health history is data collected about

    a. _____

    b. _____

    c. _____

    d. _____

    e. _____

Physical Examination

25. During the physical examination, _____ and _____ are taken and _____.

Interpreting Assessment Data and Making Nursing Judgements

26. Through a process of inferential reasoning and judgement, the nurse decides what information has meaning in relation to the client's health status.

Analysis and Interpretation

27. After collecting and validating subjective and objective data and interpreting the data, the nurse organizes the information into meaningful clusters. This depends on recognizing

    _____

28. During data clustering, you organize data and focus attention on client functions needing support and assistance for recovery.

Data Documentation

29. Identify the two essential reasons for thoroughness in data documentation.

    a. _____

    b. _____

Nursing Diagnosis

30. Define *nursing diagnosis*.

    _____
    _____

31. Define *medical diagnosis*.

    _____
    _____

32. Briefly summarize the evolution of nursing diagnosis.

    _____
    _____
    _____
    _____

33. Explain the purpose of NANDA International.

    _____
    _____
    _____

34. Explain the purpose of using nursing diagnoses.

    _____
    _____
    _____

Critical Thinking and the Nursing Diagnostic Process

35. The diagnostic process includes

    _____
    _____

36. Defining characteristics are

    _____

37. Defining characteristics that are beyond healthy norms form the basis for problem identification.

Formulation of the Nursing Diagnosis

38. Briefly explain the four types of nursing diagnoses identified by NANDA International.

a. Actual nursing diagnosis:

    _____

b. Risk nursing diagnosis:

    _____
    _____

c. Health-promotion nursing diagnosis:

    _____
    _____

d. Wellness nursing diagnosis:

    _____
    _____

Components of a Nursing Diagnosis

39. Nursing diagnoses are stated in a two-part format: the _____ followed by a _____.

40. The diagnostic label of the nursing diagnosis is

    _____
    _____

41. The related factors of the nursing diagnosis are

    _____
    _____

42. NANDA International approves a definition for each diagnosis following clinical use and testing.

43. Risk factors are

    _____
    _____

44. Nursing assessment data must support the diagnostic label.

Sources of Diagnostic Errors

45. Identify 11 ways nurses can avoid making common diagnostic errors.

    a. _____
    b. _____
    c. _____
    d. _____
    e. _____

f. _____

g. _____

h. _____

i. _____

j. _____

k. _____

Review Questions

Select the appropriate answer and cite the rationale for choosing that particular answer.

1. In most circumstances, the best source of information for nursing assessment of the adult client is the
    a. Nursing literature
    b. Physician
    c. Client
    d. Medical record

    Answer: _____   Rationale: _____
    _____
    _____

2. Reviewing the client's medical record to obtain baseline data about the client's response to illness occurs during which phase of the nursing process?
    a. Planning
    b. Nursing diagnosis
    c. Evaluation
    d. Assessment

    Answer: _____   Rationale: _____
    _____
    _____

3. A nursing diagnosis
    a. Is a statement of a client response to a health problem that requires nursing intervention
    b. Identifies health problems within the domain of nursing
    c. Is derived from the physician's history and physical examination
    d. Is not changed during the course of a client's hospitalization

    Answer: _____   Rationale: _____
    _____
    _____

4. Mr. Margauz, a 52-year-old business executive, is admitted to the coronary care unit. During his admission interview, he denies chest pain or shortness of breath. His pulse and blood pressure are normal. He appears tense and does not want you to leave his bedside. When questioned, he states that he is very nervous. At this moment, which nursing diagnosis is the most appropriate?
    a. *Alteration in comfort, chest pain*
    b. *Alteration in bowel elimination related to restricted mobility*
    c. *High risk for altered cardiac output related to heart attack*
    d. *Anxiety related to intensive care unit admission*

    Answer: _____   Rationale: _____
    _____
    _____

14

Planning and Implementing Nursing Care

Preliminary Reading

Chapter 14, pp. 178–198

Comprehensive Understanding

1. The nursing process is used to _____, _____, and _____ human responses to _____ and _____.

Establishing Priorities

2. Priority setting involves ranking nursing diagnoses in order of importance.

3. Priorities are classified as high, intermediate, or low. Give an example of each.

   High:

   _____

   Intermediate:

   _____

   Low:

   _____

Critical Thinking in Establishing Goals and Expected Outcomes

4. Once a nursing diagnosis is identified for a client, the nursing process consists of finding the best approach to address and resolve the problem.

5. Goals and expected outcomes are specific statements of the client or the nurse to achieve problem resolution.

6. Identify the two purposes for writing goals and expected outcomes.

   a. _____

   b. _____

Goals of Care

7. Define the following.

   a. Client-centred goal:

   _____

   b. Short-term goal:

   _____

   c. Long-term goal:

   _____

Expected Outcomes

8. Define *expected outcomes*.

   _____

   _____

9. Outcomes are desired responses of the client's condition in the _____, _____, _____, _____, or _____ dimensions.

10. The expected outcomes should be written in measurable behavioural terms sequentially, with time frames.

11. Identify the functions of an expected outcome.

   a. _____

   b. _____

   c. _____

   d. _____

Guidelines for Writing Goals and Expected Outcomes

12. Define and give an example of each of the seven guidelines to follow when writing goals and expected outcomes.

    a. Client centred:

    _____

    _____

    b. Singular:

    _____

    _____

    c. Observable:

    _____

    _____

    d. Measurable:

    _____

    _____

    e. Time limited:

    _____

    _____

    f. Mutual:

    _____

    _____

    g. Realistic:

    _____

    _____

13. Nursing interventions are those actions designed to assist the client in moving from the present level of health to that described in the expected outcome.

Types of Interventions

14. Interventions are based on clients' needs. Define and give an example of each of the three categories of interventions.

    a. Nurse initiated:

    _____

    _____

    b. Physician initiated:

    _____

    _____

    c. Collaborative:

    _____

    _____

Selection of Interventions

15. Identify the six factors nurses use to select nursing interventions for a specific client.

    a. _____

    b. _____

    c. _____

    d. _____

    e. _____

    f. _____

16. The advantages of the taxonomy of nursing interventions are

    a. _____

    b. _____

    c. _____

    d. _____

Planning Nursing Care

17. Define *nursing care plan*.

    _____

    _____

18. Briefly explain the purpose of a nursing care plan in relation to the following.

    a. Communication:

    _____

    b. Identification and coordination of resources:

    _____

    c. Continuity of care:

    _____

    d. Change-of-shift reports:

    _____

    e. Long-term needs of client:

    _____

    f. Expected outcome criteria:

    _____

19. The complete care plan is the blueprint for nursing action. It provides direction for implementation of the plan and a framework for evaluation of the client's response to nursing actions.

20. Briefly explain each of the following.

    a. Institutional care plans:

    _____

b. Standardized care plans:

_____

c. Care plans for community-based settings:

_____

d. Critical pathways:

_____

e. Concept maps:

_____

Consulting Other Health Care Professionals

21. Consultation is a process in which

_____

22. Consultation is based on the problem-solving approach, and the consultant is the stimulus for change.

23. The need to consult occurs when you have identified a problem that cannot be solved using personal knowledge, skills, and resources.

Implementing Nursing Care

24. Define *implementation*.

_____

25. A nursing intervention is

_____

26. Define each of the following.
    a. Direct care interventions:

    _____

    b. Indirect care interventions:

    _____

Critical Thinking in Implementation

27. When making decisions about implementing care, you need to consider the following:
    a. _____
    b. _____
    c. _____
    d. _____

Standard Nursing Interventions

28. Nursing interventions can be based on protocols and standing orders. Briefly explain each and provide an example of where they are commonly used.

a. Protocols:

_____
_____

b. Standing orders:

_____
_____
_____

Implementation Process

Reassessing the Client

29. When new data are obtained and a new need is identified, the nurse modifies nursing care.

Reviewing and Revising the Existing Nursing Care Plan

30. If the client's status has changed and the nursing diagnosis and related nursing interventions are no longer appropriate, the nursing care plan needs to be modified.

31. Identify the steps in modifying the existing care plan.
    a. _____
    b. _____
    c. _____
    d. _____

Organizing Resources and Care Delivery

32. Before implementing care, evaluate the plan to determine the need for assistance and the type of assistance required.

33. Describe how each of the following contributes to the preparation of care delivered.
    a. Equipment:

    _____

    b. Personnel:

    _____

    c. Environment:

    _____

    d. Client:

    _____

Anticipating and Preventing Complications

34. Risks to clients arise from illness, conditions, and treatment.

35. Nurses must identify the need for additional assistance, nursing skills, or both.

Direct Care

Activities of Daily Living

36. Define *activities of daily living (ADLs)*.

_____

_____

37. Conditions that result in the need for assistance with ADLs can be temporary, permanent, or rehabilitative.

Instrumental Activities of Daily Living

38. Instrumental activities of daily living (IADLs) include

_____

_____

Lifesaving Measures

39. A lifesaving measure is

_____

_____

Counselling

40. Define *counselling*.

_____

_____

41. Identify some areas in which clients or families may need counselling.

a. _____

b. _____

c. _____

Teaching

42. Define the following.

a. Teaching:

_____

_____

b. Teaching–learning process:

_____

_____

Controlling for Adverse Reactions

43. What is an adverse reaction?

_____

_____

_____

44. How do nurses control for adverse reactions?

_____

_____

_____

Indirect Care

Communicating Nursing Interventions

45. Nursing interventions are written (via the nursing care plan and medical record) or communicated orally (one nurse to another or to another health care professional).

46. Define *interdisciplinary care plan*.

_____

_____

_____

Delegating, Supervising, and Evaluating the Work of Other Staff Members

47. Give examples of tasks you could delegate to another member of the health care team.

_____

_____

_____

Review Questions

Select the appropriate answer and cite the rationale for choosing that particular answer.

1. The following statement appears on the nursing care plan for an immunosuppressed client: "The client will remain free from infection throughout hospitalization." This statement is an example of a (an)
   a. Long-term goal
   b. Short-term goal
   c. Nursing diagnosis
   d. Expected outcome

Answer: _____   Rationale: _____

_____

_____

2. The planning step of the nursing process includes which of the following activities?
   a. Assessing and diagnosing
   b. Evaluating goal achievement
   c. Setting goals and selecting interventions
   d. Performing nursing actions and documenting them

Answer: _____   Rationale: _____

_____

_____

3. The nursing care plan calls for the client, a 136 kg woman, to be turned every 2 hours. The client is unable to assist with turning. You know that you may hurt your back if you attempt to turn the client by yourself. You should
   a. Rewrite the care plan to eliminate the need for turning
   b. Ignore the intervention related to turning in the care plan
   c. Turn the client by yourself
   d. Ask another nurse to help you turn the client

Answer: _____   Rationale: _____
_____
_____

4. Mary Benoit is a client who recently received a diagnosis of diabetes. You show Mary how to administer an injection. This intervention activity is
   a. Counselling
   b. Communicating
   c. Teaching
   d. Managing

Answer: _____   Rationale: _____
_____
_____

15

Evaluation of Nursing Care

Preliminary Reading

Chapter 15, pp. 199–207

Comprehensive Understanding

1. Evaluation involves two components:
   _____ and
   _____.

Critical Thinking and Evaluation

2. Once an intervention has been performed, what types of data would you collect to see if the intervention has been successful?
   _____
   _____
   _____

3. Evaluation of care requires you to reflect on the client's responses to nursing interventions and to determine their effectiveness in promoting the client's well-being.

4. Evaluation is the step in the nursing process whereby the nurse continually redirects nursing care to meet client needs.

The Evaluation Process

5. Identify the five elements of the evaluation process.
   a. _____
   b. _____
   c. _____
   d. _____
   e. _____

Identifying Criteria and Standards

6. A goal specifies
   _____
   _____

7. Expected outcomes are
   _____
   _____

8. The purposes of the Nursing Outcomes Classification (NOC) are
   a. _____
   b. _____
   c. _____

Collecting Evaluative Data

9. Identify the two aspects of care that need to be addressed.
   a. _____
   b. _____

10. The primary source of data for evaluation is
    _____
    _____

Interpreting and Summarizing Findings

11. To objectively evaluate the success in achieving a goal, you should use the following steps.
    a. _____
    b. _____
    c. _____
    d. _____
    e. _____

12. When documenting the client's response to interventions, always include the same evaluative measures gathered during assessment.

Care Plan Revision

13. Accurate evaluation leads to the appropriate revision of ineffective care plans and discontinuation of therapy that has been successful.

Discontinuing a Care Plan

14. After determining that expected outcomes and goals have been achieved, confirm this evaluation with the client and discontinue that care plan.

Modifying a Care Plan

15. When goals are not met, identify the factors that interfered with goal achievement.

16. Lack of goal achievement may also result from an error in nursing judgement or failure to follow each step of the nursing process.

17. When a goal is not achieved, repeat the entire sequence to discover changes that need to be made to the plan or changes that have occurred in the client's condition.

18. A complete reassessment of all client factors relating to the nursing diagnosis and etiology is the first step in re-evaluating the nursing process. Briefly explain the following in relation to modifying a care plan.

    a. Reassessment:

    _____

    _____

    b. Nursing diagnosis:

    _____

    _____

    c. Goals and expected outcomes:

    _____

    _____

    d. Interventions:

    _____

    _____

    e. Evaluation:

    _____

    _____

    f. Client outcomes:

    _____

    _____

Review Questions

Select the appropriate answer and cite the rationale for choosing that particular answer.

1. Evaluation is
   a. Begun immediately before the client's discharge
   b. Necessary only if the physician orders it
   c. An integrated, ongoing nursing care activity
   d. Performed primarily by nurses in the quality assurance department

Answer: _____   Rationale: _____

_____

_____

2. Measuring the client's response to nursing interventions and his or her progress toward achieving goals occurs during which phase of the nursing process?
   a. Planning
   b. Nursing diagnosis
   c. Evaluation
   d. Assessment

Answer: _____   Rationale: _____

_____

_____

16

Documenting and Reporting

Preliminary Reading

Chapter 16, pp. 208–232

Comprehensive Understanding

1. What is documentation?

   _____

   _____

   _____

Confidentiality

2. Explain two reasons why nurses are obligated to keep information about clients confidential.

   a. _____

   b. _____

Multidisciplinary Communication Within the Health Care Team

3. Caregivers use a variety of ways to exchange information about clients. Briefly explain the following.

   a. Client record or chart:

   _____

   _____

   b. Reports:

   _____

   _____

Purposes of Records

4. Briefly explain the following purposes of a record.

   a. Communication and care planning:

   _____

   _____

   b. Legal documentation:

   _____

   _____

   c. Education:

   _____

   _____

   d. Research:

   _____

   _____

   e. Auditing–monitoring:

   _____

   _____

Guidelines for Quality Documentation and Reporting

5. Six important guidelines must be followed to ensure quality documentation and reporting. Explain each one.

   a. Factual:

   _____

   _____

   b. Accurate:

   _____

   _____

   c. Complete:

   _____

   _____

d. Current:

_____

_____

e. Organized:

_____

_____

f. Compliant with standards:

_____

_____

Common Documentation Systems

6. Narrative documentation is a storylike format that documents information specific to client conditions and nursing care. The disadvantages of this style are

a. _____

b. _____

c. _____

7. Problem-oriented medical records place emphasis on the client's problems. The method corresponds to the nursing process and facilitates communication of client needs. Explain the following major sections of the problem-oriented medical record.

a. Database:

_____

_____

b. Problem list:

_____

_____

c. Care plan:

_____

_____

d. Progress notes:

_____

_____

8. Define the acronyms and briefly explain the forms of documentation of the problem-oriented medical record.

a. SOAP or SOAPIE notes:

_____

_____

b. PIE format:

_____

_____

c. Focus charting or DAR:

_____

_____

9. Briefly explain the following forms of documentation.

a. Source records:

_____

_____

b. Charting by exception (CBE):

_____

_____

c. Critical pathways or care maps:

_____

_____

Common Record-Keeping Forms

10. Briefly explain the following formats used for record keeping.

a. Admission nursing history forms:

_____

_____

b. Flow sheets and graphic records:

_____

_____

c. Client care summary or Kardex:

_____

_____

d. Acuity records or workload measurement systems:

_____

_____

e. Standardized care plans:

_____

_____

f. Discharge summary forms:

_____

_____

Home Health Care Documentation

11. Documentation in the home health care system has different implications than it does in other areas of nursing. List two primary differences.

_____
_____
_____

12. The nurse is the pivotal person in the documentation of home health care delivery.

Long-Term Health Care Documentation

13. Because residents are stable, documentation is done using _____, and assessment may be done only _____.

Computerized Documentation

14. Explain the many benefits of computerized documentation.

_____
_____

The Electronic Health Record

15. What is an electronic health record (EHR)?

_____
_____

Reporting

16. Nurses communicate information about clients so that all members of the health care team can make informed decisions about the client and his or her care.

Change-of-Shift Reports

17. Identify the eight major areas to include in a change-of-shift report.

a. _____
b. _____
c. _____
d. _____
e. _____
f. _____
g. _____
h. _____

Telephone Reports

18. It is important that information in a telephone report be clear, accurate, and concise.

Telephone or Verbal Orders

19. List the guidelines the nurse should follow when receiving telephone orders from physicians.

a. _____
b. _____
c. _____
d. _____
e. _____
f. _____

Transfer Reports

20. List the nine major information areas in a transfer report.

a. _____
b. _____
c. _____
d. _____
e. _____
f. _____
g. _____
h. _____
i. _____

Incident Reports

21. Describe the purpose of an incident report.

_____
_____

Review Questions

Select the appropriate answer and cite the rationale for choosing that particular answer.

1. What is the primary purpose of a client's medical record?
   a. To satisfy the requirements of accreditation agencies
   b. To communicate accurate, timely information about the client
   c. To provide validation for hospital charges
   d. To provide the nurse with a defence against malpractice

Answer: _____ Rationale: _____
_____
_____

2. Which of the following is charted according to the six guidelines for quality recording?
   a. "Respirations rapid; lung sounds clear."
   b. "Was depressed today."
   c. "Crying. States she doesn't want visitors to see her like this."
   d. "Had a good day. Up and about in room."

Answer: _____   Rationale: _____
_____
_____

3. Which of the following best describes a change-of-shift report?
   a. Two or more nurses always visit all clients to review their plan of care.
   b. Nurses should exchange judgements they have made about client attitudes.
   c. The nurse should identify nursing diagnoses and clarify client priorities.
   d. Client information is communicated from a nurse on a sending unit to a nurse on a receiving unit.

Answer: _____   Rationale: _____
_____

4. What is an incident report?
   a. A legal claim against a nurse for negligent nursing care
   b. A summary report of all falls occurring on a nursing unit
   c. A report of an event inconsistent with the routine care of a client
   d. A report of a nurse's behaviour submitted to the hospital administration

Answer: _____   Rationale: _____
_____
_____

5. If an error is made while recording, what should you do?
   a. Erase it or scratch it out
   b. Obtain a new nurse's note and rewrite the entries
   c. Leave a blank space in the note
   d. Draw a single line through the error and initial it

Answer: _____   Rationale: _____
_____
_____

17

Nursing Informatics and Canadian Nursing Practice

Preliminary Reading

Chapter 17, pp. 233–244

Comprehensive Understanding

1. In an increasingly complex technological environment, long-standing routines and tools in health care are being replaced by strategic, evidence-informed practices that demand high-quality, timely health information.

Nursing Informatics and the Canadian Health Care System

2. Describe the purpose of the electronic health record.

   _____

   _____

3. In the 1980s, nursing informatics emerged as a new nursing specialty in health information management.

Defining Nursing Informatics

4. Define the most current definition of nursing informatics with the following focuses.

   a. Information technology:

      _____

      _____

   b. Conceptual:

      _____

      _____

   c. Role centred:

      _____

      _____

Evolution of Informatics in the Canadian Health Care System

5. As defined by the Canadian Organization for Advancement of Computers in Health (COACH), health informatics encompasses all health care disciplines and is the "intersection of clinical, [information management/information technology (IM/IT)] and management practices to achieve better health."

6. Define the acronym and describe the evolution of what is now known as CIHI.

   _____

   _____

   _____

   _____

   _____

7. Describe the function of the Standards Collaborative Working Groups as part of the Canada Health Infoway.

   _____

   _____

   _____

   _____

8. The events over the last 30 years have culminated in national attention to the need for timely, secure, and appropriate health information access.

9. Multiple organizations and standards development organizations operate to coordinate documentation of health information and monitoring of the Canadian health care system.

Standards in Health Informatics

Standards Development in Canada

10. Standards in health care data management refer to the established and formally endorsed coding protocols for all health information, including coding of the following aspects of health care delivery.

    a. _____

    b. _____

    c. _____

    d. _____

11. Standardization of data management also refers to standardizing forms of technology, information, or business processes.

12. List two benefits of standards in health care data management for each of the following stakeholder groups.

    a. Clients:

    _____

    _____

    b. Providers:

    _____

    _____

    c. Service delivery organizations:

    _____

    _____

    d. Educators:

    _____

    _____

    e. Researchers:

    _____

    _____

13. Standards play a role in shaping health care data in numerous ways, such as client registry standards, provider registry standards, diagnostic imaging standards, and pharmacy and laboratory standards, all of which influence how clinical practice is documented.

14. Describe the following two types of needs that can stimulate the need for a data management standard.

    a. Technical needs:

    _____

    _____

    b. Business needs:

    _____

    _____

15. Canada Health Infoway has standards for adopting, adapting, and developing a new standard that includes testing, evaluation, and retesting prior to full implementation.

16. Internationally, various standards form the basis for pan-Canadian standards. Define the following acronyms.

    a. SNOMED CT®:

    _____

    _____

    b. ICD-10-CA:

    _____

    _____

Standardizing Nursing Language

17. In the 1990s, nursing scholars began to advocate for a standardized nursing language using the following two arguments:

    ". . . if we cannot name it, we cannot control it, finance it, teach it, research it, or put it into public policy" (Clark & Lang, 1992, p. 109).

    ". . . without a language to express our concepts we cannot know whether our understanding of their meaning is the same, so we cannot communicate them with any precision to other people" (Clark, 1999, p. 42).

Health Information: Nursing Components

18. Describe what is meant by a nursing minimum data set.

    _____

    _____

    _____

19. The majority of Canadian nurses agree that the nursing components of health information known as Health Information: Nursing Components (HI:NC) are composed of the following five categories of elements. List and describe the five categories.

    a. _____

    b. _____

    c. _____

    d. _____

    e. _____

International Classification for Nursing Practice®

20. Describe the role of the International Council of Nurses in developing the International Classification for Nursing Practice (ICNP®).

   _____

   _____

   _____

   _____

21. What is the ICNP®, and what is its use?

   _____

   _____

   _____

   _____

22. The Canadian Nurses Association (CNA) endorses ICNP® as the terminology of choice for documenting professional nursing practice in Canada.

23. ICNP® uses seven axes to capture the core details of nursing practice for coding key nursing data in the electronic health record. Give an example of each of the seven axes.

   a. Focus:

   _____

   _____

   b. Judgement:

   _____

   _____

   c. Means:

   _____

   _____

   d. Action:

   _____

   _____

   e. Time:

   _____

   _____

   f. Location:

   _____

   _____

   g. Client:

   _____

   _____

Canadian Privacy Legislation

24. Although provincial standards of practice and the CNA *Code of Ethics* both address confidentiality, you also need to be aware of Canadian privacy legislation that protects client data.

25. Canadians recognize the risk of privacy violation, and many believe that personal health information is one of the most important areas in need of protection under privacy laws.

26. What are the names of the two federal legislative Acts that address the privacy of personal information?

   a. _____

   b. _____

27. Describe three examples of personal health information that is protected specifically by the *Personal Information Protection and Electronic Documents Act (PIPEDA)*.

   a. _____

   b. _____

   c. _____

National E-Nursing Strategy

28. CNA released the *E-Nursing Strategy for Canada* (2006) to direct the coordinated integration of technology into Canadian nursing practice. The strategy is intended to completely integrate information and communication technologies (ICTs) in nursing.

29. CNA identified seven key outcomes that are projected to emerge from the *E-Nursing Strategy for Canada* (2006). Describe three of these outcomes and how you have seen evidence of each in your practice to date.

   a. _____

   b. _____

   c. _____

30. The Canadian Nurses Portal known as NurseONE is a key component of the *E-Nursing Strategy* and provides such services as professional links, professional development, an online library, practice support, and discussion groups.

Clinician Engagement and Informatics Communities

31. Many Canadian and international health informatics communities exist that offer opportunities for participation, support, educational programs, and networking opportunities.

32. The following is a list of several important health informatics communities. Describe the role of each organization in influencing nursing informatics.

    a. CNA:

    _____

    _____

    _____

    b. Canadian Nursing Informatics Association (CNIA):

    _____

    _____

    _____

    c. COACH:

    _____

    _____

    _____

33. In addition to formal organizations, numerous informal communities are devoted to nursing informatics, including blogs, Wikis, listserv and discussion groups, and social networks.

Review Questions

Select the appropriate answer and cite the rationale for choosing that particular answer.

1. As a new graduate, you just started a new position and find in orientation that the EHR is often referred to. You know from your reading that this refers to the
   a. Events of health risk
   b. Electronic health record
   c. Entries of the health record
   d. Electronic histogram response

   Answer: _____ Rationale: _____

   _____

   _____

2. You have volunteered to be part of a Standards Collaborative Working Group working on delivery of care. What type of data would you most likely be developing standards on?
   a. Public health investigations

   b. Wait times
   c. Prescribing of medications
   d. Clinical observations

   Answer: _____ Rationale: _____

   _____

   _____

3. Which of the following is *not* one of the benefits of standards to clients?
   a. Enhanced client outcomes
   b. Improved coordination of care
   c. Reduced duplication of tests and procedures
   d. Accessible personal health history

   Answer: _____ Rationale: _____

   _____

   _____

4. Which of the following is *not* one of the HI:NC categories?
   a. Nursing diagnosis
   b. Client outcome
   c. Primary nurse identifier
   d. Nursing resource intensity

   Answer: _____ Rationale: _____

   _____

   _____

5. According to ICNP® terminology, nursing outcomes must contain a term from the
   a. Means and Action axes
   b. Action and Location axes
   c. Focus and Judgement axes
   d. Judgement and Client axes

   Answer: _____ Rationale: _____

   _____

   _____

6. When clients indicate to you that they are afraid that their health information will not be kept confidential, you correctly respond that all nurses are bound by confidentiality in the
   a. CNA *Code of Ethics*
   b. *PIPEDA*
   c. *Privacy Act*
   d. All of the above

   Answer: _____ Rationale: _____

   _____

   _____

18

Communication

Preliminary Reading

Chapter 18, pp. 245–264

Comprehensive Understanding

1. Communication is a lifelong process. This process allows

   _____

   _____

2. Competency in communication helps the nurse maintain and develop therapeutic relationships, promote collaboration and interdisciplinary teamwork, and meet legal, ethical, and clinical standards of care.

Communication and Interpersonal Relationships

3. Communication is the means to establishing helping–healing relationships.

4. Communication is essential to the nurse–client relationship because

   a. _____

   b. _____

5. Nurses with expertise in communication can express caring by

   _____

   _____

   _____

6. The nurse's ability to relate to others is

   _____

   _____

   _____

Developing Communication Skills

7. Briefly explain the qualities of critical thinking in relation to the communication process.

   _____

   _____

8. Critical thinking can help you overcome perceptual biases.

9. Nurses use communication skills to gather, analyze, and transmit information and to accomplish the work of each phase.

Levels of Communication

10. Summarize the following communication interactions.

    a. Intrapersonal:

       _____

       _____

    b. Interpersonal:

       _____

       _____

    c. Transpersonal:

       _____

       _____

    d. Small group:

       _____

       _____

    e. Public:

       _____

       _____

Basic Elements of the Communication Process

11. Briefly summarize the following elements of communication.

    a. Referent:

    _____

    _____

    b. Sender:

    _____

    _____

    c. Receiver:

    _____

    _____

    d. Message:

    _____

    _____

    e. Channels:

    _____

    _____

    f. Feedback:

    _____

    _____

    g. Interpersonal variables:

    _____

    _____

    h. Environment:

    _____

    _____

Forms of Communication

12. Messages are conveyed verbally, nonverbally, concretely, and symbolically.

Verbal Communication

13. Verbal communication involves spoken or written words. Verbal language is a code that conveys specific meaning as words are combined.

14. Briefly explain the important aspects of verbal communication listed below.

    a. Vocabulary:

    _____

    _____

    b. Denotative and connotative meaning:

    _____

    _____

    c. Pacing:

    _____

    _____

    d. Intonation:

    _____

    _____

    e. Clarity:

    _____

    _____

    f. Brevity:

    _____

    _____

    g. Timing and relevance:

    _____

    _____

Nonverbal Communication

15. Nonverbal communication includes

    _____

    _____

    _____

16. Nonverbal communication is much more powerful than verbal communication.

17. Nonverbal communication is communicated in a cultural context.

18. Becoming an astute observer of nonverbal behaviour takes practice, concentration, and sensitivity to others. Briefly explain the following nonverbal behaviours.

    a. Personal appearance:

    _____

    _____

    b. Posture and gait:

    _____

    _____

    c. Facial expression:

    _____

    _____

d. Eye contact:

_____

_____

e. Gestures:

_____

_____

f. Sounds:

_____

_____

g. Territoriality and personal space:

_____

_____

19. Identify the zones of personal space.

_____

_____

_____

_____

20. Identify the zones of touch.

_____

_____

_____

_____

Symbolic Communication

21. Summarize symbolic communication.

_____

_____

_____

Metacommunication

22. Define *metacommunication*.

_____

_____

Professional Nursing Relationships

23. Professional relationships are created through _____, _____, and _____.

Nurse–Client Helping Relationships

24. The relationship is therapeutic, promoting a psychological climate that facilitates positive change and growth.

25. Acceptance conveys a

_____

26. The nurse–client relationship is characterized by four goal-directed phases. Explain the phases.

a. Pre-interaction phase:

_____

_____

b. Orientation phase:

_____

_____

c. Working phase:

_____

_____

d. Termination phase:

_____

_____

27. Nurses often encourage clients to share personal stories. This is called

_____

Nurse–Family Relationships

28. Summarize the principles related to nurse–family relationships.

_____

_____

_____

Nurse–Health Care Team Relationships

29. Communication in nurse–health care team relationships is geared toward

_____

_____

_____

Nurse–Community Relationships

30. Communication within the community occurs through channels such as

_____

_____

_____

Elements of Professional Communication

31. Briefly explain the following elements of professional communication.

    a. Courtesy:

    _____

    _____

    b. Use of names:

    _____

    _____

    c. Trustworthiness:

    _____

    _____

    d. Autonomy:

    _____

    _____

    e. Assertiveness:

    _____

    _____

Communication Within the Nursing Care Process

Assessment

32. Assessment of a client's ability to communicate includes gathering data about the many contextual factors that influence communication.

33. List the contextual factors that influence communication.

    a. _____

    b. _____

    c. _____

    d. _____

    e. _____

34. Identify the psychophysiological factors that influence communication.

    _____

    _____

35. Physical barriers to communication may include _____, _____, or _____.

36. Explain how developmental factors influence communication.

    _____

    _____

    _____

37. Summarize how sociocultural factors influence communication.

    _____

    _____

    _____

38. Gender influences communication. Explain how communication differs in regard to gender.

    a. Male: _____

    b. Female: _____

Nursing Diagnosis

39. List three nursing diagnoses appropriate for a client with alterations in communication.

    a. _____

    b. _____

    c. _____

Planning

40. List three goals for effective interpersonal communication.

    a. _____

    b. _____

    c. _____

Implementation

41. Therapeutic communication techniques are specific responses that encourage the expression of feelings and ideas and convey the nurse's acceptance and respect. Briefly explain the following techniques.

    a. Active listening:

    _____

    _____

    b. Sharing observations:

    _____

    _____

    c. Sharing empathy:

    _____

    _____

    d. Sharing hope:

    _____

    _____

    e. Sharing humour:

    _____

    _____

f. Sharing feelings:

_____

_____

g. Using touch:

_____

_____

h. Using silence:

_____

_____

i. Providing information:

_____

_____

j. Clarifying:

_____

_____

k. Focusing:

_____

_____

l. Paraphrasing:

_____

_____

m. Asking relevant questions:

_____

_____

n. Summarizing:

_____

_____

o. Self-disclosure:

_____

_____

p. Confrontation:

_____

_____

42. Certain communication techniques can hinder or damage professional relationships. These techniques are referred to as *nontherapeutic*. Briefly explain the following nontherapeutic techniques.

a. Asking personal questions:

_____

_____

b. Giving personal opinions:

_____

_____

c. Changing the subject:

_____

_____

d. Automatic responses:

_____

_____

e. False reassurance:

_____

_____

f. Sympathy:

_____

_____

g. Asking for explanations:

_____

_____

h. Approval or disapproval:

_____

_____

i. Defensive responses:

_____

_____

j. Passive or aggressive responses:

_____

_____

k. Arguing:

_____

_____

43. Briefly identify the communication techniques to use with the client with special needs.

a. Clients who cannot speak clearly:

_____

_____

b. Clients who are cognitively impaired:

_____

_____

c. Clients who are hearing impaired:

_____

_____

d. Clients who are visually impaired:

_____

_____

e. Clients who are unresponsive:

_____

_____

f. Clients who do not speak English:

_____

_____

Evaluation

44. List four expected outcomes for the client with impaired communication.

a. _____

b. _____

c. _____

d. _____

Review Questions

Select the appropriate answer and cite the rationale for choosing that particular answer.

1. Transpersonal communication is
   a. Interaction that occurs within a person's spiritual domain
   b. One-to-one interaction between the nurse and the client
   c. Communication within groups
   d. Self-talk

Answer: _____   Rationale: _____

_____

_____

2. In demonstrating the method for deep-breathing exercises, you place your hands on the client's abdomen to explain diaphragmatic movement. This technique involves the use of which communication element?
   a. Feedback
   b. Tactile channel

c. Referent
d. Message

Answer: _____   Rationale: _____

_____

_____

3. Which statement about nonverbal communication is correct?
   a. It is easy for a nurse to judge the meaning of a client's facial expression.
   b. The nurse's verbal messages should be reinforced by nonverbal cues.
   c. The physical appearance of the nurse rarely influences nurse–client interaction.
   d. Words convey meanings that are usually more significant than nonverbal communication.

Answer: _____   Rationale: _____

_____

_____

4. The term referring to all of the relational aspects of a message is called
   a. Nonverbal communication
   b. Metacommunication
   c. Connotative meaning
   d. Denotative meaning

Answer: _____   Rationale: _____

_____

_____

5. The referent in the communication process is
   a. That which motivates the communication
   b. The means of conveying messages
   c. Information shared by the sender
   d. The person who initiates the communication

Answer: _____   Rationale: _____

_____

_____

19

Caring in Nursing Practice

Preliminary Reading

Chapter 19, pp. 265–275

Comprehensive Understanding

1. _____ and _____ should be a natural part of every client encounter.

Theoretical Views on Caring

2. Caring in nursing has been studied from a variety of philosophical and ethical perspectives.

Caring Is Primary

3. Benner does not try to predict or control phenomena but attempts to give nurses a rich, holistic understanding of nursing practice and caring through the interpretation of _____.

4. Briefly summarize how Benner and Wrubel described the relationship between health, illness, and disease.

   _____
   _____
   _____

The Essence of Nursing and Health

5. Explain Leininger's concept of care from a transcultural perspective.

   _____
   _____
   _____

6. Define *acts of caring* according to Leininger.

   _____
   _____
   _____

7. According to Leininger, caring is a universal phenomenon, but the expressions, processes, and patterns of caring vary among cultures.

Transpersonal Caring

8. Summarize Watson's transpersonal caring theory (transformative model).

   _____
   _____
   _____

Swanson's Theory of Caring

9. Swanson's theory of caring consists of five categories. Explain each.

   a. Knowing:

   _____
   _____

   b. Being with:

   _____
   _____

   c. Doing for:

   _____
   _____

   d. Enabling:

   _____
   _____

   e. Maintaining belief:

   _____
   _____

The Human Act of Caring

10. Roach's theory contains five concepts. Briefly describe each.

    a. Compassion

    _____

    _____

    b. Competence

    _____

    _____

    c. Confidence

    _____

    _____

    d. Conscience

    _____

    _____

    e. Committment

    _____

    _____

Summary of Theoretical Views

11. Identify the common themes among the many nursing theories.

    _____

    _____

    _____

Client's Perceptions of Caring

12. Establishing a _____, _____ _____, and _____ are recurrent caring behaviours that researchers have identified.

13. When clients sense that health care professionals are interested in them as people, clients will be more willing to follow recommendations and therapeutic plans.

14. You need to consider how clients perceive caring and the best approaches to providing care.

Ethic of Care

15. Caring is interpreted by many as being a moral imperative.

16. In any client encounter, you must know what behaviour is ethically appropriate.

17. Define *ethic of care.*

    _____

    _____

Caring in Nursing Practice

18. As you deal with health and illness in your practice, your ability to care grows.

19. Nurse behaviours that have been shown to be related to caring include

    _____

    _____

Providing Presence

20. Summarize the concept of *presence.*

    _____

    _____

21. Identify ways you can establish presence with your clients.

    _____

    _____

Touch

22. The use of touch is one comforting approach whereby the nurse reaches out to clients to communicate concern and support.

23. Give some examples of protective and task-orientated touch.

    _____

    _____

    _____

    _____

Listening

24. Listening conveys your full attention and interest. Listening to the meaning of what a client says helps create a mutual relationship.

25. You must be able to give clients your full, focused attention as they tell their stories.

26. When an ill person chooses to tell his or her story, the person is reaching out to another human being.

27. Briefly summarize Frank's view of the clinical relationship the nurse and the client share.

    _____

    _____

    _____

28. Describe what listening involves.

    _____

    _____

    _____

Knowing the Client

29. To know a client means that the nurse _____, _____, and _____.

30. Knowing the client is at the core of the process by which you make clinical decisions. By establishing a caring relationship, the mutuality that develops helps you better know the client as an individual and then choose the most appropriate and efficacious nursing therapies.

31. Describe the following nurses and how they differ in knowing their clients.

    a. Expert nurse:

    _____

    _____

    b. Novice nurse:

    _____

    _____

Spiritual Caring

32. Spiritual health is achieved when

    _____

    _____

33. Spirituality offers a sense of _____, _____, and _____.

34. When a caring relationship is established, the client and the nurse come to know one another so that both move toward a healing relationship by

    a. _____

    b. _____

    c. _____

Family Care

35. Success with nursing interventions often depends on the family's willingness to:

    _____

    _____

    _____

36. List the 10 caring behaviours that are perceived as most hopeful by families of cancer clients.

    a. _____

    b. _____

    c. _____

    d. _____

    e. _____

    f. _____

    g. _____

    h. _____

    i. _____

    j. _____

The Challenge of Caring

37. Nursing professionals can care for and assist people without medical diagnoses or new technologies and treatments.

38. Caring motivates people to become nurses, and it becomes a source of satisfaction when they know they have made a difference in their clients' lives.

39. Summarize the challenges facing nursing in today's health care system.

    _____

    _____

    _____

    _____

Review Questions

Select the appropriate answer and cite the rationale for choosing that particular answer.

1. Leininger's care theory states that the client's caring values and behaviours are derived largely from
   a. Experience
   b. Gender
   c. Culture
   d. Religious beliefs

   Answer: _____   Rationale: _____

   _____

   _____

2. The central common theme of the caring theories is
   a. Pathophysiology and self-care abilities
   b. Compensation for client disabilities
   c. The nurse–client relationship and psychosocial aspects of care
   d. Maintenance of client homeostasis

   Answer: _____   Rationale: _____

   _____

   _____

3. In order to effectively listen to the client, you need to
   a. Sit with the legs crossed
   b. Lean back in the chair
   c. Respond quickly with appropriate answers to the client
   d. Maintain good eye contact

Answer: _____   Rationale: _____

_____

_____

4. You can demonstrate caring by
   a. Helping family members become active participants in the care of the client
   b. Doing all the necessary tasks for the client
   c. Following all the physician's orders accurately
   d. Maintaining a professional distance at all times

Answer: _____   Rationale: _____

_____

_____

5. Illness is best described as
   a. A disease state that manifests as an abnormality at the cellular, tissue, or organ level
   b. An abnormal condition at the cellular, tissue, or organ level that can be acute or chronic

   c. The client's personal experience of sickness
   d. The physical experience of disease and disability

Answer: _____   Rationale: _____

_____

_____

6. One of the main concepts for the human act of caring theory is
   a. Cultivating sensitivity of oneself and others
   b. Being with and being emotionally present to the other
   c. Health is a state of being that people define acccording to their values, personality, and lifestyle
   d. Conscience is a state of moral awareness

Answer: _____   Rationale: _____

_____

_____

20

Family Nursing

Preliminary Reading

Chapter 20, pp. 276–293

Comprehensive Understanding

1. Define the concept of family nursing.

_____

_____

_____

2. Describe the goal of family nursing.

_____

_____

_____

What Is a Family?

3. The family can be defined as a _____
_____, as a _____, or as a
_____.

4. To effectively provide care, you must understand that individual attitudes about family
are deeply ingrained and deserve respect.

5. To provide individualized care, you must
understand that families take many forms and
have diverse cultural and ethnic orientations.

Current Trends in the Canadian Family

6. Summarize the various family forms.

a. Nuclear family:

_____

_____

b. Extended family:

_____

_____

c. Step-family:

_____

_____

d. Blended family:

_____

_____

e. Lone-parent family:

_____

_____

f. Other family forms:

_____

_____

7. Identify at least three current trends that
challenge the family.

a. _____

b. _____

c. _____

8. Explain the following trends and social factors that impact the structure and function of
the family.

a. Marital roles:

_____

_____

b. Economic status:

_____

_____

c. Family caregivers:

_____

_____

The Family and Health

9. The health of the family is influenced by many factors, such as

    a. _____

    b. _____

    c. _____

10. The family's beliefs, values, and practices influence the health-promoting behaviours of its members. In turn, the health status of each individual influences how the family unit functions and its ability to achieve goals.

11. Family environment is crucial because health behaviour reinforced in early life has a strong influence on later health practices.

Attributes of Healthy Families

12. The crisis-proof or effective family is able to integrate the need for stability with the need for growth and change. Explain.

    _____
    _____
    _____

13. Define *family hardiness*.

    _____
    _____

14. Define *family resiliency*.

    _____
    _____

Family Nursing Care

15. List the three things that nurses should examine when they consider how a health problem or illness affects a family and how a family affects a health problem or illness.

    a. _____

    b. _____

    c. _____

16. Briefly explain the following two focuses proposed for family nursing practice.

    a. Family as context:

    _____
    _____

    b. Family as client:

    _____
    _____

Assessing the Needs of the Family: The Calgary Family Assessment Model

17. Summarize the following three major categories of family life that the Calgary Family Assessment Model (CFAM) offers as a framework for nurses to follow when conducting family assessments.

    a. Structural dimension:

    _____
    _____

    b. Developmental dimension:

    _____
    _____

    c. Functional dimension:

    _____
    _____

Structural Assessment

18. Explain these terms.

    a. *Internal structure*:

    _____
    _____

    b. *External structure*:

    _____
    _____

    c. *Context*:

    _____
    _____

19. Explain the purpose of a genogram.

    _____
    _____
    _____

20. Explain the purpose of an ecomap.

    _____
    _____
    _____

Developmental Assessment

21. Listed below are McGoldrick and Carter's family life stages. Describe the emotional process of transition associated with each stage.

    a. Between families:

    _____
    _____

b. Joining of families:

_____
_____

c. Family with young children:

_____
_____

d. Family with adolescents:

_____
_____

e. Launching children and moving on:

_____
_____

f. Family in later life:

_____
_____

22. What does McGoldrick and Carter's model *not* address?

_____
_____

Functional Assessment

23. A functional assessment focuses mainly on how family members interact and behave toward each other.

24. Describe the two subcategories of family functioning.

a. Instrumental functioning:

_____
_____

b. Expressive functioning:

_____
_____

Family Intervention: The Calgary Family Intervention Model

25. Describe the goal of family intervention.

_____
_____
_____

26. Name the three domains of family functioning that the Calgary Family Intervention Model (CFIM) focuses on promoting and improving.

a. _____
b. _____
c. _____

Asking Interventive Questions

27. The practice of asking questions leads family members to reflect on their situation, clarify their opinions and ideas, and understand how they are affected by their family member's illness or condition.

28. Describe the two types of interventive questions.

a. Linear questions:

_____
_____

b. Circular questions:

_____
_____

Offering Commendations

29. Describe the meaning of a commendation and why it is important for nurses to make commendations to families.

_____
_____
_____

30. List five common family strengths.

a. _____
b. _____
c. _____
d. _____
e. _____

Providing Information

31. One of the roles nurses need to adopt is that of educator.

32. Family and client needs for information may be elicited through direct questioning, but they are generally

_____

33. When you assume a humble position instead of coming across as an authority on the subject, this attitude often decreases the client's _____ and invites the client to listen without feeling _____.

Validating or Normalizing Emotional Responses

34. What is the purpose of validating emotional responses?

_____
_____

Encouraging Illness Narratives

35. Describe an illness narrative.

_____

_____

Encouraging Family Support

36. You can enhance family functioning by encouraging and assisting family members to listen to each other's _____ and _____.

Supporting Family Caregivers

37. Describe the concept of reciprocity.

_____

_____

_____

38. What are some of the benefits of reciprocity?

_____

_____

_____

Encouraging Respite

39. List five community resources that may be beneficial to caregivers.

a. _____

b. _____

c. _____

d. _____

e. _____

Interviewing the Family

40. When interviewing the family, the nurse must display keen perceptual, conceptual, and executive skills. Describe each of these skills in the space provided below.

a. Perceptual skills:

_____

_____

b. Conceptual skills:

_____

_____

c. Executive skills:

_____

_____

41. Describe the four stages of family interviewing skills for nurses using the CFAM and the CFIM.

a. Stage 1:

_____

b. Stage 2:

_____

c. Stage 3:

_____

d. Stage 4:

_____

Review Questions

Select the appropriate answer and cite the rationale for choosing that particular answer.

1. Family functioning can best be described as
   a. The processes that a family uses to meet its goal
   b. The way the family members communicate with each other
   c. Interrelated with family structure
   d. Adaptive behaviours that foster health

Answer: _____   Rationale: _____

_____

_____

2. Family structure can best be described as
   a. A basic pattern of predictable stages
   b. Flexible patterns that contribute to adequate functioning
   c. The pattern of relationships and ongoing membership
   d. A complex set of relationships

Answer: _____   Rationale: _____

_____

_____

3. "Skip-generation" families (grandparents caring for grandchildren), "nonfamilies" (adults living alone), and same-sex couples (with or without children) are considered
   a. Other family forms
   b. Blended families

c. Extended families
d. Step-families

Answer: _____   Rationale: _____
_____
_____

4. The majority of families today
   a. Consist of a mother, a father, and one or more children
   b. Include stepchildren
   c. Include a mother who works outside the home
   d. Are very similar to families of the past

Answer: _____   Rationale: _____
_____
_____

5. When planning care for a client and using the concept of family as client, you
   a. Consider the developmental stage of the client and not the family
   b. Realize that cultural background is an important variable when assessing the family

c. Include only the client and his or her significant other
d. Understand that the client's family will always be a help to the client's health goals

Answer: _____   Rationale: _____
_____
_____

6. Interventions recommended by the CFIM include
   a. Providing solutions for problems as they arise
   b. Validating emotional responses, encouraging illness narratives, and encouraging the client to request help from his or her family
   c. Asking interventive questions, offering commendations, providing information, and encouraging respite
   d. Administering nursing care in a manner that provides an opportunity for change

Answer: _____   Rationale: _____
_____
_____

21

Client Education

Preliminary Reading

Chapter 21, pp. 294–311

Comprehensive Understanding

Goals of Client Education

1. Comprehensive client education includes which three important goals?

   a. _____

   b. _____

   c. _____

Maintaining and Promoting Health and Preventing Illness

2. The nurse is a visible, competent resource for clients who are intent on improving their physical and psychological well-being. In the school, home, clinic, or workplace, the nurse provides information and skills that will allow clients to practise healthier behaviours.

3. Promoting healthy behaviours through education increases _____ by allowing clients to assume more responsibility for their health.

Restoring Health

4. Injured or ill clients need _____ and _____ that will help them regain or maintain their levels of health.

5. The _____ is a vital part of a client's return to health, and family members may need as much information as the client.

6. You should not assume that the family should be involved and must first assess the client–family relationship.

Coping With Impaired Functioning

7. The family's ability to provide support can result from _____, which begins as soon as the client's needs are identified and the family displays a willingness to help.

Teaching and Learning

Role of the Nurse in Teaching and Learning

8. Nurses have an _____ responsibility to teach their clients.

9. The nurse clarifies information provided by physicians and may become the primary source of information for adjusting to health problems.

Teaching as Communication

10. The teaching process closely parallels the _____ process.

Domains of Learning

11. List the three domains in which learning occurs:

    a. _____

    b. _____

    c. _____

12. The characteristics of learning within each domain affect the teaching and evaluation methods used.

Cognitive Learning

13. Cognitive learning (Bloom 1956) classifies cognitive behaviours in an ordered hierarchy. Summarize each one.

a. Knowledge:

_____
_____

b. Comprehension:

_____
_____

c. Application:

_____
_____

d. Analysis:

_____
_____

e. Synthesis:

_____
_____

f. Evaluation:

_____
_____

Affective Learning

14. Affective learning deals with the expression of feelings and the acceptance of attitudes, opinions, and values.

15. Summarize the following hierarchy behaviours.

a. Receiving:

_____
_____

b. Responding:

_____
_____

c. Valuing:

_____
_____

d. Organizing:

_____
_____

e. Characterizing:

_____
_____

Psychomotor Learning

16. Psychomotor learning involves acquiring skills that require the integration of mental and muscular activity.

17. Summarize the following hierarchy behaviours.

a. Perception:

_____
_____

b. Set:

_____
_____

c. Guided response:

_____
_____

d. Mechanism:

_____
_____

e. Complex overt response:

_____
_____

f. Adaptation:

_____
_____

g. Origination:

_____
_____

Learning Environment

18. Factors in the physical environment where teaching takes place can make learning pleasant or difficult. List four factors to consider when selecting the learning setting.

a. _____
b. _____
c. _____
d. _____

Ability to Learn

19. Summarize how each of the following influences the ability to learn.

a. Emotional capability:

_____
_____

b. Intellectual capability:

_____

_____

c. Physical capability:

_____

_____

d. Developmental stage:

_____

_____

Learning Style and Preferences

20. Everyone has different learning preferences and styles. You should ask clients their preferred method for learning. In a group, you should

_____

_____

_____

Motivation to Learn

21. Motivation is defined as:

_____

_____

22. Briefly explain how the following distractions influence the ability to learn.

a. Physical discomfort:

_____

_____

b. Anxiety:

_____

_____

c. Environment:

_____

_____

23. Define *motivation*.

_____

_____

24. Briefly explain how the following can affect motivation.

a. Social motives:

_____

_____

b. Task mastery:

_____

_____

c. Physical motives:

_____

_____

25. Define *self-efficacy*.

_____

_____

Motivation and Transtheoretical Model of Change

26. By identifying the client's stage of change and by focusing learning activities to match the client's stage, you facilitate the learner's motivation to change and his or her transition from one stage to the next. Identify the five stages used in smoking cessation activities:

a. _____

b. _____

c. _____

d. _____

e. _____

Integrating the Nursing and Teaching Processes

27. Differentiate between the nursing process and the teaching process.

_____

_____

_____

28. The teaching process focuses on

_____

_____

_____

29. The nurse sets specific learning objectives and implements the teaching plan using teaching and learning principles to ensure

_____

_____

_____

Assessment

30. The client requires the nurse to assess the following factors. Summarize each one.

Learning Needs

a. _____

b. _____

c. _____

Ability to Learn

a. _____

b. _____

c. _____

Motivation to Learn

a. _____

b. _____

c. _____

Teaching Environment

a. _____

b. _____

c. _____

Resources for Learning

a. _____

b. _____

c. _____

d. _____

e. _____

Nursing Diagnosis

31. Classifying diagnoses by the three learning domains helps you focus specifically on subject matter and teaching methods.

Planning

32. After determining the nursing diagnoses that identify a client's learning needs, you develop a teaching plan, determine goals and expected outcomes, and involve the client in selecting learning experiences. Expected outcomes guide the

_____

_____

_____

33. A learning objective identifies the _____ of a planned learning experience and helps _____ for learning.

34. A learning objective includes the same criteria as goals or outcomes in a nursing care plan. These are

a. _____

b. _____

c. _____

d. _____

35. The principles of teaching are techniques that incorporate the principles of learning. Explain the following principles.

a. Setting priorities:

_____

_____

b. Timing:

_____

_____

c. Organizing teaching material:

_____

_____

d. Maintaining attention and promoting participation:

_____

_____

e. Building on existing knowledge:

_____

_____

f. Selecting teaching methods:

_____

_____

g. Selecting resources:

_____

_____

h. Writing teaching plans:

_____

_____

Implementation

36. Briefly explain the following teaching approaches.

a. Telling:

_____

_____

b. Selling:

_____

_____

c. Participating:

_____

_____

d. Entrusting:

_____

_____

e. Reinforcing:

_____

_____

37. Summarize the following instructional methods.

a. One-on-one discussion:

_____

_____

b. Group instruction:

_____

_____

c. Preparatory instruction:

_____

_____

d. Demonstrations:

_____

_____

e. Analogies:

_____

_____

f. Role-playing:

_____

_____

38. Identify some teaching tools to be used with the following.

a. Illiteracy and learning disability:

_____

_____

b. Cultural diversity:

_____

_____

c. Children:

_____

_____

d. Older adults:

_____

_____

Evaluation

39. Evaluation reinforces correct behaviour by the learner, helps learners realize how they should change incorrect behaviour, and helps you determine the adequacy of teaching.

40. Identify some evaluation measures.

_____

_____

_____

41. List three areas to be included when documenting client teaching.

a. _____

b. _____

c. _____

Review Questions

Select the appropriate answer and cite the rationale for choosing that particular answer.

1. An internal impulse that causes a person to take action is
   a. Anxiety
   b. Motivation
   c. Compliance
   d. Adaptation

Answer: _____   Rationale: _____

_____

_____

2. Demonstration of the principles of body mechanics used when transferring clients from bed to chair would be classified under which domain of learning?
   a. Cognitive
   b. Social
   c. Psychomotor
   d. Affective

Answer: _____   Rationale: _____

_____

_____

3. Which of the following clients is most ready to begin a client-teaching session?
   a. Ms. Benoit, who is unwilling to accept that her back injury may result in permanent paralysis
   b. Mr. Chang, a client who recently received a diagnosis of diabetes, who is complaining that he was awake all night because of his noisy roommate

c. Mrs. Ho, a client with irritable bowel syndrome, who has just returned from a morning of testing in the gastroenterology laboratory
d. Mr. Cinelli, a client who had a heart attack four days ago and now seems somewhat anxious about how this will affect his future

Answer: _____   Rationale: _____
_____
_____

4. As a nurse, you work with pediatric clients who have diabetes. Which is the youngest age group to which you can effectively teach psychomotor skills such as insulin administration?
a. Toddler
b. Adolescent
c. School age
d. Preschool

Answer: _____   Rationale: _____
_____
_____

5. Which of the following is an appropriately stated learning objective for Mr. Chang, who has just received a diagnosis of type 2 diabetes?
a. Mr. Chang will be taught self-administration of insulin by 5/2.
b. Mr. Chang will perform blood glucose monitoring with the EZ-Check Monitor by the time of discharge.
c. Mr. Chang will know the signs and symptoms of low blood sugar by 5/5.
d. Mr. Chang will understand diabetes.

Answer: _____   Rationale: _____
_____
_____

22

Developmental Theories

Preliminary Reading

Chapter 22, pp. 312–328

Comprehensive Understanding

Growth and Development

1. Define *growth*.

   _____

   _____

2. Define *development*.

   _____

   _____

Factors Influencing Growth and Development

3. Identify the major factors influencing growth and development.

   a. _____

   b. _____

   c. _____

Traditions of Developmental Theories

4. List the five traditions of developmental theories.

   a. _____

   b. _____

   c. _____

   d. _____

   e. _____

Organicism

5. Define *organicism*.

   _____

   _____

Biophysical Developmental Theories

6. Briefly summarize Gesell's theory of maturational development.

   _____

   _____

   _____

7. Identify and describe the mechanisms of Gesell's theory.

   a. _____

   b. _____

8. Briefly describe Chess and Thomas's theory of temperament development.

   _____

   _____

   _____

9. Identify and describe the three categories of temperament in Chess and Thomas's theory.

   a. _____

   b. _____

   c. _____

10. Identify and describe the mechanisms of Chess and Thomas's theory.

   _____

   _____

   _____

Cognitive Developmental Theories

11. Briefly summarize Piaget's theory of cognitive development.

   _____

   _____

   _____

12. Identify and describe the mechanisms of Piaget's theory.

   a. _____

   b. _____

13. Explain the four stages of Piaget's theory of cognitive development.

   a. Sensorimotor:

   _____

   _____

   b. Preoperational:

   _____

   _____

   c. Concrete operations:

   _____

   _____

   d. Formal operations:

   _____

   _____

Moral Developmental Theories

14. Moral developmental theories try to explain

   _____

   _____

15. Explain the three stages of Piaget's moral development theory.

   a. Premoral stage:

   _____

   _____

   b. Conventional stage:

   _____

   _____

   c. Autonomous stage:

   _____

   _____

16. Explain the six stages of Kohlberg's theory of moral development.

   a. Level I: Preconventional level

   Stage 1: _____

   Stage 2: _____

   b. Level II: Conventional level

   Stage 3: _____

   Stage 4: _____

   c. Level III: Postconventional level

   Stage 5: _____

   Stage 6: _____

17. Identify the limitations to Kohlberg's research.

   _____

   _____

   _____

18. Briefly explain Gilligan's argument against Kohlberg's theory.

   _____

   _____

   _____

Psychoanalytic and Psychosocial Tradition

19. What do theories in the psychoanalytic and psychosocial tradition describe?

   _____

   _____

20. Briefly summarize Freud's theory of personality development.

   _____

   _____

   _____

21. Identify and describe the mechanisms of Freud's theory.

   a. _____

   b. _____

   c. _____

22. Explain the five stages of Freud's theory.

   a. _____

   b. _____

   c. _____

   d. _____

   e. _____

23. Briefly summarize Erikson's theory of psychosocial development.

_____

_____

_____

24. Identify and describe the mechanisms of Erikson's theory.

a. _____

b. _____

25. Explain the following eight stages of Erikson's theory.

a. Trust versus mistrust:

_____

_____

b. Autonomy versus shame and doubt:

_____

_____

c. Initiative versus guilt:

_____

_____

d. Industry versus inferiority:

_____

_____

e. Identity versus role confusion:

_____

_____

f. Intimacy versus isolation:

_____

_____

g. Generativity versus self-absorption and stagnation:

_____

_____

h. Integrity versus despair:

_____

_____

26. Define attachment according to Crittenden's dynamic maturation model.

_____

_____

_____

27. Briefly summarize Havighurst's theory of development.

_____

_____

28. Identify a limitation to Havighurst's theory.

_____

_____

_____

29. Havighurst defined a series of essential tasks that arise from predictable and external pressures. These pressures include _____ _____, _____, and _____.

30. Briefly summarize Gould's five themes of adult development.

a. _____

b. _____

c. _____

d. _____

e. _____

Mechanistic Tradition

31. Briefly explain the mechanistic tradition.

_____

_____

Contextualism

32. Developmental theories within the contextual tradition focus on

_____

_____

Bioecological Theory

33. Briefly summarize Bronfenbrenner's theory of bioecological development.

_____

_____

_____

34. Explain the four layers of environment in Bronfenbrenner's theory.

a. _____

b. _____

c. _____

d. _____

35. Identify and describe the mechanisms of Bronfenbrenner's theory.

_____
_____
_____

Dialecticism

36. Briefly explain the dialectic tradition.

_____
_____

Keating and Hertzman's Population Health Theory

37. Briefly summarize Keating and Hertzman's population health approach.

_____
_____
_____

38. Identify and describe the mechanisms of Keating and Hertzman's theory.
    a. _____
    b. _____
    c. _____

Resilience Theory

39. Briefly describe the resilience approach to development.

_____
_____
_____

40. Identify and describe the mechanisms of resilience theory.
    a. _____
    b. _____

Review Questions

Select the appropriate answer and cite the rationale for choosing that particular answer.

1. According to Piaget, the school-age child is in the third stage of cognitive development, which is characterized by
   a. Conventional thought
   b. Concrete operations
   c. Identity versus role diffusion
   d. Postconventional thought

   Answer: _____   Rationale: _____
   _____

2. According to Bronfenbrenner's developmental theory, the individual and his or her environment are seen as mutually influential. Development of a national child care policy is an example of an intervention at which level?
   a. Microsystem
   b. Mesosystem
   c. Exosystem
   d. Macrosystem

   Answer: _____   Rationale: _____
   _____
   _____

3. According to Erikson's developmental theory, the primary developmental task of the middle adult years is to
   a. Achieve generativity
   b. Achieve intimacy
   c. Establish a set of personal values
   d. Establish a sense of personal identity

   Answer: _____   Rationale: _____
   _____
   _____

4. Which of the following behaviours is most characteristic of the concrete operations stage of cognitive development?
   a. Progression from reflex activity to imitative behaviour
   b. Inability to put oneself in another's place
   c. Thought processes become increasingly logical and coherent
   d. Ability to think in abstract terms and draw logical conclusions

   Answer: _____   Rationale: _____
   _____
   _____

5. According to Kohlberg, children develop moral reasoning as they mature. Which of the following is most characteristic of a preschooler's stage of moral development?
   a. Obeying the rules of correct behaviour
   b. Showing respect for authority is important behaviour
   c. Behaviour that pleases others is considered good
   d. Actions are determined as good or bad in terms of their consequences

   Answer: _____   Rationale: _____
   _____
   _____

23

Conception Through Adolescence

Preliminary Reading

Chapter 23, pp. 329–362

Comprehensive Understanding

1. Human growth and development are continuous, intricate, and complex processes that are often divided into stages organized by age groups.

Selecting a Developmental Framework for Nursing

2. Providing nursing care that is developmentally appropriate is easier when planning on a theoretical framework.

3. A developmental approach encourages organized care directed at the child's current level of functioning to motivate self-direction and health promotion.

Conception

4. Define the following terms or events.

   a. Nagele's rule:

   _____

   _____

   b. Fertilization:

   _____

   _____

   c. Zygote:

   _____

   _____

   d. Morula:

   _____

   _____

   e. Blastocyst:

   _____

   _____

   f. Embryo:

   _____

   _____

   g. Placenta:

   _____

   _____

   h. Implantation:

   _____

   _____

5. Explain the development process and health concerns for the following trimesters.

   a. First trimester

   Physical changes:

   _____

   _____

   Health promotion:

   _____

   _____

   Teratogens:

   _____

   _____

b. Second trimester

Physical changes:

_____

_____

Health promotion:

_____

_____

c. Third trimester

Physical changes:

_____

_____

Health promotion:

_____

_____

Transition From Intrauterine to Extrauterine Life

6. _____, _____, and _____
   changes contribute to the infant's adjustment
   to the external environment.

Physical Changes

7. An immediate assessment of the neonate's
   condition is performed because the first concern is

   _____

8. List the five physiological parameters evaluated through the Apgar assessment.

   a. _____
   b. _____
   c. _____
   d. _____
   e. _____

Psychosocial Changes

9. Which two factors are most important in
   promoting closeness of the parents and the
   neonate?

   a. _____
   b. _____

10. Define *bonding*.

   _____

Health Risks

11. Briefly explain the three most important physi-
    cal needs of the newborn in each category.

    a. Airway:

    _____

    b. Temperature:

    _____

    c. Prevention of infection:

    _____

Newborn

12. The neonatal period is defined as

    _____

    _____

Physical Changes

13. Identify the normal characteristics of the
    newborn.

    a. Height:

    _____

    b. Weight:

    _____

    c. Head circumference:

    _____

    d. Vital signs:

    _____

    e. Physical characteristics:

    _____

    f. Neurological function:

    _____

    g. Behavioural characteristics:

    _____

Cognitive Changes

14. Early cognitive development begins with
    innate behaviour, reflexes, and sensory
    functions.

15. Identify the sensory functions that contribute
    to cognitive development in the newborn.

    _____

    _____

Psychosocial Changes

16. Explain the interactions that foster deep attachment between the infant and the parents.

———————————————————————

———————————————————————

Health Risks

17. Define *hyperbilirubinemia*.

———————————————————————

———————————————————————

Health Concerns

18. Screening for inborn errors of metabolism applies to

———————————————————————

———————————————————————

19. Circumcision is a common and controversial procedure. Identify the risks of this procedure.

———————————————————————

———————————————————————

Infant

20. Infancy is the period from _____ to _____.

Physical Changes

21. Summarize the normal characteristics of the infant.
    a. Physical growth:

    ———————————————————————

    b. Vital signs:

    ———————————————————————

    c. Gross motor skills:

    ———————————————————————

    d. Fine motor skills:

    ———————————————————————

Cognitive Changes

22. Summarize the cognitive development of an infant.

———————————————————————

———————————————————————

———————————————————————

Psychosocial Changes

23. During the first year, infants begin to differentiate themselves from others as separate beings capable of acting on their own.

24. Erikson describes the psychosocial developmental crisis for the infant as trust versus mistrust.

25. Define *play*.

———————————————————————

———————————————————————

26. Identify activities appropriate at this stage of development.

———————————————————————

———————————————————————

———————————————————————

Health Risks

27. Identify the common types of injury and possible prevention strategies.

———————————————————————

———————————————————————

28. Child maltreatment includes

———————————————————————

———————————————————————

Health Concerns

29. The foundation for children's perceptions of their health status is laid early in life.

30. Internal body sensations and experiences with the outside world affect self-perceptions.

31. The quality of nutrition influences the infant's growth and development.

32. Identify the feeding alternatives for an infant.

———————————————————————

———————————————————————

33. Identify some supplementation needs of an infant.

———————————————————————

———————————————————————

34. Briefly explain health concerns related to the following.
    a. Dentition:

    ———————————————————————

    b. Immunizations:

    ———————————————————————

c. Sleep:

_____

d. Overfeeding:

_____

Toddler

35. Toddlerhood ranges from _____ to _____.

Physical Changes

36. Summarize the normal characteristics of a toddler.

   a. Self-care activities:

   _____

   b. Motor skills:

   _____

   c. Vital signs:

   _____

   d. Weight:

   _____

   e. Height:

   _____

Cognitive Changes

37. Summarize Piaget's preoperational thought stage.

   _____
   _____
   _____

38. Describe language ability at this stage.

   _____
   _____
   _____

Psychosocial Changes

39. Identify Erikson's psychosocial development stage.

   _____
   _____
   _____

40. Explain the parental implications of the following developmental states.

   a. Independence:

   _____
   _____

b. Social interactions:

_____
_____

c. Play:

_____
_____

Health Risks

41. Describe some developmental abilities for this age period.

   _____
   _____
   _____

42. Identify injury prevention strategies.

   _____
   _____
   _____

Health Concerns

43. Briefly explain the nutrition requirements for this age group.

   _____
   _____

Preschooler

44. The preschool period refers to

   _____

Physical Changes

45. Summarize the normal characteristics of the preschooler.

   a. Vital signs:

   _____

   b. Weight:

   _____

   c. Height:

   _____

   d. Coordination:

   _____

Cognitive Changes

46. Preschoolers continue to master the preoperational stage of cognition.

47. The first phase of this period (2 to 4 years) is characterized by

   _____

48. Define *artificialism*.

_____
_____
_____

49. Define *animism*.

_____
_____

50. Summarize the intuitive phase of preoperational thought (4 years).

_____
_____

51. The greatest fear of this age group is

_____
_____

52. Summarize this group's moral development.

_____
_____
_____

53. Describe the language ability for this age group.

_____
_____
_____

Psychosocial Changes

54. The preschooler's world expands beyond the family into the neighbourhood, where preschoolers meet other children and adults.

55. Identify some dependent behaviours that preschoolers may revert to during stress or illness.

_____
_____
_____

56. Summarize the pattern of play for the preschooler.

_____
_____
_____

Health Risks

57. Guidelines for injury prevention in the toddler also apply to the preschooler.

58. _____ and _____ are the top priorities for this age group.

Health Concerns

59. Parental beliefs about health, children's bodily sensations, and the ability to perform daily activities help children develop attitudes about their health.

60. Explain health concerns related to the following for this group.

    a. Nutrition:

    _____
    _____

    b. Sleep:

    _____
    _____

    c. Vision:

    _____
    _____

School-Age Child

61. The school-age years range from _____ to _____.

62. _____ signals the end of middle childhood.

63. The school and home influence growth and development, and adjustments by the parents and child are required.

64. Parents must learn to allow their child to make decisions, accept responsibility, and learn from life's experiences.

Physical Changes

65. Summarize the normal characteristics of the school-age child.

    a. Weight:

    _____

    b. Height:

    _____

    c. Cardiovascular functioning:

    _____

    d. Neuromuscular functioning:

    _____

    e. Skeletal growth:

    _____

Cognitive Changes

66. Cognitive changes provide the school-age child with the ability to think in a logical manner about the here and now. They are not yet capable of abstract thinking.

67. Define the cognitive skills that are developing in this group.

_____

_____

_____

68. Describe language development during middle childhood.

_____

_____

_____

Psychosocial Changes

69. The developmental task for school-age children is _____ versus _____.

70. Summarize psychosocial development in relation to the following.

   a. Moral development:

   _____

   _____

   b. Peer relationships:

   _____

   _____

   c. Sexual identity:

   _____

   _____

Health Risks

71. _____ and _____ are the leading causes of death or injury.

72. Infections account for the majority of all childhood illnesses; respiratory infections are the most prevalent.

73. Identify the specific health concerns of children living in poverty.

   _____

   _____

Health Concerns

74. Identify five critical functions of a school-based health promotion program.

   a. _____

   b. _____

c. _____

d. _____

e. _____

75. Accidents are the leading cause of death and injury in the school-age period. Children should be encouraged to take responsibility for their own safety.

76. Identify at least five health promotion activities that are appropriate for the school-age child.

   a. _____

   b. _____

   c. _____

   d. _____

   e. _____

77. Identify the nutritional requirements for the school-age child.

   _____

   _____

Adolescent

78. Adolescence is the period of development _____.

79. Define *puberty* and explain the changes that occur at this time.

   _____

   _____

   _____

Physical Changes

80. List the four major physical changes associated with sexual maturation.

   a. _____

   b. _____

   c. _____

   d. _____

81. The hormones responsible for the development of secondary sex characteristics are _____ and _____.

82. Summarize the weight and skeletal changes that occur during adolescence.

   _____

   _____

83. Explain the effects of physical changes on peer interactions.

_____
_____
_____

Cognitive Changes

84. Changes that occur within the mind and the widening social environment of the adolescent result in _____, the highest level of intellectual development.

85. During this period of cognitive development, the adolescent develops the ability to solve problems through logical operations.

86. For the first time, the young person can move beyond the physical or concrete properties of a situation and use reasoning powers to understand the abstract.

87. Briefly explain the cognitive abilities of this group.

_____
_____
_____

88. Describe the language skills of the adolescent.

_____
_____

Psychosocial Changes

89. The search for _____ is the major task of adolescent psychosocial development.

90. Teenagers must establish close peer relationships or risk remaining socially isolated.

91. Explain identity versus role confusion (Erikson).

_____
_____

92. Behaviours indicating a lack of resolution are _____ and _____.

93. Explain the following components of total identity.
   a. Gender identity:

   _____
   b. Group identity:

   _____
   c. Family identity:

   _____

   d. Vocational identity:

   e. Health identity:

   _____

   f. Moral identity:

   _____

Health Risks

94. Identify the leading cause of death and its sources among adolescents.

_____
_____

95. Suicide is the second leading cause of death among adolescents. List the six warning signs of suicide for this group.
   a. _____
   b. _____
   c. _____
   d. _____
   e. _____
   f. _____

96. Substance abuse is a major concern. Adolescents most at risk are those coming from _____.

97. To help adolescents form healthy habits of daily living, you need to emphasize the importance of exercise, sleep, nutrition, and stress reduction.

98. Define the two eating disorders that follow.
   a. Anorexia nervosa:

   _____
   _____

   b. Bulimia nervosa:

   _____
   _____

99. _____, _____, and _____ expectations contribute to early heterosexual and homosexual relations.

100. Briefly explain the two prominent consequences of adolescent sexual activity.
   a. Sexually transmitted infection (STI):

   _____
   _____

b. Pregnancy:

_____

_____

101. Identify health promotion interventions for the adolescent in regard to the following.

a. Unintentional injuries:

_____

_____

b. Substance abuse:

_____

_____

c. Sexual activity:

_____

_____

Health Concerns

102. Identify the health concerns of the following.

a. Adolescents in rural communities:

_____

_____

b. Minority adolescents:

_____

_____

c. Aboriginal adolescents:

_____

_____

Review Questions

Select the appropriate answer and cite the rationale for choosing that particular answer.

1. Which statement about human growth and development is accurate?
   a. Growth and development processes are unpredictable.
   b. Growth and development begin with birth and end after adolescence.
   c. All individuals progress through the same phases of growth and development.
   d. All individuals accomplish developmental tasks at the same pace.

Answer: _____   Rationale: _____

_____

2. The mother of a 2-year-old expresses concern that her son's appetite has diminished and that he seems to prefer milk to other solid foods. Which response reflects your knowledge of the principles of communication and nutrition?
   a. "Oh, I wouldn't be too worried; children tend to eat when they're hungry. I just wouldn't give him dessert unless he eats his meal."
   b. "That is not uncommon in toddlers. You might consider increasing his milk to 2 litres per day to be sure he gets enough nutrients."
   c. "Have you considered feeding him when he doesn't seem interested in feeding himself?"
   d. "A toddler's rate of growth normally slows down. It's common to see a toddler's appetite diminish in response to decreased calorie needs."

Answer: _____   Rationale: _____

_____

_____

3. Which neonatal assessment finding would be considered abnormal?
   a. Cyanosis of the hands and feet during activity
   b. Palpable anterior and posterior fontanels
   c. Soft, protuberant abdomen
   d. Absence of the rooting, grasping, and sucking reflexes

Answer: _____   Rationale: _____

_____

_____

4. To stimulate cognitive and psychosocial development of the toddler, it is important for parents to
   a. Set firm and consistent limits
   b. Foster sharing of toys with playmates and siblings
   c. Provide clarification about what is right and wrong
   d. Limit confusion by restricting exploration of the environment

Answer: _____   Rationale: _____

_____

_____

5. Which of the following statements is true of the developmental behaviours of school-age children?
   a. Formal and informal peer group membership is the key to forming self-esteem.

b. Fears centre on the loss of self-control.
c. Positive feedback from parents and teachers is crucial to development.
d. A full range of defence mechanisms is used, including rationalization and intellectualization.

Answer: _____ Rationale: _____

_____

_____

6. Adolescents have mastered age-appropriate sexuality when they feel comfortable with their sexual
a. Behaviours
b. Choices
c. Relationships
d. All of the above

Answer: _____ Rationale: _____

_____

_____

24

Young to Middle Adulthood

Preliminary Reading

Chapter 24, pp. 363–376

Comprehensive Understanding

1. Young adulthood is the period from _____ to _____.

2. Individuals in young adulthood _____ _____, _____, and _____.

3. Middle age occurs from _____ to _____.

4. Middle-age adults become aware of changes in _____ and _____ abilities. This is a time when individuals may reassess _____.

Young Adulthood

Physical Changes

5. The young adult has completed physical growth by the age of 20. List the characteristics of young adults.

   a. _____

   b. _____

   c. _____

   d. _____

6. Identify the main components of a personal lifestyle assessment of a young adult.

   _____

   _____

   _____

Cognitive Changes

7. Formal and informal education, life experiences, and work opportunities increase the young adult's _____ and _____.

8. Choosing an occupation is a _____ _____ of young adults and involves knowing their _____, _____, and _____ _____.

Psychosocial Changes

9. The emotional health of the young adult is related to the individual's ability to address and resolve personal and social tasks. Explain the patterns of change that are common in the following age groups.

   a. 23 to 28 years:

   _____

   _____

   b. 29 to 34 years:

   _____

   _____

10. _____ and _____ issues influence an adult's life and can pose challenges for nursing care.

11. Identify the six major developmental tasks of adulthood.

   a. _____

   b. _____

   c. _____

   d. _____

   e. _____

   f. _____

12. For young men and women, successful employment ensures _____ and promotes _____, _____ _____, _____, and _____.

13. Two-career marriages are _____.

14. The average age for first marriage for women is _____ years and for men is _____ years.

15. Close friends and associates of the single young adult may also be viewed as the individual's _____.

16. Identify five tasks to be completed by a couple prior to marriage.

   a. _____

   b. _____

   c. _____

   d. _____

   e. _____

17. Identify three changing norms and values in Canada related to alternative family structures.

   a. _____

   b. _____

   c. _____

Hallmarks of Emotional Health

18. During a psychological assessment of young adults, the nurse can assess for _____ of emotional health that indicate successful maturation in this developmental stage.

Health Risks

19. Briefly explain the risk factors for young adults in regard to the following.

   a. Lifestyle:

   _____

   _____

   b. Family history:

   _____

   _____

   c. Accidental death and injury:

   _____

   _____

   d. Substance abuse:

   _____

   _____

   e. Unplanned pregnancies:

   _____

   _____

   f. Sexually transmitted infections:

   _____

   _____

   g. Environmental and occupational risks:

   _____

   _____

Health Concerns

20. Give examples of nursing assessment and interventions for young adults related to the following areas of health.

   a. Infertility:

   _____

   _____

   b. Exercise:

   _____

   _____

   c. Routine health screening:

   _____

   _____

21. The psychosocial concerns of the young adult are often related to stress. Briefly explain each of the following sources of stress.

   a. Job stress:

   _____

   _____

   b. Family stress:

   _____

   _____

Pregnancy

22. Explain the health practices that you would discuss with a woman anticipating pregnancy.

   _____

   _____

   _____

   _____

   _____

23. Prenatal care is

   _____

24. Explain the physiological changes that occur during pregnancy and the puerperium.

   a. First trimester:

   _____

   _____

b. Second trimester:

_____

_____

c. Third trimester:

_____

_____

d. Puerperium:

_____

_____

25. Explain the implications for nursing associated with the following psychosocial changes that occur during pregnancy.

a. Body image:

_____

_____

b. Role changes:

_____

_____

c. Sexuality:

_____

_____

d. Coping mechanisms:

_____

_____

e. Stresses during puerperium:

_____

_____

f. Postpartum blues and depression:

_____

_____

Acute Care

26. Provide examples of when acute care might be required for young adults.

_____

_____

_____

Restorative and Continuing Care

27. Describe the effect of chronic illness and disability on the young adult.

_____

_____

_____

Middle Adulthood

28. Briefly explain the characteristics of the middle adult years.

_____

_____

Physical Changes

29. Briefly explain the major physiological changes that occur between 40 and 65 years of age.

_____

_____

_____

_____

30. Define *menopause*.

_____

_____

31. Define *sandwich generation*.

_____

_____

Psychosocial Changes

32. Summarize the psychosocial development of the middle adult in the following areas.

a. Career transition:

_____

_____

b. Sexuality:

_____

_____

c. Singlehood:

_____

_____

d. Marital changes:

_____

_____

e. Family transitions:

_____

_____

f. Care of aging parents

_____

_____

Health Concerns

33. Briefly explain each of the following physiological concerns for the middle adult and suggest appropriate nursing assessment and interventions.

a. Stress and stress reduction:

_____

_____

_____

b. Obesity:

_____

_____

_____

34. List some positive health habits that support health for the middle-aged adult.

_____

_____

_____

35. _____ and _____ are often directed at improving health habits.

36. Identify three external barriers to change.
    a. _____
    b. _____
    c. _____

37. Identify four internal barriers to change.
    a. _____
    b. _____
    c. _____
    d. _____

38. Summarize two psychosocial concerns of the middle adult and provide the appropriate nursing assessment and interventions.
    a. Anxiety:

    _____

    _____

    _____

    b. Depression:

    _____

    _____

    _____

Primary Health Care Programs

39. Primary health care programs for young and middle adults are designed to _____ _____, _____, and _____.

Acute Care

40. Identify examples of acute illnesses and injuries (similar to the young adult) that occur in middle adulthood.

_____

_____

_____

Restorative and Continuing Care

41. Identify some chronic illnesses or issues that occur in middle adulthood.

_____

_____

_____

Review Questions

Select the appropriate answer and cite the rationale for choosing that particular answer.

1. The leading cause of injury and death in the young adult population is
   a. Sexually transmitted infection
   b. Accidents
   c. Cardiovascular disease
   d. Substance abuse

Answer: _____   Rationale: _____

_____

_____

2. Psychosocial changes of pregnancy commonly involve all of the following areas *except*
   a. Altered body image
   b. Anxiety and depression
   c. Role changes
   d. Sexuality

Answer: _____   Rationale: _____

_____

_____

3. Which physiological change would be a normal assessment finding in a middle adult?
   a. Increased breast size
   b. Abdominal tenderness
   c. Increased thoracic diameter
   d. Reduced auditory acuity

Answer: _____   Rationale: _____

_____

_____

4. Which of the following is most likely to affect the overall level of health of a client in middle adulthood?
   a. Stress due to life changes
   b. Decreased visual acuity
   c. Declining sexual interest
   d. Onset of menopause

Answer: _____   Rationale: _____
_____
_____

5. In planning client education for Mrs. Higuchi, a 45-year-old woman who had an ovarian cyst removed, which of the following facts is true about the sexuality of the middle-aged adult?
   a. Menstruation ceases after menopause.
   b. Estrogen is produced after menopause.
   c. Middle-aged men are unable to produce fertile sperm.
   d. With removal of an ovarian cyst, pregnancy cannot occur.

Answer: _____   Rationale: _____
_____
_____

25

Older Adulthood

Preliminary Reading

Chapter 25, pp. 377–397

Comprehensive Understanding

1. Briefly summarize demographic trends of older Canadians.

   _____
   _____
   _____
   _____

Variability Among Older Adults

2. Briefly explain the changes of the older adult.
   a. Physiological:

   _____
   _____

   b. Cognitive:

   _____
   _____

   c. Psychosocial:

   _____
   _____

3. Explain the following terminology.
   a. Geriatrics:

   _____
   _____

   b. Gerontology:

   _____
   _____

   c. Gerontological nursing:

   _____
   _____

   d. Gerontic nursing:

   _____
   _____

Myths and Stereotypes

4. Identify at least five myths or stereotypes regarding the older adult.

   _____
   _____
   _____
   _____
   _____

5. Define *ageism*.

   _____
   _____

Nurses' Attitudes Toward Older Adults

6. The attitude of the nurse toward older adults comes in part from _____, _____, and _____.

Theories of Aging

7. Give a brief description of the following biological theories.

   a. Stochastic theories:

   _____
   _____

b. Nonstochastic theories:

_____

_____

8. Describe the three classic psychosocial theories of aging.

_____

_____

_____

_____

_____

Developmental Tasks for Older Adults

9. List the seven developmental tasks of the older adult.

a. _____

b. _____

c. _____

d. _____

e. _____

f. _____

g. _____

Community-Based and Institutional Health Care Services

10. Briefly describe the following health services that are used by the older population.

a. Assisted-living facilities:

_____

_____

b. Personal care home:

_____

_____

c. Long-term care facility:

_____

_____

Assessing the Needs of Older Adults

11. Nurses need to take into account five key points to ensure an age-specific approach.

a. _____

b. _____

c. _____

d. _____

e. _____

12. List some techniques to use for the older adult with visual impairments.

a. _____

b. _____

c. _____

13. List some techniques to use with the older adult with hearing impairment.

a. _____

b. _____

c. _____

d. _____

Physiological Changes

14. Identify the physiological changes that occur in the older adult with regard to the following.

a. General survey:

_____

_____

b. Integumentary system:

_____

_____

c. Head and neck:

_____

_____

d. Thorax and lungs:

_____

_____

e. Heart and vascular system:

_____

_____

f. Breasts:

_____

_____

g. Gastrointestinal system and abdomen:

_____

_____

h. Reproductive system:

_____

_____

i. Urinary system:

_____

_____

j. Musculoskeletal system:

_____

_____

k. Neurological system:

_____

_____

Cognitive Changes

15. The structural and physiological changes that occur in the brain during aging do not necessarily affect adaptive and functional abilities.

16. Define the following terms.

a. Dementia:

_____

_____

b. Delirium:

_____

_____

c. Depression:

_____

_____

17. Describe major differences between dementia, delirium, and depression.

_____

_____

_____

_____

18. Identify the characteristic progressive symptoms of Alzheimer's disease.

a. _____

b. _____

c. _____

Psychosocial Changes

19. Identify at least five areas that should be addressed when counselling an older adult about retirement.

a. _____

b. _____

c. _____

d. _____

e. _____

20. Briefly explain some of the reasons older adults experience social isolation.

_____

_____

_____

21. Briefly describe the sexual changes that occur in the older adult.

_____

_____

_____

22. List four factors to assess when assisting older adults with housing needs.

a. _____

b. _____

c. _____

d. _____

Addressing the Health Concerns of Older Adults

23. The two most common causes of death in the older adult are _____ and _____.

24. Health Canada's National Advisory Committee on Aging lists 7 factors to improve the health of older Canadians.

a. _____

b. _____

c. _____

d. _____

e. _____

f. _____

g. _____

Health Promotion and Maintenance: Physiological Health Concerns

25. Summarize the physiological health concerns related to each of the following.

a. Heart disease:

_____

_____

b. Cancer:

_____

_____

c. Stroke:

_____

_____

d. Smoking:

_____

_____

e. Alcohol abuse:

_____

_____

f. Nutrition:

_____

_____

g. Dental problems:

_____

_____

h. Exercise:

_____

_____

i. Arthritis:

_____

_____

j. Falls:

_____

_____

k. Sensory impairments:

_____

_____

l. Pain:

_____

_____

m. Medication use:

_____

_____

26. Briefly explain the age-related changes affecting drug therapy in adults over the age of 65.

_____

_____

Health Promotion and Maintenance: Psychosocial Health Concerns

27. Briefly describe the interventions used to maintain the psychosocial health of the older adult.

a. Therapeutic communication:

_____

_____

b. Touch:

_____

_____

c. Reality orientation:

_____

_____

d. Reminiscence:

_____

_____

e. Body-image interventions:

_____

_____

Older Adults and the Acute Care Setting

28. Older adults in the acute care setting are at increased risk for adverse events such as

a. _____

b. _____

c. _____

d. _____

e. _____

f. _____

29. Explain why the older adult is at risk for each of the following.

a. Delirium:

_____

_____

b. Dehydration:

_____

_____

c. Malnutrition:

_____

_____

d. Health care-associated infections:

_____

_____

e. Urinary incontinence:

_____

_____

f. Falls:

_____

_____

Older Adults and Restorative Care

30. Summarize the two types of ongoing care for the older adult and identify the focus of each.

_____

_____

_____

_____

Review Questions

Select the appropriate answer and cite the rationale for choosing that particular answer.

1. Which statement about older adults is accurate?
   a. Older adults are institutionalized.
   b. Most older adults live on a fixed income.
   c. Most older adults cannot learn to care for themselves.
   d. Most older adults have no sexual desire.

Answer: _____ Rationale: _____

_____

_____

2. Which statement describing *delirium* is correct?
   a. Persons with delirium may experience hallucinations.
   b. The onset of delirium is slow and insidious.

c. Symptoms of delirium are stable and unchanging.
   d. Symptoms of delirium are irreversible.

Answer: _____ Rationale: _____

_____

_____

3. Ms. Dale states that she does not need the television turned on because she cannot see very well. Normal visual changes in older adults include all of the following *except*
   a. Decreased visual acuity
   b. Decreased accommodation to darkness
   c. Double vision
   d. Sensitivity to glare

Answer: _____ Rationale: _____

_____

_____

4. Mr. DeLonghi states that he is worried about his parents' plans to retire. All of the following would be an appropriate response regarding retirement of the older adult *except*:
   a. Positive adjustment is often related to how much a person planned for the retirement.
   b. Retirement for most persons represents a sudden shock that is irreversibly damaging to self-image and self-esteem.
   c. Reactions to retirement are influenced by the importance that has been attached to the work role.
   d. Retirement may affect an individual's physical and psychological functioning.

Answer: _____ Rationale: _____

_____

_____

26

Self-Concept

Preliminary Reading

Chapter 26, pp. 398–415

Comprehensive Understanding

Nursing Knowledge Base

Development of Self-Concept

1. Each stage of development has specific activities that assist the client in developing a positive self-concept. Identify some activities for each stage.

   a. 0 to 1 year:

   _____

   _____

   b. 1 to 3 years:

   _____

   _____

   c. 3 to 6 years:

   _____

   _____

   d. 6 to 12 years:

   _____

   _____

   e. 12 to 20 years:

   _____

   _____

   f. Mid-20s to mid-40s:

   _____

   _____

   g. Mid-40s to mid-60s:

   _____

   _____

   h. Late 60s on:

   _____

   _____

2. Self-concept is a dynamic perception that is based on the following:

   a. _____

   b. _____

   c. _____

   d. _____

   e. _____

   f. _____

   g. _____

   h. _____

   i. _____

   j. _____

   k. _____

   l. _____

   m. _____

Components and Interrelated Terms of Self-Concept

3. A healthy self-concept has a high degree of stability and generates positive or negative feelings toward the self.

4. Briefly explain the four significant components of self-concept.

   a. Identity:

   _____

   _____

b. Body image:

_____

_____

c. Self-esteem:

_____

_____

d. Role performance:

_____

_____

5. List the processes through which a child learns appropriate behaviours.

a. _____

b. _____

c. _____

d. _____

e. _____

Stressors Affecting Self-Concept

6. Stressors challenge a person's adaptive capacities.

7. A self-concept stressor is any

_____

_____

8. Being able to adapt to stressors is likely to lead to a positive sense of self, whereas failure to adapt often leads to a negative sense of self.

9. Any change in health can be a stressor that affects self-concept.

10. A physical change in the body leads to an altered body image. Identity and self-esteem can also be affected.

11. A crisis occurs when a person cannot overcome obstacles with the usual methods of problem solving and adapting.

12. Define *identity*.

_____

_____

13. Stressors throughout life affect identity. Give an example of a stressor for each developmental stage.

a. Adolescence:

_____

_____

b. Adulthood:

_____

_____

c. Retirement:

_____

_____

14. Changes in the appearance, structure, or function of a body part will require a change in body image. Identify at least five stressors that affect body image.

a. _____

b. _____

c. _____

d. _____

e. _____

15. Transitions within one's roles may lead to the following. Explain.

a. Role conflict:

_____

_____

b. Role ambiguity:

_____

_____

c. Role strain:

_____

_____

d. Role overload:

_____

_____

The Family's Effect on Development of Self-Concept

16. The family plays a key role in creating and maintaining its members' self-concepts.

17. Children learn from their parents and siblings a basic sense of who they are and how they are expected to live.

The Nurse's Effect on the Client's Self-Concept

18. A nurse's acceptance of a client with an altered self-concept helps stimulate positive rehabilitation.

19. List five areas you must clarify and assess about yourself in order to promote a positive self-concept in clients.

a. _____

b. _____

c. _____

d. _____

e. _____

Self-Concept and the Nursing Process

Assessment

20. In assessing self-concept, you should focus on each component of self-concept; behaviours suggestive of _____, actual and potential self-concept _____ _____, and _____ patterns.

21. Much of the data regarding self-concept are most effectively gathered through observation of a client's nonverbal behaviour and by paying attention to the content of the client's conversation rather than through direct questioning.

22. The nursing assessment should include consideration of previous coping behaviours: the _____, _____; and _____ ____ of the stressors; and the client's _____ _____ and _____ resources.

23. As the nurse identifies previous coping patterns, it is useful to consider if these patterns have contributed to healthy functioning or created more problems.

24. Exploring resources and strengths, such as helpful significant others or prior use of community resources, can be important in formulating a realistic and effective plan.

25. Asking the client how he or she believes interventions will make a difference in the problem can provide useful information regarding the client's expectations and can provide an opportunity to discuss the client's goals. Give an example.

_____

_____

Nursing Diagnosis

26. Accurate development of a nursing diagnosis requires discussing the problem with the client and the family.

Planning

27. The nurse, client, and family need to plan care directed at helping the client regain or maintain a healthy self-concept.

28. Interventions focus on helping the client and on coping methods.

29. The nurse looks for strengths in both the individual and the family and provides resources and education to turn limitations into strengths.

30. Before involving the family, you need to consider the _____ and _____.

Implementation

Health Promotion

31. List some healthy lifestyle measures that contribute to a healthy self-concept.

_____

_____

_____

_____

Acute Care

32. In acute care, the nurse is likely to encounter clients who are experiencing _____ to their self-concept due to the nature of the treatment and diagnostic procedure.

33. Identify ways a nurse can assist a client in the adjustment to a change in physical appearance.

_____

_____

_____

Restorative Care

34. Identify goals to help a client attain a more positive self-concept.

a. _____

b. _____

c. _____

d. _____

e. _____

35. Identify seven nursing interventions for the client to engage in self-exploration.

a. _____

b. _____

c. _____

d. _____

e. _____

f. _____

g. _____

Evaluation

36. Client care evaluates the actual care delivered by the health team based on expected outcomes. Briefly explain the expected outcomes for a self-concept disturbance.

_____

_____

37. Client expectations evaluate care from the client's perspective. Give an example.

_____

_____

Review Questions

Select the appropriate answer and cite the rationale for choosing that particular answer.

1. Which developmental stage is particularly crucial for identity development?
   a. Infancy
   b. Preschool age
   c. Adolescence
   d. Young adulthood

Answer: _____   Rationale: _____

_____

_____

2. Which of the following statements about body image is correct?
   a. Physical changes are quickly incorporated into a person's body image.
   b. Body image refers only to the external appearance of a person's body.
   c. Body image involves attitudes related to the body, including physical appearance, structure, or function.
   d. Perceptions by other persons have no influence on a person's body image.

Answer: _____   Rationale: _____

_____

_____

3. Sandeep, who is 2 years old, is praised for using his potty instead of wetting his pants. This is an example of learning a behaviour by
   a. Identification
   b. Imitation
   c. Substitution
   d. Reinforcement–extinction

Answer: _____   Rationale: _____

_____

_____

4. Mrs. Watson has just undergone a radical mastectomy. You are aware that Mrs. Watson will probably have considerable anxiety over
   a. Role performance
   b. Self-identity
   c. Body image
   d. Self-esteem

Answer: _____   Rationale: _____

_____

_____

5. Which of the following statements demonstrates that your self-concept is positively affecting the client?
   a. "You've got to take a more active part in caring for your ostomy."
   b. "I know your ostomy is difficult to look at, but you will get used to it in time."
   c. (While grimacing) "Ostomy care isn't so bad."
   d. "Let me show you how to place the bag on your stoma."

Answer: _____   Rationale: _____

_____

_____

Critical Thinking Model for Nursing Care Plan for Disturbed Body Image

Imagine that you are the student nurse in the Nursing Care Plan on page 410 of your text. Complete the *assessment phase* of the critical thinking model by writing in the appropriate boxes on the model shown. Think about the following:

- In developing Ms. Johnson's plan of care, what knowledge did you apply?
- In what way might your previous experience apply in this case?
- What intellectual or professional standards were applied to Ms. Johnson?
- What critical thinking attitudes were used in assessing Ms. Johnson?
- As you review your assessment, what key areas did you cover?

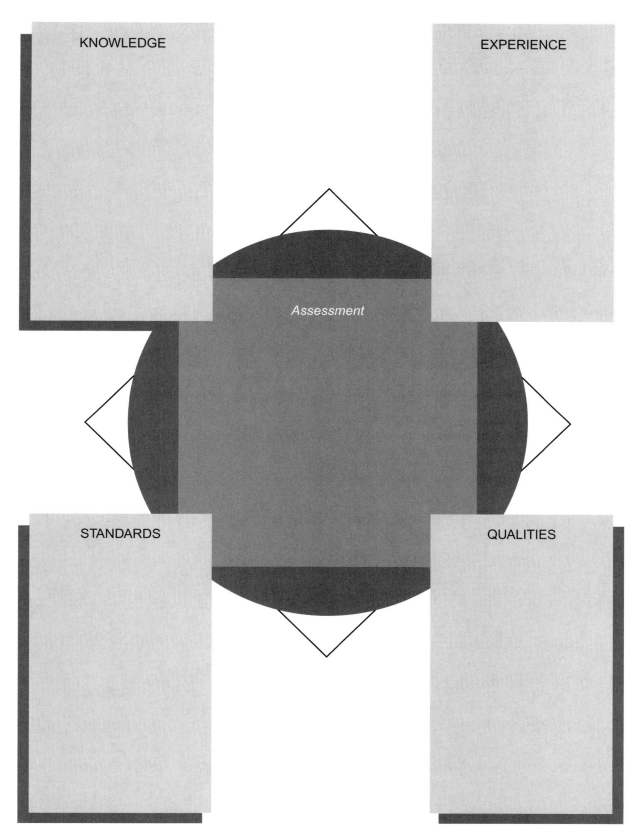

KNOWLEDGE

EXPERIENCE

Assessment

STANDARDS

QUALITIES

CHAPTER 26 Critical Thinking Model for Nursing Care Plan for *Disturbed Body Image*
See answers on page 528.

27

Sexuality

Preliminary Reading

Chapter 27, pp. 416–433

Comprehensive Understanding

Scientific Knowledge Base

Sexual and Gender Identity

1. Define the following.

   a. *Sexual identity*:

   _____

   _____

   b. *Gender identity*:

   _____

   _____

   c. *Transsexuality*:

   _____

   _____

Sexual Orientation

2. Define *sexual orientation*.

   _____

   _____

3. Define *heterosexuality*.

   _____

   _____

4. Define *homosexuality*.

   _____

   _____

5. Define *bisexuality*.

   _____

   _____

6. You must not assume that you know your clients' gender identity or sexual orientation.

7. If you learn of a client's sexual orientation, you should not assume that you may tell anyone else or include it in the medical record without the client's knowledge.

8. Define *homophobia*.

   _____

   _____

9. The nurse who is nonjudgemental and equipped with an appropriate knowledge base can help address the problems of homophobia and provide nursing care that does not discriminate against the client's sexual orientation.

Sexual Development

10. Each stage of development brings changes in sexual functioning and the role of sexuality in relationships. Explain each stage.

    a. Infancy and childhood:

    _____

    _____

    b. Puberty/adolescence:

    _____

    _____

    c. Adulthood:

    _____

    _____

d. Older adulthood:

_____

_____

Sexual Response Cycle

11. The four phases of the sexual response cycle are _____, _____, _____, and _____.

12. These phases are the result of vasocongestion and myotonia (muscle contraction). Explain each of these physiological responses.

    a. Female:

    _____

    _____

    b. Male:

    _____

    _____

Sexual Behaviour

13. Sexual behaviour comprises the broad array of sexual activities people participate in. It is difficult to say what is "normal" or "abnormal" because what is unusual or atypical varies between cultures and from one period to another.

High-Risk Sexual Behaviour

14. Define *safer sex*.

    _____

    _____

15. List three examples of unsafe sex practices.

    a. _____

    b. _____

    c. _____

Sexually Transmitted Infections

16. A major problem in dealing with sexually transmitted infections (STIs) is

    _____

    _____

17. List the prevalent STIs.

    a. _____

    b. _____

    c. _____

    d. _____

    e. _____

    f. _____

18. People most likely to be infected with an STI are those who

    a. _____

    b. _____

    c. _____

19. The predominant routes of infection for human immunodeficiency virus (HIV) are

    _____, _____, and _____.

Contraception

20. Numerous contraceptive options are available. Briefly list the options available under the following categories.

    a. Nonprescriptive methods:

    _____

    _____

    b. Methods requiring a health care professional:

    _____

    _____

21. Emergency contraception pills (ECPs) are most effective up to ___ days following intercourse and are recommended to

    _____

    _____

    _____

Abortion

22. Since 1988, Canada has been one of the few countries without any criminal law restricting abortion.

23. Two-thirds of abortions are performed in hospitals; the remaining one-third are done in abortion clinics and health centres.

24. Health care professionals must reflect on personal values related to abortion. The health care professional is entitled to personal views and should not be forced to participate in counselling or procedures contrary to his or her beliefs or values.

Nursing Knowledge Base

Sociocultural Dimensions of Sexuality

25. Global cultural diversity creates considerable variability in sexual norms and represents a wide spectrum of beliefs and values.

26. Common areas of diversity include the following:

    a. _____

    b. _____

    c. _____

    d. _____

    e. _____

    f. _____

Discussing Sexual Issues

27. Identify the issues regarding the difficulty the nurse has in discussing sexuality with clients.

    a. _____

    b. _____

    c. _____

    d. _____

Alterations in Sexual Health

28. Explain the following issues.

    a. Infertility:

    _____

    _____

    b. Sexual abuse:

    _____

    _____

    c. Sexual dysfunction:

    _____

    _____

Clients With Particular Sexual Health Concerns

29. Describe the possible sexual concerns that should be considered for each of the following clients.

    a. Pregnant and postpartum women:

    _____

    _____

    b. Clients recovering from surgery:

    _____

    _____

    c. Clients with illness or disability:

    _____

    _____

Sexuality and the Nursing Process

30. A person's sexuality has physical, psychological, social, and cultural elements.

Assessment

31. Briefly explain the following factors that affect sexuality.

    a. Physical:

    _____

    _____

    b. Self-concept:

    _____

    _____

    c. Relationship:

    _____

    _____

    d. Self-esteem:

    _____

    _____

32. List the questions you may use to elicit a brief sexual history from an adult.

    a. _____

    b. _____

    c. _____

    d. _____

33. Explain how you can anticipate when a client is at risk for sexual dysfunction.

    _____

    _____

34. Briefly explain the physical assessment in evaluating the cause of sexual concerns or problems.

    a. Female:

    _____

    _____

    b. Male:

    _____

    _____

Nursing Diagnosis

35. Identify clues that may signal risk for or an actual nursing diagnosis related to sexuality.

    a. _____

    b. _____

c. _____
d. _____
e. _____

Planning

36. The PLISSIT model developed by Annon (1974) guides the planning phases. Explain each of the following.

a. P:

_____
_____

b. LI:

_____
_____

c. SS:

_____
_____

d. IT:

_____
_____

Implementation

Health Promotion

37. Topics of education vary depending on the defining characteristics and related factors. Describe some situations.

_____
_____

Acute Care

38. Nursing interventions that address alterations in sexuality are aimed at _____, _____, _____ _____, or _____.

39. The client should be encouraged to investigate and acknowledge social and ethical values and analyze the role of sexuality in his or her self-concept.

40. Identify situational and developmental crises that prompt education.

_____
_____

Restorative Care

41. In the home, it is important to assist individuals in creating an environment comfortable for sexual activity.

42. In the long-term care setting, facilities should make proper arrangements for privacy during residents' sexual experiences.

Evaluation

43. Client care evaluates the actual care delivered by the health care team based on the expected outcomes.

44. Client or spouse verbalizations determine if goals and outcomes have been achieved.

45. Sexuality is felt more than observed, and sexual expression requires an intimacy not amenable to observation.

46. All people involved may need to be reminded of the individual nature of sexual expression and the multiple factors that affect perceptions and responses.

47. Client expectations evaluate care from the client's perspective. Briefly explain the client's perspective with respect to resolution of his or her sexual concerns.

_____
_____

Review Questions

Select the appropriate answer and cite the rationale for choosing that particular answer.

1. At what developmental stage is it particularly important for children reared in lone-parent families to be exposed to same-sex adults?
a. Infancy
b. Toddlerhood and preschool years
c. School age
d. Adolescence

Answer: _____   Rationale: _____
_____
_____

2. In the school-age child, learning and reinforcement of gender-appropriate behaviours are most commonly derived from
a. Parents
b. Teachers

c. Siblings

d. Peers

Answer: _____   Rationale: _____

_____

_____

3. Why is it often more difficult to discuss sexuality issues with older clients?
   a. Older people are less likely to be sexually active.
   b. They are more likely to have complex causes for sexual problems.
   c. They may have more difficulty discussing intimate issues.
   d. They are frequently deaf, and it is difficult to talk about this in a loud voice.

Answer: _____   Rationale: _____

_____

_____

4. The least effective means of preventing pregnancy is
   a. Coitus interruptus
   b. Calendar (rhythm) method
   c. Body temperature method
   d. Mucus method

Answer: _____   Rationale: _____

_____

_____

5. The only 100% effective method to avoid contracting a disease through sex is
   a. Using condoms
   b. Avoiding sex with partners at risk
   c. Knowing the sexual partner's health history
   d. Abstinence

Answer: _____   Rationale: _____

_____

_____

Critical Thinking Model for Nursing Care Plan for Sexual Dysfunction

Imagine that you are Jack, the nursing student in the Nursing Care Plan on page 430 of your text. Complete the *assessment phase* of the critical thinking model by writing your answers in the appropriate boxes of the model shown. Think about the following:

- In developing Mr. Clements's plan of care, what knowledge did you apply?

- In what way might your previous experience assist in this case?

- What intellectual or professional standards were applied to Mr. Clements?

- What critical thinking attitudes did you utilize in assessing Mr. Clements?

- As you review your assessment, what key areas did you cover?

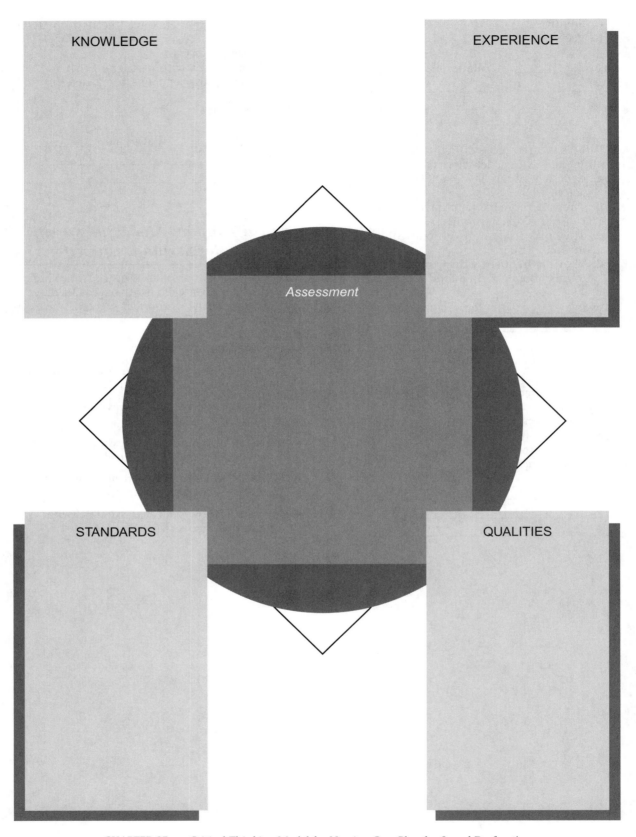

KNOWLEDGE

EXPERIENCE

Assessment

STANDARDS

QUALITIES

CHAPTER 27   Critical Thinking Model for Nursing Care Plan for *Sexual Dysfunction*
See answers on page 529.

28

Spiritual Health

Preliminary Reading

Chapter 28, pp. 434–451

Comprehensive Understanding

1. Define *spirituality*.

   _____

   _____

   _____

Scientific Knowledge Base

2. Describe the association between spirituality and health.

   _____

   _____

   _____

Nursing Knowledge Base

Historical Perspectives

3. Identify four historical milestones related to spirituality and nursing.

   _____

   _____

   _____

   _____

4. Some scholars are challenging what is perceived as _____ of spirituality.

5. Absence of an idealized spiritual state does not dictate some _____.

6. We need to be cautious about creating ____ _____, especially those based on _____.

Theoretical Perspectives

7. Describe spiritual care according to two nursing theories.

a. Systems model (Neuman):

   _____

   _____

   _____

b. Theory of human caring (Watson):

   _____

   _____

   _____

Traditional Concepts Associated With Spiritual Health

8. The concepts of _____, _____, _____, and _____ give direction in understanding the views each individual has of life and its value.

9. Individuals' definitions of spirituality are influenced by their own _____, _____, _____, _____, and _____.

10. Identify the central characteristic of spirituality in nursing.

    _____

    _____

    _____

11. Briefly describe spiritual care.

    _____

    _____

    _____

    _____

12. It is not unusual for youth who have been reared in a religious tradition to _____ as they search for _____.

13. Evidence of healthy spirituality is _____ _____ for others and self.

14. A _____ may help protect older adults from _____ and _____ that occur with aging.

15. Explain how the following view spirituality.

    a. Atheists:

    _____
    _____
    _____

    b. Agnostics:

    _____
    _____
    _____

16. Explain the concept of faith.

    _____
    _____
    _____

17. The belief that comes with faith involves _____, or an awareness of that which one cannot see or know in ordinary ways.

18. Define *religion*.

    _____
    _____
    _____

19. Explain the differences between the terms *spirituality* and *religion*.

    _____
    _____
    _____
    _____

20. Summarize the concept of hope.

    _____
    _____
    _____

Spiritual Challenges

21. Define *spiritual distress*.

    _____
    _____
    _____

22. Briefly explain each of the following causes of spiritual distress.

    a. Acute illness:

    _____
    _____
    _____

    b. Chronic illness:

    _____
    _____
    _____

    c. Terminal illness:

    _____
    _____
    _____

23. Knowledge about spirituality begins with

    _____
    _____

Spiritual Health and the Nursing Process

24. Spiritual care goes beyond assessing a client's

    _____

25. Briefly explain shared community and compassion.

    _____
    _____
    _____

26. It is important for nurses to sort out value judgements about other people's belief systems.

27. The nurse must be willing to share and discover another person's meaning and purpose in life, sickness, and health.

28. A nurse must learn to look beyond _____ _____ when establishing a client relationship, which can be done by identifying _____.

Assessment

29. The assessment should focus on aspects of spirituality most likely to be influenced by life experiences, events, and questions in the case of illness and hospitalization.

30. A key to success in conducting a spiritual assessment is _____ throughout the course of the client's stay.

31. The JAREL Spiritual Well-Being Scale provides nurses and other health care professionals with a tool for assessing client's spiritual well-being. Briefly summarize the three dimensions.

    a. Faith and belief:

    b. Life and self-responsibility:

    c. Life satisfaction and self-actualization:

32. Explain how the following can affect a client's spiritual health.

    a. Fellowship and community:

    b. Ritual and practice:

    c. Vocation:

Planning

33. In order to develop an individualized plan of care, the nurse integrates knowledge gathered from the assessment with knowledge relating to resources and therapies available for spiritual care.

34. Identify three examples of goals and outcomes for spiritual caregiving.

    a.

    b.

    c.

Implementation

Health Promotion

35. Spiritual care should be a central theme in promoting an individual's overall well-being.

36. Briefly explain the following interventions and how they are helpful in maintaining or promoting a client's spiritual health.

    a. Establishing presence:

    b. Supporting a healing relationship:

Acute Care

37. Within acute care settings, clients experience multiple stressors that threaten to overwhelm their coping resources.

38. Explain how the following interventions are helpful in the client's therapeutic plan.

    a. Support systems:

    b. Diet therapies:

    c. Supporting rituals:

    d. Prayer:

    e. Supporting grief work:

Evaluation

Client Care

39. Client care evaluates the actual care delivered by the health team based on the expected outcomes. Give some examples.

Client Expectations

40. A client's expectation evaluates care from the client perspective. Give some examples.

_____

_____

_____

Review Questions

Select the appropriate answer and cite the rationale for choosing that particular answer.

1. When planning care to include spiritual needs for a client of the Hindu faith, the religious practices you should understand include all of the following, *except*
   a. Public prayer is important
   b. Modesty is important
   c. Religious symbols should not be removed
   d. Same-sex caregivers are preferred

Answer: _____   Rationale: _____

_____

_____

2. When consulting with the dietary department regarding meals for a client of the Hindu religion, which of the following dietary items would *not* be included on the meal trays?
   a. Meats
   b. Dairy products
   c. Vegetable entrees
   d. Fruits

Answer: _____   Rationale: _____

_____

_____

3. A client who is an Orthodox Jew may
   a. Keep a cross and prayer beads at the bedside
   b. Refuse treatment on the Sabbath
   c. Prefer to have pork with meals
   d. Choose death over breaking kosher

Answer: _____   Rationale: _____

_____

_____

4. In death, Muslims prepare the body by
   a. Having the staff wash the body with lavender prior to sending it to the morgue
   b. Chanting prayers over the body to sing the soul to heaven
   c. Having family members wash the body and wrap it in a white cloth with the head turned to the right shoulder
   d. Not touching the body with their bare hands

Answer: _____   Rationale: _____

_____

_____

5. Mr. Lanois recently received a diagnosis of a malignant tumour. Staff have observed him crying on several occasions, and now he cries as he reads from his Bible. Interventions to help Mr. Lanois cope with his illness would include
   a. Asking the parish nurse from his congregation to visit him
   b. Engaging Mr. Lanois in diversional activities to reduce feelings of hopelessness
   c. Sitting at Mr. Lanois' bedside and listening to him with an encouraging yet realistic attitude
   d. Praying with Mr. Lanois as often as possible

Answer: _____   Rationale: _____

_____

_____

Critical Thinking Model for Nursing Care Plan for Spiritual Distress

Imagine that you are Leah, the nurse in the Nursing Care Plan on page 446 of your text. Complete the *planning phase* of the critical thinking model by writing your answers in the appropriate boxes of the model shown. Think about the following:

1. In developing James's plan of care, what knowledge did you apply?

2. In what way might your previous experience assist in developing a plan of care for James?

3. When developing a plan of care, what intellectual and professional standards were applied?

4. What critical thinking attitudes might have been applied when developing James's plan?

5. How will you accomplish the goals?

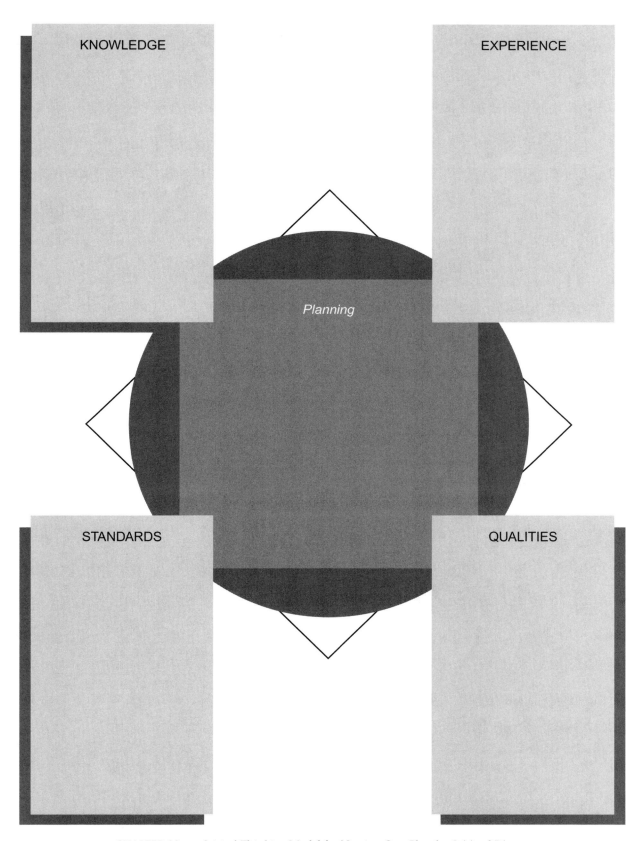

KNOWLEDGE

EXPERIENCE

Planning

STANDARDS

QUALITIES

CHAPTER 28   Critical Thinking Model for Nursing Care Plan for *Spiritual Distress*
See answers on page 530.

29

The Experience of Loss, Death, and Grief

Preliminary Reading

Chapter 29, pp. 452–475

Comprehensive Understanding

Scientific Knowledge Base

Loss

1. Give an example of the five categories of loss.

   a. Necessary loss:

   _____

   _____

   _____

   b. Actual loss:

   _____

   _____

   _____

   c. Perceived loss:

   _____

   _____

   _____

   d. Maturational loss:

   _____

   _____

   _____

   e. Situational loss:

   _____

   _____

   _____

Grief

2. Describe the following terms.

   a. *Grief*:

   _____

   _____

   b. *Bereavement*:

   _____

   _____

Theories of Grief

3. List the phases of the grieving process proposed by each of the theorists listed below.

   Kübler-Ross's Stages of Dying

   a. _____

   b. _____

   c. _____

   d. _____

   e. _____

   Bowlby's Phases of Mourning

   a. _____

   b. _____

   c. _____

   d. _____

   Worden's Four Tasks of Mourning

   a. _____

   b. _____

   c. _____

   d. _____

Types of Grief

4. Briefly describe the following types of grief.

   a. Normal grief:

   _____

   _____

b. Anticipatory grief:

_____

_____

c. Complicated grief:

_____

_____

d. Disenfranchised grief:

_____

_____

Nursing Knowledge Base

5. Briefly explain the factors that influence loss and grief.
   a. Human development:

   _____

   _____

   b. Psychosocial perspectives:

   _____

   _____

   c. Socioeconomic status:

   _____

   _____

   d. Personal relationships:

   _____

   _____

   e. Nature of the loss:

   _____

   _____

   f. Culture and ethnicity:

   _____

   _____

   g. Spiritual beliefs:

   _____

   _____

Coping With Grief and Loss

6. Explain how the mechanism of hope is used to cope with grief and loss.

   _____

   _____

   _____

The Nursing Process and Grief

Assessment

7. You should avoid assuming that a particular behaviour indicates grief; rather, you should allow clients to share what is happening in their own ways.

8. It is important for you to assess how a client is reacting rather than how the client *should be* reacting. A single behaviour can represent various types of grief. Therefore, the identification of the type and stage of grief should be used only to guide your assessment and not to judge the outcomes of the grieving process.

9. Identify some symptoms of normal grief feelings.

   _____

   _____

10. Briefly explain end-of-life decisions.

    _____

    _____

11. Assess your own experience with grief.

    _____

    _____

Nursing Diagnosis

12. List four possible nursing diagnoses for clients or families experiencing grief.
    a. _____
    b. _____
    c. _____
    d. _____

Planning

13. When caring for the dying client, it is important to devise a plan that helps a client die with dignity and offers family members the assurance that their loved one is cared for compassionately.

14. List three goals appropriate for a client dealing with loss.
    a. _____
    b. _____
    c. _____

15. Briefly explain how to prioritize the needs of the grieving client.

_____

_____

_____

Implementation

Health Promotion

16. Nurses help clients and families deal with loss, make decisions about the client's health care, and adjust to any disappointment, frustration, and anxiety created by their loss.

17. Describe five therapeutic communication strategies you can use to help clients discuss and work through their loss.

    a. _____

    b. _____

    c. _____

    d. _____

    e. _____

18. Give an example of a nursing strategy to promote hope for each dimension.

    a. Affective dimension:

    _____

    _____

    b. Cognitive dimension:

    _____

    _____

    c. Behavioural dimension:

    _____

    _____

    d. Affiliative dimension:

    _____

    _____

    e. Temporal dimension:

    _____

    _____

    f. Contextual dimension:

    _____

    _____

19. Identify the nursing strategies to facilitate mourning for the client.

    a. _____

    b. _____

c. _____

d.

e. _____

f. _____

g. _____

Acute Care

Palliative Care

20. According to the World Health Organization, when health care professionals deliver palliative care, they do the following:

    a. _____

    b. _____

    c. _____

    d. _____

    e. _____

    f. _____

    g. _____

21. Give examples of how the following contribute to comfort for the dying client.

    a. Symptom control:

    _____

    _____

    b. Maintaining dignity and self-esteem:

    _____

    _____

    c. Preventing abandonment and isolation:

    _____

    _____

    d. Providing a comfortable and peaceful environment:

    _____

    _____

Hospice Care

22. Identify the components of hospice care.

    a. _____

    b. _____

    c. _____

    d. _____

    e. _____

    f. _____

    g. _____

    h. _____

Care After Death

23. Care after death includes caring for the body with dignity and sensitivity and in a manner consistent with the client's religious or cultural beliefs.

24. Explain how you can support the family through the organ and tissue request or donation process.

_____

_____

_____

Evaluation

Client Care

25. Grieving is an individual process, and resolution of loss does not follow a set schedule.

26. The care of the dying client requires you to evaluate the client's level of comfort with illness and the client's quality of life.

Client Expectations

27. The client expects individualized care, including relief of symptoms, preservation of dignity, and support of the family to maximize quality of life.

Review Questions

Select the appropriate answer and cite the rationale for choosing that particular answer.

1. Which statement about loss is accurate?
   a. Loss is experienced only when something valued is actually absent.
   b. The more an individual has invested in what is lost, the less the feeling of loss.
   c. Loss may be maturational, situational, or both.
   d. The degree of stress experienced is unrelated to the type of loss.

Answer: _____   Rationale: _____

_____

_____

2. A hospice program emphasizes
   a. Curative treatment and alleviation of symptoms
   b. Palliative treatment and control of symptoms

   c. Hospital-based care
   d. Prolongation of life

Answer: _____   Rationale: _____

_____

_____

3. Trying uncertain forms of complementary therapy is a behaviour that is characteristic of which stage of dying?
   a. Anger
   b. Depression
   c. Bargaining
   d. Acceptance

Answer: _____   Rationale: _____

_____

_____

4. All of the following are crucial needs of the dying client *except*
   a. Control of pain
   b. Preservation of dignity and self-worth
   c. Love and belonging
   d. Freedom from decision making

Answer: _____   Rationale: _____

_____

_____

Critical Thinking Model for Nursing Care Plan for Ineffective Coping

Imagine that you are the student nurse in the Nursing Care Plan on pages 464–465 of your text. Complete the *evaluation phase* of the critical thinking model by writing your answers in the appropriate boxes of the model shown. Think about the following:

• In evaluating Mrs. Miller's plan of care, what knowledge did you apply?

• In what way might your previous experience influence your evaluation of Mrs. Miller's care?

• During evaluation, what intellectual and professional standards were applied to Mrs. Miller's care?

• In what way do critical thinking attitudes play a role in how you approach evaluation of Mrs. Miller's care?

• How might you adjust Mrs. Miller's care?

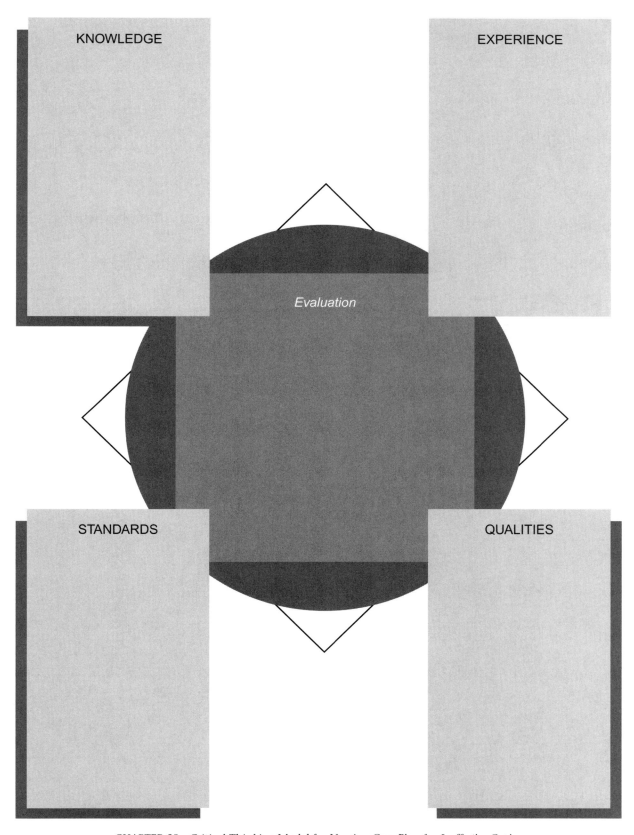

KNOWLEDGE

EXPERIENCE

Evaluation

STANDARDS

QUALITIES

CHAPTER 29   Critical Thinking Model for Nursing Care Plan for *Ineffective Coping*
See answers on page 531.

30

Stress and Adaptation

Preliminary Reading

Chapter 30, pp. 476–492

Comprehensive Understanding

1. Stress is

_____

_____

_____

2. Stressors are

_____

_____

_____

Conceptualizations of Stress

3. Explain the fight-or-flight response to stress.

_____

_____

_____

4. List (in sequence) and briefly describe the three stages of the general adaptation syndrome.

   a. _____

   b. _____

   c. _____

5. Define *homeostasis*.

_____

_____

_____

6. Explain the following terms.

   a. *Primary appraisal*:

_____

_____

   b. *Secondary appraisal*:

_____

_____

   c. *Coping*:

_____

_____

7. Explain the two types of crisis.

   a. Developmental crisis:

_____

_____

   b. Situational crisis:

_____

_____

Stress Response Systems

8. Explain how the following areas of the brain are involved in the stress response.

   a. Medulla oblongata:

_____

_____

   b. Reticular formation:

_____

_____

   c. Pituitary gland:

_____

_____

The Relationship Between Type of Stressor and Health

9. Distinguish between the two different types of stress.

   a. Distress:

   _____

   _____

   b. Eustress:

   _____

   _____

10. Explain post-traumatic stress disorder.

   _____

   _____

   _____

Nursing Knowledge Base

11. Summarize the following models related to stress and coping.

   a. Neuman's systems model:

   _____

   _____

   b. Pender et al.'s health promotion model:

   _____

   _____

12. The following factors can potentially be stressors. Explain.

   a. Situational factors:

   _____

   _____

   b. Maturational factors:

   _____

   _____

   c. Sociocultural factors:

   _____

   _____

Nursing Process

Assessment

13. When assessing a client's stress level and coping resources, you must ask the client to share personal and sensitive information. Therefore, you must first establish a trusting nurse–client relationship.

14. Give an example of each of the following factors to assess.

   a. Perception of stressor:

   _____

   b. Available coping resources:

   _____

   c. Maladaptive coping used:

   _____

   d. Adherence to healthy practices:

   _____

15. Identify six physical indicators of stress.

   a. _____
   b. _____
   c. _____
   d. _____
   e. _____
   f. _____

Nursing Diagnosis

16. Stress can result in multiple diagnostic statements.

17. Give two examples of nursing diagnostic statements related to stress.

   _____

   _____

Planning

18. Desirable outcomes for persons experiencing stress are

   a. _____
   b. _____
   c. _____
   d. _____

Implementation

Health Promotion

19. Identify the primary modes of intervention for stress.

   a. _____
   b. _____
   c. _____

20. Explain how the following methods reduce stressors.

    a. Time management:

    _____
    _____
    _____

    b. Regular exercise:

    _____
    _____
    _____

    c. Guided imagery and visualization:

    _____
    _____
    _____

    d. Support systems:

    _____
    _____
    _____

    e. Progressive muscle relaxation:

    _____
    _____
    _____

    f. Assertiveness training:

    _____
    _____
    _____

    g. Journal writing:

    _____
    _____
    _____

    h. Stress management in your workplace:

    _____
    _____
    _____

Acute Care

21. Crisis intervention is

    _____
    _____
    _____

22. Crises occur

    _____
    _____

Restorative and Continuing Care

23. Briefly explain when recovery from stress occurs.

    _____
    _____
    _____

Evaluation

24. Briefly explain the client's care in relation to
    a. Client's perceptions of stress:

    _____
    _____
    _____

    b. Client's expectations:

    _____
    _____
    _____

Review Questions

Select the appropriate answer and cite the rationale for choosing that particular answer.

1. Which definition does *not* characterize stress?
   a. Any situation in which a nonspecific demand requires an individual to respond or take action
   b. A phenomenon affecting social, psychological, developmental, spiritual, and physiological dimensions
   c. A condition eliciting an intellectual, behavioural, or metabolic response
   d. Efforts to maintain relative constancy within the internal environment

Answer: _____   Rationale: _____
_____
_____

2. Which statement about homeostasis is *not* accurate?
   a. Homeostatic mechanisms provide long-term and short-term control over the body's equilibrium.
   b. Homeostatic mechanisms are self-regulatory.

c. Homeostatic mechanisms function through negative feedback.
d. Illness may inhibit normal homeostatic mechanisms.

Answer: _____   Rationale: _____
_____
_____

3. Major homeostatic mechanisms are controlled by all of the following *except*
a. Thymus gland
b. Medulla oblongata
c. Reticular formation
d. Pituitary gland

Answer: _____   Rationale: _____
_____
_____

4. Which of the following is a stage of the general adaptation syndrome?
a. Alarm reaction
b. Fight-or-flight response
c. Coping mechanisms
d. Inflammatory response

Answer: _____   Rationale: _____
_____
_____

5. Crisis intervention is a specific measure used for helping a client resolve a particular, immediate stress problem. This approach is based on
a. The ability of the nurse to solve the client's problems
b. An in-depth analysis of a client's situation
c. Teaching the client how to help make the mental connection between the stressful event and his or her reaction to it.
d. Effective communication between the nurse and the client

Answer: _____   Rationale: _____
_____
_____

Critical Thinking Model for Nursing Care Plan for Caregiver Role Strain

Imagine that you are the nurse in the Nursing Care Plan on pages 486–487 of your text. Complete the evaluation phase of the critical thinking model by writing your answers in the appropriate boxes of the model shown. Think about the following:

- In evaluating the care of Carl and Evelyn, what knowledge did you apply?

- In what way might your previous experience influence the evaluation of Carl's care?

- During evaluation, what intellectual and professional standards were applied to Carl's care?

- In what way do critical thinking attitudes play a role in how you approach the evaluation of Carl's care?

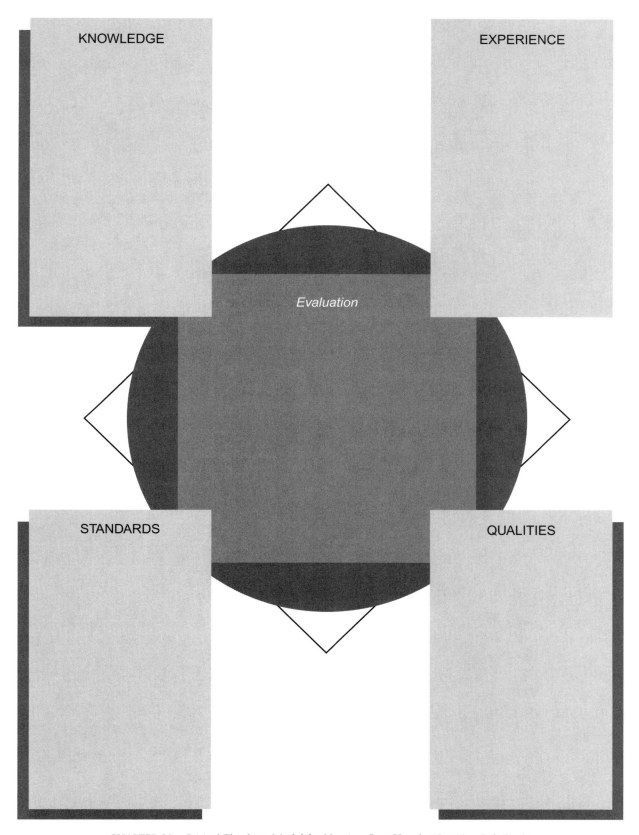

KNOWLEDGE

EXPERIENCE

Evaluation

STANDARDS

QUALITIES

CHAPTER 30   Critical Thinking Model for Nursing Care Plan for *Caregiver Role Strain*
See answers on page 532.

31

Vital Signs

Preliminary Reading

Chapter 31, pp. 493–539

Comprehensive Understanding

Guidelines for Measuring Vital Signs

1. Identify the guidelines that assist you to incorporate vital sign measurement into practice.

   a. _____

   b. _____

   c. _____

   d. _____

   e. _____

   f. _____

   g. _____

   h. _____

   i. _____

   j. _____

   k. _____

Body Temperature

Physiology

2. The body temperature is the difference between the _____ and the _____.

3. Define *core temperature*.

   _____

   _____

4. Define *thermoregulation*.

   _____

   _____

5. Briefly summarize how neural and vascular mechanisms control body temperature.

   _____

   _____

   _____

6. List four sources, or mechanisms, for heat production.

   a. _____

   b. _____

   c. _____

   d. _____

7. Explain the following mechanisms of body heat loss and give an example of each.

   a. Radiation:

   _____

   _____

   _____

   b. Conduction:

   _____

   _____

   _____

   c. Convection:

   _____

   _____

   _____

d. Evaporation:

_____

_____

_____

e. Diaphoresis:

_____

_____

_____

8. Briefly explain the skin's role in temperature regulation.

a. Insulation of the body:

_____

_____

b. Vasoconstriction:

_____

_____

c. Temperature sensation:

_____

_____

9. Identify four factors that must be present for a person to control body temperature.

a. _____

b. _____

c. _____

d. _____

Factors Affecting Body Temperature

10. Changes in body temperature within the normal range occur when the relationship between heat production and heat loss is altered by physiological or behavioural variables. Summarize the following variables.

a. Age:

_____

_____

b. Exercise:

_____

_____

c. Circadian rhythm:

_____

_____

d. Stress:

_____

_____

e. Environment:

_____

_____

11. Temperature alterations can be related to _____, _____, _____, _____, or any combination of these alterations.

12. Pyrexia, or fever, occurs because

_____

_____

13. Explain how a fever works as an important defence mechanism.

_____

_____

14. Explain how a fever serves a diagnostic purpose.

_____

_____

15. Explain how a fever affects metabolism.

_____

_____

16. Define the following terms.

a. Hyperthermia:

_____

_____

b. Malignant hyperthermia:

_____

_____

17. Define and explain the causes of heatstroke.

_____

_____

_____

18. Define and explain the causes of heat exhaustion.

_____

_____

_____

19. Define and explain the causes of hypothermia.

_____

_____

_____

20. Frostbite occurs when

_____

_____

_____

Assessment

21. List the routine assessment sites for intermittent temperature measurement.

    a. _____

    b. _____

    c. _____

    d. _____

22. State the formulas for the following conversions.

    a. Fahrenheit to Celsius:

    _____

    b. Celsius to Fahrenheit:

    _____

23. Identify three types of thermometers and list advantages and disadvantages of each.

    a. _____

    _____

    _____

    b. _____

    _____

    _____

    c. _____

    _____

    _____

Nursing Diagnosis

24. Identify three nursing diagnoses related to thermoregulation.

    a. _____

    b. _____

    c. _____

Planning and Implementation

Health Promotion

25. Health promotion for clients at risk of altered temperature is directed toward

    _____

    _____

    _____

26. Identify the risk factors for hypothermia.

    _____

    _____

    _____

Acute Care

27. The procedures used to intervene and treat an elevated temperature depend on the fever's cause; its adverse effects; and its strength, intensity, and duration.

28. Explain the differences related to febrile states in each of the following.

    a. Children:

    _____

    _____

    _____

    b. Hypersensitivity to drugs:

    _____

    _____

    _____

29. Give three examples of each type of fever therapy.

    Pharmacological

    a. _____

    b. _____

    c. _____

    Nonpharmacological

    a. _____

    b. _____

    c. _____

30. Identify an independent and a dependent nursing intervention to control shivering.

    _____

    _____

    _____

31. First aid treatment for heatstroke includes

    _____

    _____

    _____

32. Summarize the treatment for hypothermia.

    _____

    _____

    _____

Restorative and Continuing Care

33. Summarize the client teaching in regard to the treatment of a fever.

    _____

    _____

Evaluation

Pulse

34. Define *pulse*.

_____

_____

Physiology and Regulation

35. Define the following terms.

a. *Stroke volume*:

_____

_____

b. *Cardiac output*:

_____

_____

Assessment of Pulse

36. Identify the two most common peripheral pulse sites to assess.

a. _____

b. _____

37. Identify the five major parts of the stethoscope.

a. _____

b. _____

c. _____

d. _____

e. _____

Character of the Pulse

38. List four characteristics to identify during peripheral pulse assessment. Using an asterisk, specify the two characteristics to identify when assessing an apical pulse.

a. _____

b. _____

c. _____

d. _____

39. Define the following.

a. Tachycardia:

_____

_____

b. Bradycardia:

_____

_____

c. Dysrhythmia:

_____

_____

d. Pulse deficit:

_____

_____

Respiration

40. Define the following.

a. Ventilation:

_____

_____

b. Diffusion:

_____

_____

c. Perfusion:

_____

_____

Physiological Control

41. Breathing is a passive process. The respiratory centre in the brain stem regulates the involuntary control of respirations.

42. Ventilation is controlled by levels of _____ _____, _____, and _____ in the arterial blood.

43. The most important factor in the control of ventilation is the level of _____.

44. *Hypoxemia* occurs

_____

_____

_____

Mechanics of Breathing

45. Briefly summarize the process of inspiration.

_____

_____

_____

46. Define the following terms.

a. Tidal volume:

_____

_____

b. Eupnea:

_____

_____

_____

Assessment of Ventilation

47. Accurate measurement requires _____ and _____ of chest wall movement.

48. List three objective measurements used in respiratory status assessment.

    a. _____

    b. _____

    c. _____

49. Define the following alterations in breathing patterns.

    a. Bradypnea:

    b. Tachypnea:

    c. Hyperpnea:

    d. Apnea:

    e. Hypoventilation

    f. Hyperventilation:

    g. Cheyne-Stokes respiration:

    h. Kussmaul's respiration:

    i. Biot's respiration:

Assessment of Diffusion and Perfusion

50. The respiratory processes of diffusion and perfusion can be evaluated by measuring the oxygen saturation of the blood.

51. The percentage of saturation of arterial blood is _____ and of venous blood is _____.

52. Explain the purpose of a pulse oximeter.

    _____

53. List three things that can affect the accuracy of an oxygen saturation reading.

    a. _____

    b. _____

    c. _____

Blood Pressure

54. Define the following terms.

    a. *Blood pressure*:

    b. *Systolic*:

    c. *Diastolic*:

55. The difference between the systolic and diastolic pressure is the _____.

Physiology of Arterial Blood Pressure

56. Blood pressure reflects the interrelationships of the following. Briefly explain each.

    a. Cardiac output:

    b. Peripheral vascular resistance:

    c. Blood volume:

    d. Blood viscosity:

    e. Artery elasticity:

Factors Influencing Blood Pressure

57. List six factors that influence blood pressure.

a. _____

b. _____

c. _____

d. _____

e. _____

f. _____

Hypertension

58. Identify the criteria for the diagnosis of hypertension in an adult.

_____

_____

_____

59. Briefly summarize the physiology of hypertension.

_____

_____

_____

60. List five risk factors that are linked to hypertension.

a. _____

b. _____

c. _____

d. _____

e. _____

Hypotension

61. Identify the criteria for the diagnosis of hypotension in an adult.

_____

_____

62. Explain the physiology of hypotension and its causes.

_____

_____

_____

63. Orthostatic hypotension occurs when

_____

_____

_____

64. Explain how you would assess a client for orthostatic hypotension.

_____

_____

_____

Measurement of Blood Pressure

65. Identify two methods for measuring blood pressure.

a. _____

b. _____

66. Identify the two types of sphygmomanometers and list their advantages and disadvantages.

a. _____

b. _____

67. The sounds heard over an artery distal to the blood pressure cuff are Korotkoff sounds. Describe each.

a. First:

_____

_____

b. Second:

_____

_____

c. Third:

_____

_____

d. Fourth:

_____

_____

e. Fifth:

_____

_____

68. During the initial assessment, you should obtain and record the blood pressure in both arms. Pressure differences between the arms greater than _____ mm Hg indicate vascular problems.

69. Identify five common mistakes in blood pressure assessment.

a. _____

b. _____

c. _____

d. _____

e. _____

70. Identify four reasons why the measurement of blood pressure in infants and children is difficult.

    a. _____

    b. _____

    c. _____

    d. _____

71. Explain the rationale for the use of an ultra-sonic stethoscope.

    _____

    _____

    _____

72. Identify the method you may use to assess blood pressure when Korotkoff sounds are not audible with the standard stethoscope.

    _____

73. Define *auscultatory gap*.

    _____

    _____

    _____

74. Give an example of when you would assess a client's blood pressure using the client's lower extremities.

    _____

    _____

    _____

75. Identify the advantages and disadvantages of using automatic blood pressure devices.

    _____

    _____

    _____

76. List the benefits of blood pressure self-measurement.

    a. _____

    b. _____

    c. _____

    d. _____

Health Promotion and Vital Signs

77. Identify at least two variations that are unique to the older adult.

    a. Temperature:

    _____

    _____

    b. Pulse rate:

    _____

    c. Blood pressure:

    _____

    _____

    d. Respirations:

    _____

    _____

Review Questions

Select the appropriate answer and cite the rationale for choosing that particular answer.

1. The skin plays a role in temperature regulation by
   a. Insulating the body
   b. Constricting blood vessels
   c. Sensing external temperature variations
   d. All of the above

   Answer: _____   Rationale: _____

   _____

   _____

2. You bathe the client who has a fever with cool water. You do this to increase heat loss by means of
   a. Radiation
   b. Convection
   c. Condensation
   d. Conduction

   Answer: _____   Rationale: _____

   _____

   _____

3. You are assessing a client suspected of having the nursing diagnosis *hyperthermia related to vigorous exercise in hot weather*. In reviewing the data, you know that the most important sign of heatstroke is
   a. Confusion
   b. Hot, dry skin
   c. Excess thirst
   d. Muscle cramps

   Answer: _____   Rationale: _____

   _____

   _____

4. When taking a client's radial pulse, you note a dysrhythmia. The most appropriate action is to
   a. Inform the physician immediately
   b. Wait 5 minutes and retake the radial pulse
   c. Take the pulse apically for 1 full minute
   d. Check the client's record for the presence of a previous dysrhythmia

Answer: _____   Rationale: _____
_____
_____

5. You are auscultating Mrs. McKinnon's blood pressure. You inflate the cuff to 180 mm Hg. At 156 mm Hg, you hear the onset of a tapping sound. At 130 mm Hg, the sound changes to a murmur or swishing. At 100 mm Hg, the sound momentarily becomes sharper, and at 92 mm Hg, it becomes muffled. At 88 mm Hg, the sound disappears. Mrs. McKinnon's blood pressure is
   a. 180/92
   b. 180/130
   c. 156/88
   d. 130/88

Answer: _____   Rationale: _____
_____
_____

32

Health Assessment and Physical Examination

Preliminary Reading

Chapter 32, pp. 540–634

Comprehensive Understanding

Purposes of Physical Examination

1. Physical assessment skills allow you to _____ _____ and _____.

2. Your success in providing care depends on your ability to recognize a change in the client's status and to modify therapies so that the client gains the most desirable outcome.

3. Whether a complete or partial physical assessment is performed, an examination should be integrated into routine care.

4. List the five nursing purposes for performing a physical assessment.

   a. _____

   b. _____

   c. _____

   d. _____

   e. _____

Analyzing Signs and Symptoms

5. The main objective of the nurse–client interaction is for the nurse to find out what is central to the client's concerns and to help the client find solutions.

6. A complete assessment is needed to form a definitive diagnosis.

7. You learn to group significant findings into patterns of data that reveal actual or high-risk nursing diagnoses.

8. The baseline is

   _____

   _____

   _____

General Inspection

9. Summarize at least 14 specific observations of the client's general appearance and behaviour.

   a. _____

   b. _____

   c. _____

   d. _____

   e. _____

   f. _____

   g. _____

   h. _____

   i. _____

   j. _____

k. _____

l. _____

m. _____

n. _____

Physical Examination Modes

Inspection

10. Define *inspection*.

_____
_____
_____

11. List six principles to facilitate accurate inspection of body parts.

a. _____

b. _____

c. _____

d. _____

e. _____

f. _____

Palpation

12. Define *palpation*.

_____
_____
_____

13. Identify the parts of the hand used to assess each of the following.

a. Temperature:

_____

b. Pulsations:

_____

c. Vibrations:

_____

d. Turgor:

_____

14. Briefly explain the following.

a. Light palpation:

_____
_____

b. Deep palpation:

_____
_____

Percussion

15. Identify the information obtained through percussion.

_____
_____
_____

16. Explain the two types of percussion.

a. Direct:

_____
_____

b. Indirect:

_____
_____

17. Percussion produces five types of sounds. Identify the type and where in the body the sound is found.

a. _____

b. _____

c. _____

d. _____

e. _____

Auscultation

18. Define *auscultation*.

_____
_____
_____

19. Briefly explain the following characteristics of sound.

a. Frequency:

_____
_____

b. Loudness:

_____
_____

c. Quality:

_____
_____

d. Duration:

_____
_____

Preparation for Physical Examination

20. Briefly explain the following pre-examination preparations.

    a. Physical:

    _____

    _____

    b. Positioning:

    _____

    _____

    c. Psychological:

    _____

    _____

21. List at least six variations in the nurse's individual style that are appropriate when examining children.

    a. _____
    b. _____
    c. _____
    d. _____
    e. _____
    f. _____

22. List at least five variations in the nurse's individual style that are appropriate when examining older adults.

    a. _____
    b. _____
    c. _____
    d. _____
    e. _____

23. List at least three environmental factors that you should attempt to control before performing a physical examination.

    a. _____
    b. _____
    c. _____

24. Examination techniques cause you to contact body fluids and discharge. Standard precautions/routine practices should be used throughout the examination.

25. Handwashing is done before equipment preparation and before the examination.

26. All equipment should be checked to see that it functions properly.

27. List eight principles to follow for a well-organized examination.

    a.
    b. _____
    c. _____
    d. _____
    e. _____
    f. _____
    g. _____
    h. _____

28. Assessment of vital signs is the first part of the physical assessment.

Height, Weight, and Circumference

29. A person's general level of health can be reflected in the ratio of height and weight.

30. List three actions that should be taken to ensure accurate weight measurement of a hospitalized client.

    a. _____
    b. _____
    c. _____

31. In the infant, a chest circumference can be compared with the head circumference to rule out problems in head or chest size.

Assessing Mental and Emotional Status

32. An alteration in mental or emotional status may reflect a disturbance in cerebral functioning.

33. List three factors that may change cerebral function.

    a. _____
    b. _____
    c. _____

34. Define *delirium* and list the clinical criteria for it.

    _____
    _____
    _____
    _____

Level of Consciousness

35. The level of consciousness exists along a continuum, from full awakening, alertness, and cooperation to unresponsiveness to any form of external stimuli.

36. Identify the tool and the three factors to assess consciousness.

_____

_____

_____

_____

Behaviour and Appearance

37. Behaviour, moods, hygiene, grooming, and choice of dress reveal pertinent information about mental status.

Language

38. Explain the function of the cerebral cortex in language.

_____

_____

39. List 3 things you should do to assess the client's language capabilities.

   a. _____

   b. _____

   c. _____

Intellectual Function

40. Intellectual function includes the following. Briefly explain how each is assessed.

   a. Abstract thinking:

   _____

   _____

   b. Judgement:

   _____

   _____

   c. Memory:

   _____

   _____

   d. Knowledge:

   _____

   _____

Assessing Sensory and Motor Functions

Sensory Function

41. The sensory pathways of the central nervous system conduct sensations of _____, _____, _____, _____, and _____.

42. Summarize how you would assess the client's sensory function.

_____

_____

_____

_____

Motor Function

43. Which primary motor pathways mediate things such as muscle tone, posture, muscular activity, reflex activity, balance, coordination, gait and equilibrium?

_____

_____

_____

Assessing the Integumentary System

44. The physical assessment skills of _____ _____ and _____ are used to assess the integument's function and integrity.

Skin

45. Assessment of the skin can reveal a variety of conditions including changes in _____ _____, _____, _____, _____, and _____.

46. The skin provides the body's _____ _____ and acts as a sensory organ for _____, _____, _____, and _____.

47. Define the following terms.

   a. *Melanoma*:

   _____

   _____

   b. *Basal cell carcinoma*:

   _____

   _____

48. List at least four risks for skin lesions in the hospitalized client.

   a. _____

   b. _____

   c. _____

   d. _____

49. For each skin colour variation in the following table, identify the mechanism that produces colour change, the common causes of the variation, and the optimal sites for assessment.

Skin Colour	Mechanisms	Causes	Assessment Sites
Cyanosis			
Pallor			
Jaundice			
Erythema			

50. Petechiae are

_____

_____

_____

51. When a lesion is detected, it is inspected for

_____, _____, _____, _____, _____, _____, and _____.

52. Define *moisture*.

_____

_____

_____

53. Excessive dryness can worsen skin conditions such as _____ and _____.

54. The temperature of the skin depends on the amount of _____ circulating through the dermis.

55. The character of the skin's surface and the feel of deeper portions are its _____.

56. Define *skin turgor* and describe normal findings.

_____

_____

_____

57. Identify the two causes of edema.

_____

_____

58. Briefly describe the following primary skin lesions.

a. Macule:

_____

_____

b. Papule:

_____

_____

c. Nodule:

_____

_____

d. Tumour:

_____

_____

e. Wheal:

_____

_____

f. Vesicle:

_____

_____

g. Pustule:

_____

_____

h. Ulcer:

_____

_____

i. Atrophy:

_____

_____

59. Explain the following terms related to lesions.

a. *Senile keratosis*:

_____

_____

_____

b. *Cherry angiomas*:

_____

_____

Hair and Scalp

60. When inspecting the hair, you note the _____, _____, _____, _____, _____ and _____.

61. Define the following.

a. Alopecia:

_____

_____

b. Hirsutism:

_____

_____

62. Name the three types of lice.

a. _____

b. _____

c. _____

Nails

63. When inspecting the nail bed, you note the _____, _____, and _____.

64. You palpate the nail base to determine

_____

_____

_____

65. Briefly describe clubbing.

_____

_____

_____

Assessing the Head and the Neck

Head

66. For each procedure in the following table, identify the steps that should be taken in assessing the head.

Inspection	Palpation	Percussion	Auscultation

Eyes

67. For each procedure in the following table, identify the steps that should be taken in assessing the eyes.

Inspection	Palpation	Percussion	Auscultation
Visual acuity			
Visual fields			
Extraocular movements			

Inspection of External Eye Structures

68. For each procedure in the following table, identify the steps that should be taken in assessing the external eye structures.

Inspection	Palpation	Percussion	Auscultation
Eyebrows			
Eyelids			
Lacrimal apparatus			
Conjunctivae and sclerae			
Corneas, pupils, and irises			

69. Define the following common eye and visual abnormalities.

   a. Exophthalmos:

   _____

   _____

   b. Strabismus:

   _____

   _____

   c. Nystagmus:

   _____

   _____

Inspection and Internal Eye Structures

70. Identify the six structures you would assess in the internal eye.

   a. _____

   b. _____

   c. _____

   d. _____

   e. _____

   f. _____

Ears

71. For each procedure in the following table, identify the steps that should be taken in assessing the ears.

Inspection	Palpation	Percussion	Auscultation
External ear			
Middle ear			
Inner ear			

72. Identify the mechanisms for sound transmission.

   a. _____

   b. _____

   c. _____

   d. _____

   e. _____

73. Identify the types of problems that affect the ear.

   a. _____

   b. _____

   c. _____

   d. _____

74. The three types of hearing loss are _____ _____, _____, and _____.

75. Define *ototoxicity*.

   _____

   _____

   _____

76. Briefly explain how a tuning fork works.

   _____

   _____

   _____

77. Define *Weber test*.

_____

_____

_____

78. Define *Rinné test*.

_____

_____

_____

Nose

79. For each procedure in the following table, identify the steps that should be taken in assessing the nose.

Inspection	Palpation	Percussion	Auscultation

Paranasal Sinuses

80. For each procedure in the following table, identify the steps that should be taken in assessing the sinuses.

Inspection	Palpation	Percussion	Auscultation

Mouth and Pharynx

81. For each procedure in the following table, identify the steps that should be taken in assessing the mouth and pharynx.

Inspection	Palpation	Percussion	Auscultation
Lips			
Buccal mucosa, gums, and teeth			
Tongue and floor of mouth			

… *continued*

Inspection	Palpation	Percussion	Auscultation
Palates			
Pharynx			

Neck

82. For each procedure in the following table, identify the steps that should be taken in assessing the neck.

Inspection	Palpation	Percussion	Auscultation
Neck muscles			
Lymph nodes			
Thyroid gland			
Carotid artery and jugular vein			
Trachea			

Assessing the Thorax and Lungs

83. For each procedure in the following table, identify the steps that should be taken in assessing the thorax and lungs.

Inspection	Palpation	Percussion	Auscultation
Posterior thorax			
Lateral thorax			
Anterior thorax			

84. Accurate physical assessment of the thorax and lungs requires review of the ventilatory and respiratory functions of the lung.

85. Define *tactile fremitus*.

_____
_____
_____

86. Define kyphosis:

_____
_____

87. Identify the normal breath sounds and where they are located.

_____
_____
_____

88. Complete the following table of adventitious breath sounds.

Sound	Auscultation Site	Cause	Character
Crackles			
Rhonchi			

Sound	Auscultation Site	Cause	Character
Wheezes			
Pleural friction rub			

Assessing the Heart

89. Assessment of heart function involves a review of signs and symptoms from the nursing history, pulse assessment, and direct examination of the heart.

90. Define what occurs during the two phases of the cardiac cycle.
    a. Systole:

    b. Diastole:

91. Define the following heart sounds.
    S_1: _____
    S_2: _____
    S_3: _____
    S_4: _____

92. Define *dysrhythmia*.

93. Define *murmur*.

94. List the six factors to assess when a murmur is detected.
    a. _____
    b. _____

c. _____
d. _____
e. _____
f. _____

95. Define *thrill*.

96. Answer the following questions regarding the point of maximal impulse (PMI).
    a. What is the PMI?

    b. Where is the PMI normally located in the infant and young child?

    c. Where is the PMI located in the older child and adult?

    d. What techniques may be used to locate the PMI?

Assessing the Breasts

97. For each procedure in the following table, identify the steps that should be taken in assessing the breasts.

Inspection	Palpation	Percussion	Auscultation

98. It is important to examine the breasts of female and male clients.

99. The American Cancer Society (2008) recommends the following guidelines for early detection of breast cancer.

    a. _____

    b. _____

    c. _____

    d. _____

    e. _____

100. Briefly explain the proper technique for palpating breast tissue.

    _____

    _____

    _____

101. List seven characteristics that should be included when describing an abnormal breast mass.

    a. _____

    b. _____

    c. _____

    d. _____

    e. _____

    f. _____

    g. _____

102. Define the following terms.

    a. Metastasize:

    _____

    _____

    b. Fibrocystic breast disease:

    _____

    _____

Assessing the Abdomen

103. The abdominal examination includes an assessment of the lower gastrointestinal tract in addition to the liver, stomach, uterus, ovaries, kidneys, and bladder.

104. Describe four techniques used to help the client relax during assessment of the abdomen.

    a. _____

    b. _____

    c. _____

    d. _____

105. For each procedure in the following table, identify the steps that should be taken in assessing the abdomen.

Inspection	Palpation	Percussion	Auscultation
Abdomen			
Liver			

106. Define the following.
    a. Hernias:
    _____
    _____

    b. Distension:
    _____
    _____

    c. Peristalsis:
    _____
    _____

    d. Paralytic ileus:
    _____
    _____

    e. Borborygmi:
    _____
    _____

    f. Aneurysm:
    _____
    _____

Assessing the Female Genitalia and Reproductive Tract

107. For each procedure in the following table, identify the steps that should be taken in assessing the female genitalia and reproductive tract.

Inspection	Palpation	Percussion	Auscultation
External genitalia			
Cervix			
Vagina			

108. Briefly explain the preparation of a client for a complete examination of the genitalia and reproductive tract.
_____
_____
_____
_____

109. Define the following terms.
    a. Chancres:
    _____
    _____

    b. Cystocele:
    _____
    _____

    c. Rectocele:
    _____
    _____

110. Speculum examination of the internal genitalia includes
_____
_____
_____

Assessing Male Genitalia

111. For each procedure in the following table, identify the steps that should be taken in assessing the male genitalia.

Inspection	Palpation	Percussion	Auscultation
Penis			
Scrotum			
Inguinal ring and canal			
Rectum and anus			

112. An examination of the male genitalia includes assessment of the external genitalia and the inguinal ring and canal.

113. Summarize how you would assess sexual maturity.

_____

_____

_____

Assessing the Anus, Rectum, and Prostate

114. The purpose of digital palpation is

_____

_____

_____

Assessing the Extremities

115. The assessment of musculoskeletal function focuses on determining the range of joint motion, muscle strength and tone, and joint and muscle condition.

116. Describe the manoeuvres used to assess balance and gross motor function.

a. _____

b. _____

c. _____

Assessing the Upper and Lower Extremities

117. For each procedure in the following table, identify the steps that should be taken in assessing the upper and lower extremities.

Inspection	Palpation	Coordination	Sensory System	Reflexes
Upper extremities				
Lower extremities				

118. Define the following.

   a. Hypertonicity:

   _____

   _____

   b. Osteoporosis:

   _____

   _____

Review Questions

Select the appropriate answer and cite the rationale for choosing that particular answer.

1. The component that should receive the highest priority before a physical examination is
   a. Preparation of the environment
   b. Preparation of the equipment
   c. Physical preparation of the client
   d. Psychological preparation of the client

Answer: _____   Rationale: _____

_____

2. The nurse assesses the skin turgor of the client by
   a. Grasping a fold of skin on the back of the forearm and releasing
   b. Palpating the skin with the dorsum of the hand
   c. Pressing the skin for 5 seconds, releasing, and noting each centimetre of depth
   d. Inspecting the buccal mucosa with a penlight

Answer: _____   Rationale: _____

_____

_____

3. While examining Mr. Polanzsky, you note a circumscribed elevation of skin filled with serous fluid on his upper lip. The lesion is 0.4 cm in diameter. This type of lesion is called a
   a. Macule
   b. Nodule
   c. Vesicle
   d. Pustule

Answer: _____   Rationale: _____

_____

_____

4. When assessing the client's thorax, you should
    a. Complete the left side and then the right side
    b. Change the position of the stethoscope between inspiration and expiration
    c. Compare symmetrical areas from side to side
    d. Begin with the posterior lobes on the right side

Answer: _____   Rationale: _____
_____
_____

5. In a client with pneumonia, you hear high-pitched, continuous musical sounds over the bronchi on expiration. These sounds are called
    a. Crackles
    b. Rhonchi
    c. Wheezes
    d. Friction rubs

Answer: _____   Rationale: _____
_____
_____

6. The second heart sound (S_2) occurs when
    a. The mitral and tricuspid valves close
    b. There is rapid ventricular filling
    c. Systole begins
    d. The aortic and pulmonic valves close

Answer: _____   Rationale: _____
_____
_____

33

Infection Control

Preliminary Reading

Chapter 33, pp. 635–674

Comprehensive Understanding

Scientific Knowledge Base

1. An infection is

_____

_____

_____

2. Define *communicable*.

_____

_____

_____

Chain of Infection

3. Development of an infection occurs in a cycle that depends on the following elements:

a. _____

b. _____

c. _____

d. _____

e. _____

f. _____

4. Microorganisms include _____, _____, _____, and _____.

5. Define the following.

a. Virulence:

_____

_____

b. Immunocompromised:

_____

_____

6. The potential for microorganisms to cause disease depends on four factors. Name them.

a. _____

b. _____

c. _____

d. _____

7. Define *reservoir*.

_____

_____

_____

8. Define *carriers*.

_____

_____

_____

9. To thrive, organisms require the following. Briefly explain each one.

a. Food:

_____

_____

b. Oxygen (or no oxygen):

_____

_____

c. Water:

_____

_____

d. Temperature:

_____

_____

e. pH:

_____

_____

f. Minimal light:

_____

_____

10. What is a portal of exit? Give examples.

_____

_____

_____

11. List the major modes of transmission of microorganisms from the reservoir to the host.

_____

_____

The Infectious Process

12. The severity of the client's illness depends on the _____, the _____ _____, and the _____ _____.

13. Describe the two types of infections.

a. Localized:

_____

_____

b. Systemic:

_____

_____

Defences Against Infection

14. The immune response is

_____

_____

15. Explain the normal body defences against infection.

a. Normal flora:

_____

_____

_____

b. Body system defences:

_____

_____

_____

c. Inflammation:

_____

_____

_____

16. For each body system or organ in the grid that follows, identify at least one defence mechanism and the primary action to prevent infection.

System/Organ	Defence Mechanism	Action
Skin		
Mouth		
Respiratory tract		
Urinary tract		
Gastrointestinal tract		

17. The inflammatory response includes the following. Explain each briefly.

    a. Vascular and cellular responses:

    _____
    _____
    _____

    b. Inflammatory exudates:

    _____
    _____
    _____

    c. Tissue repair:

    _____
    _____
    _____

18. Briefly explain the following vascular and cellular responses.

    a. Edema:

    _____
    _____
    _____

    b. Phagocytosis:

    _____
    _____
    _____

Health Care–Acquired Infections

19. Define *health care–acquired infection (HAI)/ nosocomial infection.*

    _____
    _____
    _____

20. Define the following types of nosocomial infections (HAIs).

    a. Exogenous:

    _____
    _____

    b. Endogenous:

    _____
    _____

21. Identify at least three factors that increase a hospitalized client's risk of acquiring a health care-associated infection (HAI).

    a. _____
    b. _____
    c. _____

22. Identify the major sites for nosocomial infection (HAI).

    _____
    _____

Nursing Process in Infection Control

Assessment

23. Nurses assess the client's defence mechanisms, suscesptibility, and knowledge of infections.

24. Knowing the factors that increase the client's susceptibility or risk for infection, you are better able to plan preventive therapy that includes aseptic technique.

25. Any reduction in the body's primary or secondary defences against infection places a client at risk. List at least four risk factors of each.

    a. Inadequate primary defences:

    _____
    _____
    _____
    _____

    b. Inadequate secondary defences:

    _____
    _____
    _____
    _____

26. The following factors influence client susceptibility to infection. Explain each one.

    a. Age:

    _____
    _____

    b. Nutritional status:

    _____
    _____

    c. Stress:

    _____
    _____

    d. Disease process:

    _____
    _____

    e. Medical therapy:

    _____
    _____

Clinical Appearance

27. Describe the signs and symptoms of each type of infection.

    a. Local:

    _____

    _____

    b. Systemic:

    _____

    _____

28. Describe how an infection is manifested in an older adult.

    _____

    _____

    _____

Laboratory Data

29. List at least five laboratory values that may indicate infection.

    a. _____
    b. _____
    c. _____
    d. _____
    e. _____

Clients With Infection

30. The ways in which infection can affect the client's and family's needs may be _____ ___, _____, _____, or _____.

Nursing Diagnosis

31. You may diagnose a risk for infection or make diagnoses that result from the effects of infection on health status.

Planning

32. List four common goals for the client with an actual or potential risk for infection.

    a. _____
    b. _____
    c. _____
    d. _____

Implementation

Health Promotion

33. List five ways you may prevent an infection from developing or spreading.

    a. _____

    b. _____
    c. _____
    d. _____
    e. _____

34. List preventive interventions to protect a client from invasion by pathogens.

    _____

    _____

    _____

Asepsis

35. Explain the following methods of controlling or eliminating infectious agents.

    a. Cleaning:

    _____

    _____

    b. Disinfection:

    _____

    _____

    c. Sterilization:

    _____

    _____

    d. Control or elimination of reservoirs:

    _____

    _____

    e. Control of portals of exit:

    _____

    _____

    f. Control of transmission:

    _____

    _____

    g. Hand hygiene:

    _____

    _____

36. Describe the Centers for Disease Control and Prevention (CDC) guidelines on handwashing and the use of alcohol-based waterless antiseptics.

    a. _____
    b. _____
    c. _____
    d. _____
    e. _____

f. _____

g. _____

h. _____

i. _____

37. Many measures that control the exit of microorganisms also control the entrance of pathogens. Give at least five examples.

a. _____

b. _____

c. _____

d. _____

e. _____

38. A client's resistance to infection improves as the nurse protects the body's normal defences against infection. Explain.

_____

_____

_____

39. Standard precautions/routine practices call for the appropriate use of protective devices and clothing, including _____, _____, _____, _____, and _____.

40. Barrier protection is indicated for use with all clients because every client has the potential to

_____

41. The CDC's (1996) and Health Canada's (1999) isolation guidelines contain a two-tiered approach. Explain.

a. Standard precautions (tier one):

_____

_____

b. Transmission-based (isolation) precautions (tier two):

_____

_____

42. List some basic principles common to all categories of isolation precautions.

_____

_____

_____

43. Briefly summarize the psychological implications of isolation.

_____

_____

44. Explain the techniques for collecting specimens from the client with a suspected infection.

a. Wound:

_____

_____

b. Blood:

_____

_____

c. Stool:

_____

_____

d. Urine:

_____

_____

45. Explain Health Canada's recommendations for bagging waste or linen.

_____

_____

46. Describe how you would transport a client with an infection.

_____

_____

_____

Role of the Infection-Control Professional

47. List eight responsibilities of the infection-control professional.

a. _____

b. _____

c. _____

d. _____

e. _____

f. _____

g. _____

h. _____

Client Education

48. List six topics you need to discuss with the client in relation to infection-control practices.

a. _____

b. _____

c. _____

d. _____

e. _____

f. _____

Surgical Asepsis

49. Briefly explain what is meant by the concepts of *surgical asepsis* and *medical asepsis*.

_____

_____

_____

50. Explain when surgical asepsis must be used.

_____

_____

_____

51. List three teaching points that reduce the risk of client-associated contamination during sterile procedures or treatments.

a. _____

b. _____

c. _____

52. List the seven principles of surgical asepsis.

a. _____

b. _____

c. _____

d. _____

e. _____

f. _____

g. _____

53. List and briefly explain the eight steps in performing a sterile procedure.

a. _____

b. _____

c. _____

d. _____

e. _____

f. _____

g. _____

h. _____

Evaluation

54. The success of infection-control techniques is measured by determining whether the goals for reducing or preventing infection are achieved.

55. Two important skills in evaluation are the ability to correctly assess wounds for healing and the ability to conduct a physical assessment of body systems.

56. A clear description of any signs and symptoms of systemic or local infection is necessary to give all nurses a baseline for comparative evaluation.

57. The client at risk for infection must understand the measures needed to reduce or prevent microorganism growth and spread.

Review Questions

Select the appropriate answer and cite the rationale for choosing that particular answer.

1. Of the following, which is not an element in the chain of infection?
   a. Infectious agent or pathogen
   b. Reservoir for pathogen growth
   c. Mode of transmission
   d. Formation of immunoglobulin

   Answer: _____　Rationale: _____

   _____

   _____

2. Pathogenic organisms include all of the following *except*
   a. Bacteria
   b. Leukocytes
   c. Viruses
   d. Fungi

   Answer: _____　Rationale: _____

   _____

   _____

3. The severity of a client's illness will depend on all of the following *except*
   a. Extent of infection
   b. Pathogenicity of the microorganism
   c. Susceptibility of the host
   d. Incubation period

   Answer: _____　Rationale: _____

   _____

   _____

4. Which of the following best describes an iatrogenic infection or health care–acquired infection (HAI)?
   a. It results from a diagnostic or therapeutic procedure.
   b. It occurs when clients are infected with their own organisms as a result of immunodeficiency.

c. It involves an incubation period of 3 to 4 weeks before it can be detected.

d. It results from an extended infection of the urinary tract.

Answer: _____ Rationale: _____

_____

_____

5. The nurse sets up a sterile field on the client's over-bed table. In which of the following instances is the field contaminated?

a. The nurse keeps the top of the table above his or her waist.

b. Sterile saline solution is spilled on the field.

c. Sterile objects are kept within a 2.5-cm border of the field.

d. The nurse, who has a cold, wears a double mask.

Answer: _____ Rationale: _____

_____

_____

6. When a client on airborne or droplet isolation precautions must be transported to another part of the hospital, which of the following is *not* required of you as the nurse?

a. Place a mask on the client before leaving the room.

b. Obtain a physician's order to prohibit the client from being transported.

c. Advise personnel in diagnostic or procedural areas that the client is under isolation precautions.

d. Provide the client with tissues and a bag for proper disposal of secretions.

Answer: _____ Rationale: _____

_____

_____

34

Medication Administration

Preliminary Reading

Chapter 34, pp. 675–755

Comprehensive Understanding

Scientific Knowledge Base

1. A medication is a substance used in the diagnosis, treatment, cure, relief, or prevention of health alterations.

Pharmacological Concepts

2. A single medication may have three different names. Define each one.

   a. Chemical name:

   _____

   _____

   b. Generic name:

   _____

   _____

   c. Trade name:

   _____

   _____

3. A medication classification indicates:

   _____

   _____

4. The form of the medication determines its

   _____

   _____

Medication Legislation and Standards

5. Briefly summarize the role of the federal government in drug regulation.

   _____

   _____

   _____

6. Describe the *Food and Drug Act*.

   _____

   _____

7. The Health Protection Branch is responsible for

   _____

   _____

8. Summarize the role of the provincial government in drug regulation.

   _____

   _____

   _____

9. Summarize the role of health care institutions.

   _____

   _____

   _____

10. Describe why it is important for registered nurses to be aware of both federal and provincial regulations affecting drug administration in their practice.

    _____

    _____

    _____

    _____

Pharmacokinetics as the Basis of Medication Actions

11. Pharmacokinetics is the study of

    _____

    _____

Absorption

12. Define *absorption*.

_____

_____

13. Briefly explain the following factors that influence drug absorption.

a. Route of administration:

_____

_____

b. Ability of a medication to dissolve:

_____

_____

c. Blood flow to the area of absorption:

_____

_____

d. Body surface area:

_____

_____

e. Lipid solubility of a medication:

_____

_____

Distribution

14. The rate and extent of distribution depend on the physical and chemical properties of the drug and on the physiological makeup of the person taking the drug.

15. Explain how each of the following affect the rate and extent of medication distribution.

a. Circulation:

_____

_____

b. Membrane permeability:

_____

_____

c. Protein binding:

_____

_____

Metabolism

16. Define *biotransformation* and identify where it occurs.

_____

_____

17. Explain why biotransformation is an important concept for registered nurses to understand.

_____

_____

_____

Excretion

18. After drugs are metabolized, they exit the body through the following routes:

_____

19. Identify the primary organ for drug excretion and explain what happens if this organ's function declines.

_____

_____

Types of Medication Action

20. Define the following predicted or unintended effects of drugs and provide a nursing practice example.

a. Therapeutic effects:

_____

_____

b. Side effects:

_____

_____

c. Adverse effects:

_____

_____

d. Toxic effects:

_____

_____

e. Idiosyncratic reactions:

_____

_____

f. Allergic reactions:

_____

_____

g. Anaphylactic reactions:

_____

_____

Medication Interactions

21. Describe the process of a medication interaction and provide an example from nursing practice.

_____

_____

_____

22. Describe the concept of a "synergistic effect" and provide an example from nursing practice.

_____

_____

_____

Medication Dose Responses

23. When a medication is prescribed, the goal is to achieve a constant blood level within a safe therapeutic range.

24. Repeated doses are required to achieve a constant therapeutic concentration of a medication because a portion of a drug is always being excreted.

25. Define the following.

   a. Serum concentration:

   _____

   _____

   b. Serum half-life:

   _____

   _____

26. Using the concepts of serum concentration and serum half-life, explain why it is important for both clients and nurses to follow regular dosage schedules and adhere to prescribed doses and dose intervals.

_____

_____

_____

27. Explain the following time intervals of medication actions.

   a. Onset of drug action:

   _____

   _____

   b. Trough:

   _____

   _____

   c. Duration of action:

   _____

   d. Plateau:

   _____

   _____

Routes of Administration

28. The route prescribed for a drug's administration depends on its properties, the desired effect, and the client's physical and mental condition.

Oral Routes

29. The oral route is the easiest and the most commonly used route.

30. Identify the types of oral routes, explain how the oral routes are used, and identify the effects of using these routes.

_____

_____

_____

Parenteral Routes

31. The parenteral route involves administering a drug through injection into body tissues.

32. List the four major sites of parenteral injections.

   a. _____
   b. _____
   c. _____
   d. _____

33. Define the following advanced techniques of medication administration.

   a. Epidural:

   _____

   _____

   b. Intrathecal:

   _____

   _____

   c. Intraosseous:

   _____

   _____

   d. Intraperitoneal:

   _____

   _____

e. Intrapleural:

_____

_____

f. Intra-arterial:

_____

_____

g. Intracardiac:

_____

_____

h. Intra-articular:

_____

_____

Topical Administration

34. Medications that are applied to the skin and mucous membranes generally have local effects.

35. Identify five methods for applying medications to mucous membranes.

a. _____
b. _____
c. _____
d. _____
e. _____

Inhalation Route

36. Describe the three passages through which inhalations can be administered.

a. Nasal:

_____

_____

b. Oral:

_____

_____

c. Endotracheal or tracheal:

_____

_____

Intraocular Route

37. Describe the process of intraocular medication delivery.

_____

_____

Systems of Medication Measurement

38. The following are measurements used in drug therapy. Briefly explain their basic units.

a. Metric system:

_____

_____

b. Household measurements

_____

_____

39. A solution is

_____

_____

Nursing Knowledge Base

Clinical Calculations

Conversions Within One System

40. Indicate which direction the decimal point is moved for the following mathematical calculations in the metric system and provide a rationale.

a. Division:

_____

_____

b. Multiplication:

_____

_____

Conversion Between Systems

41. To make actual drug calculations, it is necessary to work with units in the same measurement system.

42. Before making a conversion, the nurse compares the measurement system available with the measurement system ordered.

43. Complete the following measurement equivalents.

Metric	Household
1 mL	_____ drops
_____ mL	1 tablespoon
30 mL	_____ tablespoon(s)
_____ mL	1 cup
_____ mL	1 pint
_____ mL	1 quart

44. Complete the following conversions.

   a. 100 mg = _____ g

   b. 2.5 L   = _____ mL

   c. 500 mL = _____ L

   d. 15 mg   = _____ g

   e. 30 gtt = _____ mL

   f. g 1/6   = _____ mg

Dose Calculations

45. Write out the formula used to determine the correct dose when preparing solid or liquid forms of medications.

46. Define the following.

   a. Dose ordered:

   b. Dose on hand:

   c. Amount on hand:

Pediatric Doses

47. Write out the formula applied to accurately calculate safe pediatric doses.

48. Explain why calculating children's medication doses requires caution.

49. The nurse who is administering the medications is accountable for

Prescriber's Role

50. Identify the primary responsibilities of the prescriber in giving medications to clients.

51. Identify recommendations to reduce medication errors associated with both verbal medication orders and prescriptions.

Types of Orders

52. Briefly explain the five common types of medication orders.

   a. Routine:

b. PRN:

_____

_____

c. Single (one-time):

_____

_____

d. STAT:

_____

_____

e. Now:

_____

_____

53. List the six parts of a prescription.

a. _____

b. _____

c. _____

d. _____

e. _____

f. _____

Pharmacist's Role

54. Identify the primary responsibility of the pharmacist in the administration of medications.

_____

Distribution Systems

55. List the three medication distribution systems and identify the advantages and disadvantages of each.

a. _____

b. _____

c. _____

Nurse's Role

56. Summarize the nurse's primary responsibilities when administering medications and explain why these responsibilities are important in nursing practice.

_____

_____

_____

_____

Critical Thinking

Knowledge

57. Summarize the knowledge needed from other disciplines to safely administer medications.

_____

_____

Experience

58. Psychomotor skills, the client's attitudes, knowledge, physical and mental status, and responses can make medication administration a complex experience.

Cognitive and Behavioural Attributes

59. Demonstrating accountability and responsibility when administering medications means that the nurse

_____

_____

60. A medication error is

_____

_____

61. Identify steps that registered nurses can take to prevent medication errors.

_____

_____

62. Explain what steps you should take if a medication error occurs.

_____

_____

_____

Standards

63. List the "seven rights" of medication administration and briefly explain each one.

a. _____

b. _____

c. _____

d. _____

e. _____

f. _____

g. _____

64. Briefly summarize seven client rights related to medication administration.

_____

_____

_____

65. Explain the importance of adhering to agency policies and procedures when administering medications.

_____

_____

_____

Nursing Process and Medication Administration

Assessment

66. Describe the following elements of nursing assessment and explain each element's significance as related to safe medication administration.

   a. History:

   _____

   _____

   b. History of allergies:

   _____

   _____

   c. Medication data:

   _____

   _____

   d. Diet history:

   _____

   _____

   e. Client's perceptual or coordination problems:

   _____

   _____

   f. Client's current condition:

   _____

   _____

   g. Client's attitude toward medication use:

   _____

   _____

   h. Client's knowledge and understanding of medication therapy:

   _____

   _____

   i. Client's learning needs:

   _____

   _____

Nursing Diagnosis

67. Assessment provides data on the client's condition, ability to self-administer medications, and medication use patterns. This information can be used to determine actual or potential problems with medication therapy.

68. Identify potential nursing diagnoses that apply to the process of medication administration.

_____

_____

_____

Planning

69. Organize nursing care activities to ensure the safe administration of medications.

70. Identify a goal and related outcomes that the nurse or client needs to meet before the administration of medications, and provide the rationale for each goal and outcome.

_____

_____

_____

_____

_____

Implementation

Health Promotion

71. Identify factors that can influence the client's compliance with the medication regimen and provide the rationale for your answers.

_____

_____

_____

72. Identify important information that you should provide to the client and family in relation to medications and provide the rationale for your answers.

_____

_____

_____

Acute Care

73. Identify the necessary components of medication orders.

_____

_____

_____

74. Explain why the following interventions are essential for safe and effective medication administration.

    a. Receiving and reconciling medication orders:

    _____

    _____

    b. Correct transcription and communication of orders:

    _____

    _____

    c. Accurate dose calculation and measurement:

    _____

    _____

    d. Correct administration, adhering to the seven rights of medication administration:

    _____

    _____

    e. Recording medication administration:

    _____

    _____

Restorative Care

75. Regardless of the type of medication activity and environment, you are responsible for

    _____

    _____

Special Considerations for Administering Medications to Specific Age Groups

Infants and Children

76. Identify strategies to address children's psychosocial preparation prior to administering medications.

    _____

    _____

Older Adults

77. Identify special considerations for older adults when administering medication and provide rationales.

    _____

    _____

    _____

78. Describe the difference between rational and irrational polypharmacy.

    _____

    _____

    _____

Evaluation

79. You must know the therapeutic action and common side effects of each medication in order to monitor a client's response to that medication.

80. Many different evaluation measures can be used in the context of medication administration. Identify various measures used in practice to evaluate medication administration processes.

    _____

    _____

    _____

    _____

81. The most common type of measurement is

    _____

    _____

Medication Administration

Oral Administration

82. The easiest and most desirable way to administer medications is by mouth.

83. The primary contraindication to giving oral medications is

    _____

    _____

84. To protect the client against possible aspiration, what nursing assessments should be conducted? What nursing interventions should be implemented? Provide rationales for your answers.

    _____

    _____

    _____

    _____

Topical Medication Applications

85. Topical medications are applied locally, most often to intact skin. They can also be applied to mucous membranes.

Skin Applications

86. Explain the procedure for administering the following skin applications.

    a. Ointment:

    _____

    _____

    b. Lotion:

    _____

    _____

    c. Powder:

    _____

    _____

    d. Transdermal patch:

    _____

    _____

Nasal Instillation

87. Summarize the rationale for nasal instillations.

    _____

    _____

    _____

Eye Instillation

88. List three principles for administering eye instillations.

    a. _____

    b. _____

    c. _____

89. Summarize the procedure for administering ophthalmic medications and provide rationales for steps specific to ophthalmic medication delivery.

    _____

    _____

    _____

    _____

Ear Instillation

90. Explain the procedure for administering ear instillations.

    a. Adult:

    _____

    _____

    b. Children:

    _____

    _____

91. Identify the significant differences between adults and children when administering ear medications.

    _____

    _____

    _____

Vaginal Instillation

92. Vaginal medications are available as _____, _____, _____, or _____.

Rectal Instillation

93. Explain the differences between vaginal and rectal suppositories and the reason for these differences.

    _____

    _____

    _____

94. Summarize the procedure for administering rectal suppositories and provide rationales for steps specific to rectal suppository administration.

    _____

    _____

    _____

    _____

Administering Medications by Inhalation

95. Identify the common demographics of clients who are prescribed medications via the inhalation route.

    _____

    _____

96. Summarize the procedure for teaching clients to self-administer medications via a metered-dose inhaler and provide the rationale.

    _____

    _____

Administering Medications by Irrigations

97. Identify the principles you must adhere to when when performing irrigations and provide rationales for your answers.

    _____

    _____

    _____

Administering Parenteral Medications

98. Each type of injection requires certain skills to ensure that the drug reaches the proper location.

99. When medications are administered parenterally, it is an invasive procedure that must be performed using aseptic techniques.

Equipment

100. Identify the two major types of syringes.

a. _____

b. _____

101. Identify three factors that must be considered when selecting a needle for an injection.

a. _____

b. _____

c. _____

102. Identify the advantages of using the Tubex or Carpuject injection systems.

_____

_____

Preparing an Injection From an Ampule

103. An ampule is

_____

104. Summarize the procedure for withdrawing medication from an ampule and provide the rationale for each step.

_____

_____

_____

Preparing an Injection From a Vial

105. A vial is a

_____

106. The vial is a closed system, and air must be injected into it to permit easy withdrawal of the solution.

107. Summarize the procedure for withdrawing medication from a vial and provide a rationale for each step.

_____

_____

_____

108. Describe the difference between withdrawing medication from a vial as compared to withdrawing medication from an ampule (provide a rationale for your answer).

_____

_____

_____

_____

Mixing Medications

109. If two medications are compatible, it is possible to mix two drugs together into one injection if the total dosage is within accepted limits.

110. List the three principles to follow when mixing medications from two vials.

a. _____

b. _____

c. _____

111. When mixing medications from an ampule and a vial, which medication should be prepared first? Provide the rationale for your answer.

_____

_____

_____

Insulin Preparation

112. Insulin is

_____

_____

113. Explain why insulin must be administered by injection.

_____

_____

114. Insulin is classified by

_____

_____

115. Summarize the procedure for mixing two kinds of insulin in the same syringe.

_____

_____

_____

Administering Injections

116. The characteristics of the tissues injected influence the

_____

_____

_____

117. List the techniques used to minimize client discomfort associated with injections, and provide rationales for your answers.

a. _____

b. _____

c. _____

d. _____

e. _____

f. _____

g. _____

Subcutaneous Injections

118. Subcutaneous injections involve placing the medications into the loose connective tissue under the dermis.

119. Explain the differences in absorption between a subcutaneous and an intramuscular injection.

120. The best sites for subcutaneous injections include _____, _____, and _____.

121. The site chosen for a subcutaneous injection should be free of _____, _____, _____, and _____.

122. Identify the maximum amount of water-soluble medication given by the subcutaneous route.

    _____

    _____

    _____

123. Identify the factors to consider when determining if a subcutaneous injection should be given at a 90- or 45-degree angle.

    _____

    _____

    _____

Intramuscular Injections

124. Identify the major risk of using the IM route (provide the rationale for your answer).

    _____

    _____

    _____

125. The angle of insertion for an IM injection is _____ degrees.

126. Indicate the maximum volume of medication for IM injection in each of the following groups (provide rationales for your answers).

    a. Well-developed adult:

    _____

    _____

    _____

    b. Older children, older adults, or thin adults:

    _____

    _____

    c. Older infants and small children:

    _____

    _____

    _____

Sites

127. List the assessment criteria for selecting an IM site.

    a. _____

    b. _____

    c. _____

    d. _____

128. Describe the characteristics, advantages, and disadvantages of the following injection sites.

    a. Vastus lateralis:

    _____

    _____

    _____

    b. Ventrogluteal:

    _____

    _____

    _____

    c. Dorsogluteal:

    _____

    _____

    _____

    d. Deltoid:

    _____

    _____

    _____

Technique for Intramuscular Injections

129. Describe the Z-track technique for administering IM injections. Explain the rationale for using the Z-track method of injection.

    _____

    _____

    _____

    _____

Intradermal Injections

130. Explain the rationale for using the intradermal route to administer medication.

    _____

    _____

    _____

Safety in Administering Medications by Injection

131. Explain the rationale for the use of a needleless device.

    _____

    _____

Intravenous Administration

132. The nurse administers medications intravenously by the following methods.

    _____

    _____

    _____

133. Identify the advantage and disadvantage of the large-volume infusion method (provide rationales for your answers).

    _____

    _____

    _____

134. Explain the advantage and disadvantage of the IV bolus route of administration (provide rationales for your answers).

    _____

    _____

    _____

135. List the advantages of using volume-controlled infusions.

    a. _____

    b. _____

    c. _____

136. Describe the set-up and purpose of a piggyback set.

    _____

    _____

    _____

137. Describe the set-up and purpose of a tandem set.

    _____

    _____

    _____

138. Describe the set-up and purpose of a volume-control administration set.

    _____

    _____

    _____

139. Describe the set-up and purpose of a mini-infusion pump.

    _____

    _____

    _____

140. List two advantages of using intermittent venous access devices.

    a. _____

    b. _____

Administration of IV Therapy in the Home

141. When receiving home intravenous therapy, client education should include

    _____

    _____

Review Questions

Select the appropriate answer and cite the rationale for choosing that particular answer.

1. The study of how drugs enter the body, reach their sites of action, are metabolized, and exit from the body is called
   a. Pharmacology
   b. Pharmacokinetics
   c. Pharmacopoeia
   d. Biopharmaceutica

   Answer: _____   Rationale: _____

   _____

   _____

2. Which statement correctly characterizes drug absorption?
   a. Many drugs must enter the systemic circulation to have a therapeutic effect.
   b. Mucous membranes are relatively impermeable to chemicals, making absorption slow.
   c. Oral medications are absorbed more quickly when administered with meals.

d. Drugs administered subcutaneously are absorbed more quickly than those injected intramuscularly.

Answer: _____   Rationale: _____

_____

_____

3. The onset of drug action is the time it takes for a drug to
   a. Produce a response
   b. Accelerate the cellular process
   c. Reach its highest effective concentration
   d. Produce blood serum concentration and maintenance

Answer: _____   Rationale: _____

_____

_____

4. Which of the following is *not* a parenteral route of administration?
   a. Buccal
   b. Subcutaneous
   c. Intramuscular
   d. Intradermal

Answer: _____   Rationale: _____

_____

_____

5. Using the body surface area formula, what dose of drug X should a child who weighs 12 kg (body surface area = 0.54 m^2) receive if the normal adult dose of drug X is 300 mg?
   a. 50 mg
   b. 95 mg
   c. 100 mg
   d. 200 mg

Answer: _____   Rationale: _____

_____

_____

6. The nurse is preparing an insulin injection in which both short-acting (clear) and long-acting (cloudy) insulin will be mixed. Into which vial should the nurse inject air first?
   a. The vial of long-acting insulin
   b. The vial of short-acting insulin
   c. Either vial, as long as long-acting insulin is drawn up first
   d. Neither vial; it is not necessary to put air into vials before withdrawing medication

Answer: _____   Rationale: _____

_____

_____

35

Complementary and Alternative Therapies

Preliminary Reading

Chapter 35, pp. 756–773

Comprehensive Understanding

Complementary and Alternative Medicine Therapies in Health Care

1. Describe the difference between the following terms.

   a. Complementary therapies:

   _____

   _____

   _____

   b. Alternative therapies:

   _____

   _____

   _____

2. Explain the following alternative medical systems and give an example of each.

   a. Acupuncture:

   _____

   _____

   _____

   b. Ayurveda:

   _____

   _____

   _____

   c. Homeopathic medicines:

   _____

   _____

   _____

   _____

   d. Latin American practices:

   _____

   _____

   _____

   e. Traditional Aboriginal medicine:

   _____

   _____

   _____

   f. Naturopathic medicine:

   _____

   _____

   _____

   g. Traditional Chinese medicine:

   _____

   _____

   _____

3. Describe *integrative medical programs*.

   _____

   _____

   _____

Nursing-Accessible Therapies

Relaxation Therapy

4. Define the *stress response*.

5. *Relaxation* is

6. *Progressive relaxation* training helps to

7. *Passive relaxation* involves teaching

8. Relaxation techniques can lower _____ _____, decrease _____ _____, improve _____, and reduce _____.

9. The type of relaxation intervention should be matched to

10. Identify the limitations of relaxation therapy.

Meditation and Breathing

11. *Meditation* is

12. Identify the clinical applications of meditation.

13. Identify the limitations of meditation.

Imagery

14. *Imagery* is

15. *Creative visualization* is

16. Identify the clinical applications of imagery.

17. Identify the limitations of imagery.

Training-Specific Therapies

Biofeedback

18. *Biofeedback* is

19. Identify the clinical applications of biofeedback.

20. Identify the limitations of biofeedback.

Therapeutic Touch

21. *Therapeutic touch* is

22. Therapeutic touch consists of five phases. Explain each.

    a. Centring:

    b. Assessment:

    c. Unruffling:

    d. Treatment:

e. Evaluation:

_____

_____

23. Identify the physiological indicators of energy imbalance.

_____

_____

24. Identify the clinical applications of therapeutic touch.

_____

_____

25. Identify the limitations of therapeutic touch.

_____

_____

Chiropractic Therapy

26. *Chiropractic therapy* is

_____

_____

27. Describe the clinical applications of chiropractic therapy.

_____

_____

28. Identify the limitations of chiropractic therapy.

_____

_____

Traditional Chinese Medicine

29. Traditional Chinese medicine (TCM) comprises several healing modalities, including

_____

_____

30. Explain the concept of *yin and yang*.

_____

_____

31. *Qi* is

_____

_____

32. Traditional Chinese medicine classifies disease into three categories. State the influences of each.

a. External causes:

_____

b. Internal causes:

_____

_____

c. Nonexternal, noninternal causes:

_____

_____

33. Define *meridians*.

_____

_____

Acupuncture

34. *Acupuncture* is

_____

_____

35. Describe the clinical applications of acupuncture.

_____

_____

36. Identify the limitations of acupuncture.

_____

_____

Role of Nutrition in Disease Prevention and Health Promotion

Herbal Therapies

37. The goal of herbal therapy is

_____

_____

38. Describe the clinical applications of herbal therapy.

_____

_____

39. Explain what a natural product number (NPN) is.

_____

_____

40. Identify the limitations of herbal therapy.

_____

_____

41. Herbal products should be avoided or used cautiously by

   _____

   _____

Nursing Role in Complementary and Alternative Therapies

42. Summarize the role of the nurse regarding complementary and alternative medicine therapies.

   _____

   _____

   _____

Review Questions

Select the appropriate answer and cite the rationale for choosing that particular answer.

1. Clients choose to use unconventional therapies because
   a. They are willing to pay more to feel better.
   b. It is now widely accepted by Health Canada's Office of Natural Health Products.
   c. They are dissatisfied with conventional medicine.
   d. They want religious approval for the remedies they use.

   Answer: _____   Rationale: _____

   _____

   _____

2. An herb considered safe for the treatment of mild depression is
   a. Milk thistle
   b. St. John's wort

   c. Pokeroot
   d. Hawthorn

   Answer: _____   Rationale: _____

   _____

   _____

3. You can best assess your client's use of alternative therapies by
   a. Asking the client true/false questions about his or her health
   b. Asking for a thorough medical history
   c. Reviewing laboratory studies that assess levels of certain herbs
   d. Asking open-ended questions on alternative therapies

   Answer: _____   Rationale: _____

   _____

   _____

4. Which of the following steps should you take to be better informed about alternative therapies?
   a. Keep abreast of the current research on alternative therapies.
   b. Familiarize yourself with recent case studies on alternative therapies.
   c. Familiarize yourself with general principles of phytotherapy.
   d. Review herb manufacturers' literature on specific herbs.

   Answer: _____   Rationale: _____

   _____

   _____

36

Activity and Exercise

Preliminary Reading

Chapter 36 pp. 774–795

Comprehensive Understanding

Scientific Knowledge Base

1. *Body mechanics* include

_____

_____

_____

Overview of Body Mechanics, Exercise, and Activity

2. Define *body alignment*.

_____

_____

_____

3. Body balance is achieved when

_____

_____

_____

4. Define *centre of gravity*.

_____

_____

5. Proper body alignment and posture are maintained by using the following two simple techniques.

a. _____

b. _____

6. Define *friction*.

_____

_____

_____

7. List two techniques that minimize friction.

a. _____

b. _____

8. *Activity tolerance* is

_____

_____

_____

9. There are three categories of exercises. Briefly explain and give an example of each.

a. Isotonic contraction:

_____

_____

b. Isometric contraction:

_____

_____

c. Resistive isometric:

_____

_____

Regulation of Movement

10. List three systems responsible for coordinating body movements.

a. _____

b. _____

c. _____

11. List five functions of the skeletal system.

    a. _____

    b. _____

    c. _____

    d. _____

    e. _____

12. Describe the following.

    a. Joints:

    _____

    _____

    b. Cartilaginous joint:

    _____

    _____

    c. Fibrous joint:

    _____

    _____

    d. Synovial joint:

    _____

    _____

    e. Ligaments:

    _____

    _____

    f. Cartilage:

    _____

    _____

    g. Tendons:

    _____

    _____

13. Briefly describe how skeletal muscles affect movement.

    _____

    _____

14. Briefly explain the work of muscles concerned with

    a. Movement:

    _____

    _____

    b. Posture:

    _____

    _____

15. The nervous system regulates and coordinates the following different muscle groups. Briefly explain each.

    a. Antagonistic muscles:

    _____

    _____

    b. Synergistic muscles:

    _____

    _____

    c. Antigravity muscles:

    _____

    _____

16. Briefly describe how movement and posture are regulated by the nervous system.

    _____

    _____

    _____

17. Define *proprioception*.

    _____

    _____

    _____

18. The structures in the ear that assist in maintaining balance are the

    _____

Principles of Body Mechanics

19. List five principles of body mechanics.

    a. _____

    b. _____

    c. _____

    d. _____

    e. _____

Pathological Influences on Body Mechanics

20. Briefly explain how the following pathological conditions may affect body alignment and mobility.

    a. Congenital abnormalities:

    _____

    _____

    _____

    b. Disorders of bones, joints, and muscles:

    _____

    _____

    _____

    c. Central nervous system damage:

    _____

    _____

    _____

d. Musculoskeletal trauma:

_____

_____

_____

Nursing Knowledge Base

Developmental Changes

21. The greatest change and impact on the maturational process is observed _____.

22. Identify the descriptive characteristics of body alignment and mobility for the following age groups.

   a. Infants:

_____

_____

   b. Toddlers:

_____

_____

   c. Adolescents:

_____

_____

   d. Young to middle-age adults:

_____

_____

   e. Older adults:

_____

_____

Behavioural Aspects

23. Clients are more likely to incorporate an exercise program into their daily life if this choice is _____ and _____.

Environmental Issues

24. Explain the exercise and activity issues related to the following sites.

   a. Work:

_____

_____

   b. Schools:

_____

_____

c. Community:

_____

Cultural and Ethnic Influences

25. The nurse must consider what motivates and what is deemed appropriate and enjoyable when developing a physical fitness program for culturally diverse populations. Briefly describe a comprehensive fitness program that would be suitable for an ethnocultural group with which you interact.

_____

_____

_____

_____

Family and Social Support

26. Briefly explain how a family may be a motivational tool in regard to physical fitness.

_____

_____

_____

Nursing Process

Assessment

27. Briefly explain how the assessment of body alignment and posture is carried out.

   a. Standing:

_____

_____

   b. Sitting:

_____

_____

   c. Recumbent:

_____

_____

28. There are three components to assess in regard to mobility. Explain each.

   a. Range of motion:

_____

_____

   b. Gait:

_____

_____

   c. Exercise:

_____

_____

29. Identify 3 factors that affect activity tolerance.

    a. _____

    b. _____

    c. _____

Nursing Diagnosis

30. Assessment of the client's _____, _____, _____, and _____ provides clusters of data or defining characteristics that can lead you to a nursing diagnosis.

31. Give five examples of nursing diagnoses related to exercise and activity.

    a. _____

    b. _____

    c. _____

    d. _____

    e. _____

Planning

32. The plan should include consideration of

    a. _____

    b. _____

    c. _____

    d. _____

    e. _____

Implementation

Health Promotion

33. List the five recommendations for exercise.

    a. _____

    b. _____

    c. _____

    d. _____

    e. _____

34. Explain how to calculate the client's maximum heart rate (MHR).

    _____

    _____

35. An exercise program should include the following. Explain each.

    a. Aerobic exercise:

    _____

    _____

    b. Stretching and flexibility exercises:

    _____

    _____

    c. Resistance training:

    _____

    _____

36. Briefly explain proper lifting techniques.

    _____

    _____

    _____

Acute Care

37. The musculoskeletal system can be maintained by encouraging the use of stretching and isometric-type exercises.

38. Briefly explain the technique of stretching exercises.

    _____

    _____

    _____

39. Explain how you would help a client to maintain or improve joint mobility.

    _____

    _____

    _____

40. Explain how walking affects joint mobility.

    _____

    _____

41. Explain how you would assist the client to walk.

    _____

    _____

Restorative and Continuing Care

42. Explain how the nurse would implement a plan of care to increase activity and exercise in the following specific disease conditions.

    a. Coronary heart disease:

    _____

    _____

    _____

    b. Hypertension:

    _____

    _____

    _____

c. Chronic obstructive pulmonary disease:

_____

_____

_____

d. Diabetes mellitus:

_____

_____

_____

Evaluation

Client Care

43. This phase of the nursing process evaluates the actual care delivered by the health care team based on the expected outcomes.

44. Comparisons are made with baseline measures that include _____, _____ _____, _____, _____, and _____.

Client Expectations

45. You need to know your client's expectations concerning activity and exercise.

Review Questions

Select the appropriate answer and cite the rationale for choosing that particular answer.

1. Which of the following is true of body mechanics?
   a. The narrower the base of support, the greater your stability.
   b. The higher the centre of gravity, the greater your stability.
   c. When friction is reduced between the object to be moved and the surface on which it is moved, less force is required to move it.
   d. Rolling, turning, or pivoting requires more work than lifting.

Answer: _____   Rationale: _____

_____

_____

2. White, shiny, flexible bands of fibrous tissue binding joints together and connecting various bones and cartilage types are known as
   a. Muscles
   b. Ligaments

c. Joints
d. Tendons

Answer: _____   Rationale: _____

_____

_____

3. The nurse would expect all of the following physiological effects of exercise on the body systems except
   a. Decreased cardiac output
   b. Increased respiratory rate and depth
   c. Increased muscle tone, size, and strength
   d. Change in metabolic rate

Answer: _____   Rationale: _____

_____

_____

4. Which of the following is a possible nursing diagnosis related to activity and exercise?
   a. Altered thought processes
   b. Altered oral mucous membrane
   c. Relocation stress syndrome
   d. Impaired gas exchange

Answer: _____   Rationale: _____

_____

_____

Critical Thinking Model for Nursing Care Plan for Activity Intolerance

Imagine that you are Eric, the nurse in the Care Plan on page 788 of your text. Complete the *planning phase* of the critical thinking model by writing your answers in the appropriate boxes of the model shown. Think about the following:

* In developing Mrs. Wertenberger's plan of care, what knowledge did Eric apply?

* In what way might Eric's previous experience assist in developing a plan of care for Mrs. Wertenberger?

* When developing a plan of care, what intellectual or professional standards were applied to Mrs. Wertenberger?

* What critical thinking attitudes might have been applied in developing Mrs. Wertenberger's plan?

* How will Eric accomplish his goals?

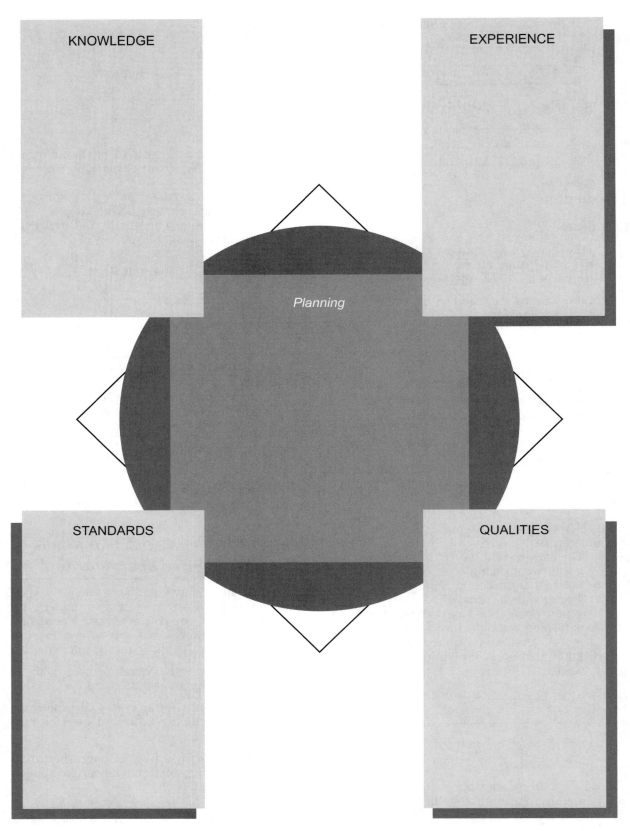

KNOWLEDGE

EXPERIENCE

Planning

STANDARDS

QUALITIES

CHAPTER 36   Critical Thinking Model for Nursing Care Plan for *Activity Intolerance*
See answers on page 533.

37

Client Safety

Preliminary Reading

Chapter 37, pp. 796–828

Comprehensive Understanding

Scientific Knowledge Base

Environmental Safety

1. A client's environment includes

   _____

   _____

   _____

2. List five characteristics of a safe environment.

   a. _____

   b. _____

   c. _____

   d. _____

   e. _____

3. Give an example of the four basic physiological needs that influence a person's safety.

   a. Oxygen:

      _____

      _____

   b. Nutrition:

      _____

      _____

   c. Temperature:

      _____

      _____

   d. Humidity:

      _____

      _____

4. Physical hazards in the community and health care settings place clients at risk for accidental injury and death. List four physical hazards that contribute to accidental injury.

   a. _____

   b. _____

   c. _____

   d. _____

5. A *poison* is

   _____

   _____

6. Define *pathogen*.

   _____

   _____

   _____

7. Identify the most effective method for limiting the transmission of pathogens.

   _____

   _____

8. Define *immunization*.

   _____

   _____

   _____

9. Describe the two types of immunity.

   a. Active:

      _____

      _____

b. Passive:

_____

_____

10. Describe how the human immunodeficiency virus (HIV) is transmitted and who is at risk to contract it.

_____

_____

_____

11. A healthy environment is free from pollution.

12. A *pollutant* is

_____

_____

13. Define the following types of pollution.
    a. Air:

    _____

    _____

    b. Land:

    _____

    _____

    c. Water:

    _____

    _____

    d. Noise:

    _____

    _____

Nursing Knowledge Base

14. In addition to being knowledgeable about the environment, to minimize threats to client safety, nurses must be familiar with
    a. _____
    b. _____
    c. _____
    d. _____
    e. _____

Risks at Developmental Stages

15. Identify at least three threats to safety in the following developmental stages.
    a. Infant, toddler, preschooler:

    _____

    _____

    _____

b. School-age:

_____

_____

_____

c. Adolescent:

_____

_____

_____

d. Adult:

_____

_____

_____

e. Older adult:

_____

_____

_____

Individual Risk Factors

16. Explain how the following risk factors threaten safety.
    a. Lifestyle:

    _____

    _____

    b. Impaired mobility:

    _____

    _____

    c. Sensory or communication impairment:

    _____

    _____

    d. Lack of safety awareness:

    _____

    _____

Risks in the Health Care Agency

17. List the four major risks to client safety in the health care environment.
    a. _____
    b. _____
    c. _____
    d. _____

Safety and the Nursing Process

Assessment

18. To conduct a thorough client assessment, consider possible threats to the client's safety, including the client's immediate environment, as well as any individual risk factors.

19. Identify the specific assessments you need to make in the following settings.

    a. The client's home:

    _____

    _____

    b. A health care environment:

    _____

    _____

20. Explain the following health care environment risks.

    a. Risk for falls:

    _____

    _____

    b. Risk for medical errors:

    _____

    _____

Nursing Diagnosis

21. Identify four actual or potential nursing diagnoses for safety risks.

    a. _____
    b. _____
    c. _____
    d. _____

Planning

22. Identify three common goals that focus on the client's need for safety.

    a. _____
    b. _____
    c. _____

Implementation

Health Promotion

23. Nursing interventions are directed toward ensuring a client's safety in all settings and include health promotion, developmental interventions, environmental interventions, and limiting specific risks to client safety.

24. Identify at least four interventions for each of the following developmental age groups.

    a. Infant, toddler, preschooler:

    _____

    _____

    b. School-age:

    _____

    c. Adolescent:

    _____

    _____

    d. Adult:

    _____

    _____

    e. Older adult:

    _____

    _____

Environmental Interventions

25. Describe four fire-containment guidelines.

    a. _____
    b. _____
    c. _____
    d. _____

Limiting Specific Risks to Client Safety

26. List eight measures to prevent falls in the health care setting.

    a. _____
    b. _____
    c. _____
    d. _____
    e. _____
    f. _____
    g. _____
    h. _____

27. A *physical restraint* is

    _____

    _____

28. The immobility imposed by restraining a client can lead to the following complications.

    a. Physical:

    _____

    _____

    b. Psychological:

    _____

    _____

29. Use of restraints must meet the following objectives.
    a. _____
    b. _____
    c. _____
    d. _____

30. Explain why an Ambularm is used.
    _____
    _____

31. Explain the use of side rails.
    _____
    _____

32. List five teaching strategies for prevention of electrical shocks.
    a. _____
    b. _____
    c. _____
    d. _____
    e. _____

Evaluation

Client Care

33. The nurse continually assesses the client and family's need for additional support services such as _____, _____, _____, and _____.

Client Expectations

34. The expected outcomes include a _____ and _____ environment.

Review Questions

Select the appropriate answer and cite the rationale for choosing that particular answer.

1. Which of the following would most threaten an individual's safety?
   a. 70% humidity
   b. Carbon dioxide
   c. Unrefrigerated fresh vegetables
   d. Lack of a clean water supply

Answer: _____ Rationale: _____
_____

2. The developmental stage that carries the highest risk of an injury from a fall is
   a. Preschool
   b. School-age
   c. Adulthood
   d. Older adulthood

Answer: _____ Rationale: _____
_____
_____

3. Mrs. Gupta falls asleep while smoking in bed and drops the burning cigarette on her blanket. When she awakens, her bed is on fire, and she quickly calls the nurse. On observing the fire, the nurse should immediately
   a. Report the fire
   b. Attempt to extinguish the fire
   c. Assist Mrs. Gupta to a safe place
   d. Close all windows and doors to contain the fire

Answer: _____ Rationale: _____
_____
_____

4. Sixteen-year-old Simon is admitted to an adolescent unit with a diagnosis of substance abuse. The nurse examines Simon and finds that he has bloodshot eyes, slurred speech, and an unstable gait. He smells of alcohol and is unable to answer questions appropriately. The appropriate nursing diagnosis would be
   a. Self-care deficit related to alcohol abuse
   b. Altered thought processes related to sensory overload
   c. Knowledge deficit related to alcohol abuse
   d. High risk for injury related to impaired sensory perception

Answer: _____ Rationale: _____
_____
_____

5. If a client receives an electric shock, your first action should be to
   a. Assess the client's airway, breathing, and circulation (pulse)
   b. Assess the client for thermal injury
   c. Notify the physician
   d. Notify the maintenance department

Answer: _____ Rationale: _____
_____
_____

Critical Thinking Model for Nursing Care Plan for Risk for Injury

Imagine that you are Mr. Key, the nurse in the Care Plan on page 806 of your text. Complete the *assessment phase* of the critical thinking model by writing your answers in the appropriate boxes of the model shown. Think about the following:

- In developing Ms. Cohen's plan of care, what knowledge did Mr. Key apply?

- In what way might Mr. Key's previous experience assist in this case?

- What intellectual or professional standards were applied to Ms. Cohen's case?

- What critical thinking attitudes might have been applied in this case?

- As you review your assessment, what key areas did you cover?

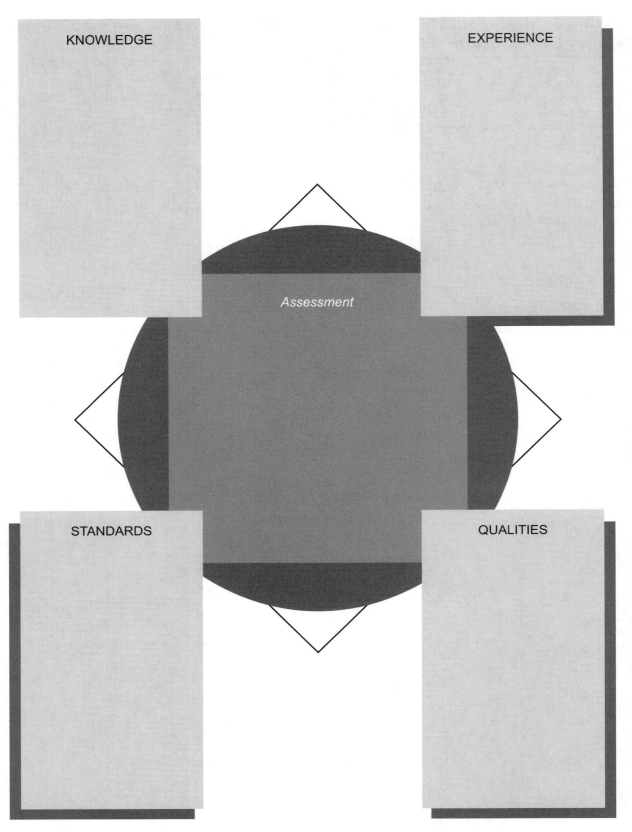

KNOWLEDGE

EXPERIENCE

Assessment

STANDARDS

QUALITIES

CHAPTER 37   Critical Thinking Model for Nursing Care Plan for *Risk for Injury*
See answers on page 534.

38

Hygiene

Preliminary Reading

Chapter 38, pp. 829–878

Comprehensive Understanding

Scientific Knowledge Base

1. Proper hygiene care requires an understanding of the anatomy and physiology of the integument, oral cavity, eyes, ears, nose, hands, feet, and nails.

The Skin

2. Identify the functions of the skin.

   _____

   _____

3. Define the three primary layers.

   a. Epidermis:

   _____

   _____

   b. Dermis:

   _____

   _____

   c. Subcutaneous:

   _____

   _____

The Feet, Hands, and Nails

4. Define the following terms.

   a. Cuticle:

   _____

   _____

   b. Lunula:

   _____

   _____

The Oral Cavity

5. Three pairs of salivary glands secrete about one litre of saliva per day.

6. The buccal glands are

   _____

   _____

7. Teeth are organs of chewing, or _____, and are designed to _____

   _____.

8. Regular oral hygiene is necessary to maintain the integrity of tooth surfaces and to prevent

   _____

   _____

The Hair

9. Identify the factors that can affect the hair's characteristics.

   _____

   _____

The Eyes, Ears, and Nose

10. Cleansing of the sensitive sensory tissues should be done to prevent injury and client discomfort.

Nursing Knowledge Base

11. Briefly explain each of the following factors influencing hygiene habits.

    a. Social practices:

    _____

    _____

b. Personal preferences:

_____

_____

c. Body image:

_____

_____

d. Socioeconomic status:

_____

_____

e. Health beliefs and motivation:

_____

_____

f. Cultural variables:

_____

_____

g. Physical condition:

_____

_____

The Nursing Process

Assessment

Physical Examination

The Skin

12. When inspecting the skin, the nurse thoroughly examines

   a. _____
   b. _____
   c. _____
   d. _____
   e. _____
   f. _____

13. Common skin problems can affect how hygiene is administered. Describe the hygiene provided for the following.

   a. Dry skin:

   _____

   _____

   b. Acne:

   _____

   _____

   c. Skin rashes:

   _____

   _____

d. Contact dermatitis:

_____

_____

e. Psoriasis

_____

_____

f. Abrasion:

_____

_____

14. Briefly explain the six conditions that place clients at risk for impaired skin integrity.

   a. Immobilization:

   _____

   _____

   b. Reduced sensation:

   _____

   _____

   c. Nutrition and hydration alterations:

   _____

   _____

   d. Secretions and excretions on the skin:

   _____

   _____

   e. Vascular insufficiency:

   _____

   _____

   f. External devices:

   _____

   _____

The Feet and Nails

15. Assessment of the feet involves a thorough examination of all skin surfaces, including the soles of the feet and the areas between the toes.

16. Inspection of the feet for lesions includes noting areas of

   a. _____
   b. _____
   c. _____

17. Define *neuropathy*.

   _____

   _____

18. Describe a nursing assessment for neuropathy.

    _____
    _____
    _____

19. Identify the characteristics of the following foot and nail problems.

    a. Calluses:

       _____
       _____

    b. Corns:

       _____
       _____

    c. Plantar warts:

       _____
       _____

    d. Athlete's foot:

       _____
       _____

    e. Ingrown nails:

       _____
       _____

    f. Ram's horn nails:

       _____
       _____

    g. Paronychia:

       _____
       _____

    h. Foot odour:

       _____
       _____

The Oral Cavity

20. The nurse inspects all areas of the oral cavity for

    a. _____
    b. _____
    c. _____
    d. _____

The Hair

21. Describe the characteristics of the following hair and scalp conditions.

    a. Dandruff:

       _____
       _____

    b. Ticks:

       _____

    c. Pediculosis capitis:

       _____
       _____

    d. Pediculosis corporis:

       _____
       _____

    e. Pediculosis pubis:

       _____
       _____

    f. Alopecia:

       _____
       _____

The Eyes, Ears, and Nose

22. Identify the normal assessment findings for the following.

    a. Eyes:

       _____
       _____

    b. Nose:

       _____
       _____

    c. Ears:

       _____
       _____

Developmental Changes

The Skin

23. For each developmental stage, briefly describe normal conditions that create a high risk for impaired skin integrity.

    a. Neonate:

       _____
       _____

    b. Toddler:

       _____
       _____

    c. Adolescent:

       _____
       _____

    d. Older adult:

       _____
       _____

The Feet and Nails

24. Identify the common foot problems of the older adult.

_____

_____

The Oral Cavity

25. Identify the factors associated with aging that can result in poor oral care.

_____

_____

_____

Self-Care Ability

26. Identify the factors that are assessed to determine a client's ability to perform routine hygiene.

_____

_____

Cultural Factors

27. Explain how culture affects a client's hygiene needs.

_____

_____

_____

Clients at Risk for Hygiene Problems

28. Provide examples of clients at risk for the following.

a. Oral problems:

_____

_____

b. Skin problems:

_____

_____

c. Foot problems:

_____

_____

d. Eye care problems:

_____

_____

Special Considerations in Hygiene Assessment

29. Explain how footwear may predispose a client to foot and nail problems.

_____

_____

Nursing Diagnosis

30. List four possible nursing diagnoses that apply to clients in need of hygiene care.

a. _____

b. _____

c. _____

d. _____

Planning

31. List factors to consider when planning hygiene care.

_____

_____

Implementation

Health Promotion

32. List four guidelines for educating clients about hygiene care.

a. _____

b. _____

c. _____

d. _____

Bathing and Skin Care

33. A complete bed bath is

_____

_____

34. A partial bed bath involves

_____

_____

35. Identify guidelines the nurse should follow when assisting or providing a client with any type of bath.

_____

_____

36. Explain bag baths and identify the advantages of this method.

_____

_____

37. Define _perineal care_ and identify the clients at risk for skin breakdown in the perineal area.

_____

_____

_____

38. A back rub promotes
   a. _____
   b. _____
   c. _____
   d. _____
   e. _____

39. Morning care involves
   a. _____
   b. _____
   c. _____
   d. _____
   e. _____
   f. _____
   g. _____
   h. _____

Foot and Nail Care

40. List at least eight guidelines to include when advising clients with peripheral neuropathy or vascular insufficiency about foot care.
   a. _____
   b. _____
   c. _____
   d. _____
   e. _____
   f. _____
   g. _____
   h. _____

Oral Hygiene

41. Oral hygiene helps maintain:
   _____
   _____

42. Briefly explain the following interventions in relation to oral hygiene.
   a. Diet:
   _____
   _____

   b. Brushing and flossing:
   _____
   _____

   c. Oral care for the unconscious or debilitated client:
   _____
   _____

   d. Denture care:
   _____

Hair and Scalp Care

43. Briefly describe the rationale for the following.
   a. Brushing and combing:
   _____

   b. Shampooing:
   _____
   _____

   c. Shaving:
   _____
   _____

   d. Moustache and beard care:
   _____
   _____

Care of the Eyes, Ears, and Nose

44. Care focuses on preventing infection and maintaining normal sensory function.

45. Describe basic eye care for a client.
   _____
   _____

46. Describe the correct procedure for cleaning eyeglasses.
   _____
   _____

47. Briefly describe proper contact lens care technique.
   _____
   _____

48. Describe each of the following techniques necessary in caring for an artificial eye.
   a. Removal:
   _____
   _____

   b. Cleansing:
   _____
   _____

   c. Reinsertion:
   _____
   _____

   d. Storage:
   _____
   _____

Ear Care

49. Describe the procedure for removing cerumen from the ear.

    _____

    _____

50. Describe the following types of hearing aids.

    a. In-the-canal (ITC):

    _____

    b. In-the-ear (ITE):

    _____

    c. Behind-the-ear (BTE):

    _____

Nasal Care

51. Describe three interventions used to remove secretions from the nose.

    a. _____

    b. _____

    c. _____

Client's Room Environment

Maintaining Comfort

52. Identify four factors the nurse can control to create a more comfortable environment.

    a. _____

    b. _____

    c. _____

    d. _____

Room Equipment

53. A typical hospital room contains the following basic pieces of furniture.

    a. _____

    b. _____

    c. _____

    d. _____

    e. _____

54. A client's bed must be frequently inspected to ensure the linens are _____, _____, and _____.

55. Identify the factors a nurse considers when making a client's bed.

    _____

    _____

Evaluation

Client Care

56. Evaluation of hygiene measures occurs both before, during, and after each particular skill.

57. The standards for evaluation are the expected outcomes established in the planning stage of the client's care.

Client Expectations

58. The client's expectations are important guidelines in determining client satisfaction.

Review Questions

Select the appropriate answer and cite the rationale for choosing that particular answer.

1. Mr. Ng is a 19-year-old client in the rehabilitation unit. He is completely paralyzed below the neck. The most appropriate bath for Mr. Ng is a
   a. Partial bed bath
   b. Complete bed bath
   c. Sitz bath
   d. Tepid bath

   Answer: _____   Rationale: _____

   _____

   _____

2. All of the following will help maintain skin integrity in the older adult except
   a. Environmental air that is cold and dry
   b. Use of warm water and mild cleansing agents for bathing
   c. Bathing every other day
   d. Drinking 8 to 10 glasses of water a day

   Answer: _____   Rationale: _____

   _____

   _____

3. When preparing to give complete morning care to a client, what would the nurse do first?
   a. Gather the necessary equipment and supplies.
   b. Remove the client's gown or pajamas while maintaining privacy.

c. Assess the client's preferences for bathing practices.
d. Lower the side rails and assist the client to assume a comfortable position.

Answer: _____ Rationale: _____

_____

_____

4. Mrs. Veech has diabetes. Which intervention should be included in her teaching plan regarding foot care?
   a. Use a pumice stone to smooth corns and calluses.
   b. File toenails straight across and square.
   c. Apply powder to dry areas along the feet and between the toes.
   d. Wear elastic stockings to improve circulation.

Answer: _____ Rationale: _____

_____

_____

5. Assessment of the hair and scalp reveals that a client has pediculosis capitis. An appropriate intervention would be
   a. Shave hair off the affected area
   b. Place oil on the hair and scalp until all of the lice are dead

c. Use a medicated shampoo and repeat 7 to 10 days later
d. Shampoo with regular shampoo and dry with the hair-dryer set at the hottest setting

Answer: _____ Rationale: _____

_____

_____

Critical Thinking Model for Nursing Care Plan for Ineffective Tissue Perfusion, Improper Foot Care and Hygiene

You are the nurse in the Care Plan on page 844 of your text. Complete the *planning phase* of the critical thinking model by writing your answers in the appropriate boxes of the model shown. Think about the following:

• In developing Mr. James's plan of care, what knowledge did you apply?

• In what way might your previous experience assist in developing a plan of care for Mr. James?

• When developing a plan of care, what intellectual and professional standards were applied?

• What critical thinking attitudes might have been applied in developing Mr. James's plan of care?

• How will you accomplish the goals?

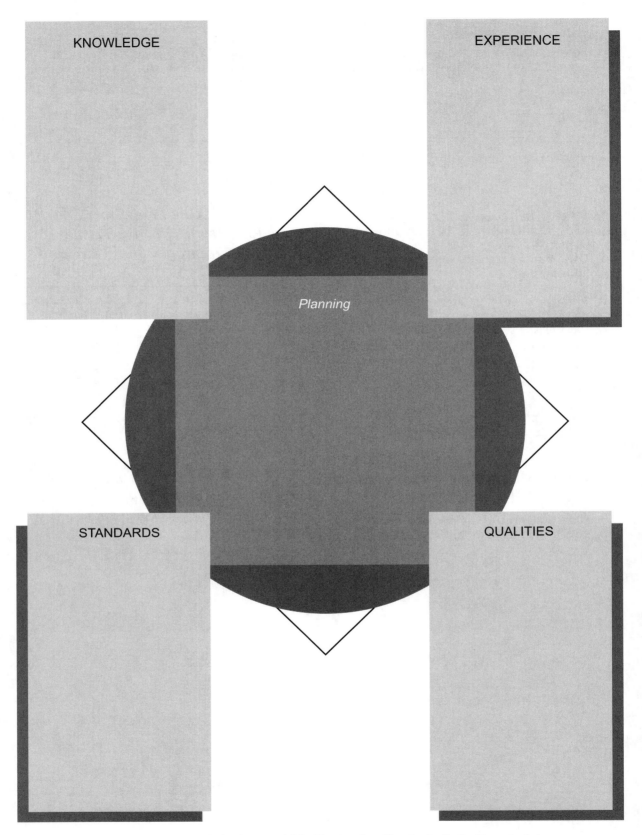

KNOWLEDGE

EXPERIENCE

Planning

STANDARDS

QUALITIES

CHAPTER 38   Critical Thinking Model for Nursing Care Plan for *Ineffective Tissue Perfusion,*
Improper Foot Care and Hygiene
See answers on page 535.

39

Cardiopulmonary Functioning and Oxygenation

Preliminary Reading

Chapter 39, pp. 879–932

Comprehensive Understanding

Scientific Knowledge Base

Cardiovascular Physiology

1. Cardiopulmonary physiology involves delivery of _____ to the right side of the heart and to the pulmonary circulation, and _____ from the lungs to the left side of the heart and the tissues.

2. The cardiac system delivers _____, _____, and other _____ to the tissues, and removes the _____ _____ through the _____, _____ _____, and the _____.

3. The right ventricle pumps blood through the _____. The left ventricle pumps blood to the _____.

4. The four chambers of the heart fill with blood during _____ and empty during _____.

5. Describe the Frank–Starling law of the heart.

   _____

   _____

   _____

6. Briefly describe the flow of blood through the heart.

   _____

   _____

   _____

7. Describe the following types of circulation.

   a. Coronary artery:

      _____

   b. Systemic:

      _____

8. Describe the following terms related to blood flow regulation.

   a. Cardiac output:

      _____

      _____

   b. Cardiac index:

      _____

      _____

   c. Stroke volume:

      _____

      _____

   d. Preload:

      _____

      _____

   e. Afterload:

      _____

      _____

   f. Myocardial contractility:

      _____

      _____

9. Describe how the following affect the conduction system of the heart.

   a. Sympathetic nerve fibres:

   _____

   _____

   _____

   b. Parasympathetic nerve fibres:

   _____

   _____

   _____

10. Diagram and label the electrical conduction system of the heart in the box below.

11. Diagram and label the components of the ECG waveform for normal sinus rhythm (NSR) in the box below.

Respiratory Physiology

12. The three steps in the process of oxygenation are_____, _____, and _____.

13. The _____, _____ _____, _____, and _____ are essential for ventilation, perfusion, and exchange of respiratory gases.

14. Define *ventilation*.

   _____

   _____

15. Define the following terms related to the work of breathing.

   a. Surfactant:

   _____

   _____

   b. Accessory muscles:

   _____

   _____

   c. Compliance:

   _____

   _____

d. Airway resistance:

_____

_____

16. Spirometry is used to

_____

_____

17. Variations in lung volumes may be associated with health states such as _____, _____, _____, or _____ and _____ conditions of the lungs.

18. The amount of _____, _____ _____, and _____ can affect pressures and volumes within the lungs.

19. Briefly describe the pulmonary circulation.

_____

_____

20. Identify the normal distribution of pressures within the pulmonary circulation.

_____

_____

21. Respiratory gases are exchanged in the ____ _____ and the _____ of the body tissues.

22. Define *diffusion*.

_____

_____

23. How can the rate of diffusion be affected?

_____

_____

24. List four factors required for oxygen transport and delivery.

a. _____

b. _____

c. _____

d. _____

25. Describe the breakdown of carbon dioxide as it is diffused into the red blood cells.

_____

_____

26. Explain the two regulators that control the process of respiration.

    a. Neural:

    _____

    _____

    b. Chemical:

    _____

    _____

Factors Affecting Oxygenation

27. List the four factors that influence oxygenation.

    a. _____

    b. _____

    c. _____

    d. _____

28. Explain the following factors that affect the body's ability to meet oxygen demands. Give examples of each.

    a. Decreased carrying capacity:

    _____

    _____

    b. Decreased inspired oxygen concentration:

    _____

    _____

    c. Hypovolemia:

    _____

    _____

    d. Increased metabolic rate:

    _____

    _____

29. Explain how the following conditions affect chest wall movement.

    a. Pregnancy:

    _____

    _____

    b. Obesity:

    _____

    _____

    c. Musculoskeletal abnormalities:

    _____

    _____

    d. Trauma:

    _____

    _____

    e. Neuromuscular diseases:

    _____

    _____

    f. Central nervous system alterations:

    _____

    _____

    g. Influences of chronic disease:

    _____

    _____

Alterations in Cardiac Functioning

30. Illnesses and conditions that affect _____ _____, _____, _____, _____, and _____ cause alterations in cardiac functioning.

31. Define *dysrhythmias*.

    _____

    _____

32. Briefly describe the following dysrhythmias.

    a. Asystole:

    _____

    _____

    b. Sinus bradycardia:

    _____

    _____

    c. Sinus tachycardia:

    _____

    _____

    d. Dysrhythmia:

    _____

    _____

    e. A-Fib:

    _____

    _____

    f. Ventricular tachycardia:

    _____

    _____

    g. Ventricular fibrillation:

    _____

    _____

33. Failure of the myocardium to eject sufficient volume to the systemic and pulmonary circulations can result in left-sided and right-sided heart failure. Complete the grid below.

Type of Failure	Clinical Findings
Left-Sided	
Right-Sided	

34. Define each of the following.
   a. Valvular heart disease:

   _____
   _____

   b. Stenosis:

   _____
   _____

   c. Regurgitation:

   _____
   _____

   d. Myocardial ischemia:

   _____
   _____

   e. Angina pectoris:

   _____
   _____

   f. Myocardial infarction:

   _____
   _____

35. Describe the chest pain associated with myocardial infarction.

   _____
   _____
   _____

36. Briefly explain acute coronary syndrome (ACS).

   _____
   _____

Alterations in Respiratory Functioning

37. The three primary alterations in respiratory function are _____, _____, and _____.

38. Complete the grid below.

Alterations	Causes	Signs and Symptoms
Hyperventilation		
Hypoventilation		
Hypoxia		

39. Define the following terms.

    a. Atelectasis:

    _____

    _____

    b. Cyanosis:

    _____

    _____

Nursing Knowledge Base

Developmental Factors

40. Identify at least one physiological factor influencing tissue oxygenation for each developmental level listed.

    a. Infants and toddlers:

    _____

    _____

    b. School-age children and adolescents:

    _____

    _____

    c. Young and middle-aged adults:

    _____

    _____

    d. Older adults:

    _____

    _____

Lifestyle Risk Factors

41. Briefly describe how the following lifestyle factors influence respiratory function.

    a. Poor nutrition:

    _____

    _____

    b. Inadequate exercise:

    _____

    _____

    c. Smoking:

    _____

    _____

    d. Substance abuse:

    _____

    _____

    e. Stress:

    _____

    _____

Environmental Factors

42. List four occupational pollutants.

    a. _____

    b. _____

    c. _____

    d. _____

Nursing Process

Assessment

43. The nursing assessment of a client's cardiopulmonary functioning should include data from the following areas. Briefly explain each.

    a. Health history:

    _____

    _____

    _____

    b. Physical examination:

    _____

    _____

    _____

    c. Diagnostic tests:

    _____

    _____

    _____

44. Define the following terms.

    a. Fatigue:

    _____

    _____

    b. Dyspnea:

    _____

    _____

    c. Orthopnea:

    _____

    _____

    d. Cough:

    _____

    _____

    e. Productive cough:

    _____

    _____

    f. Hemoptysis:

    _____

    _____

g. Wheezing:

_____

_____

45. Briefly explain the following techniques used during the physical examination to assess tissue oxygenation.

   a. Inspection:

   _____

   _____

   _____

   b. Palpation:

   _____

   _____

   c. Percussion:

   _____

   _____

   d. Auscultation:

   _____

   _____

   _____

46. Describe the following tests that determine myocardial contraction and blood flow.

   a. Echocardiography:

   _____

   _____

   b. Scintigraphy:

   _____

   _____

   c. Cardiac catheterization and angiography:

   _____

   _____

   _____

47. Describe the following diagnostic tests used to determine the adequacy of the cardiac conduction system.

   a. Electrocardiogram:

   _____

   _____

   b. Holter monitor:

   _____

   _____

c. ECG exercise stress test:

_____

_____

d. Electrophysiological studies:

_____

_____

48. Describe the following tests used to measure the adequacy of ventilation and oxygenation.

   a. Pulmonary function tests:

   _____

   _____

   b. CT scan:

   _____

   _____

   c. Arterial blood gases:

   _____

   _____

   d. Pulse oximetry:

   _____

   _____

   e. Chest X-ray examination:

   _____

   _____

   f. Lung scan:

   _____

   _____

49. Describe the following tests used to determine abnormal cells or infection in the respiratory tract.

   a. Bronchoscopy:

   _____

   _____

   b. Sputum specimens:

   _____

   _____

   c. Thoracentesis:

   _____

   _____

Nursing Diagnosis

50. Clients with an altered level of oxygenation can have nursing diagnoses that are primarily from a cardiovascular or pulmonary origin.

Planning

51. List four goals appropriate for a client with actual or potential oxygenation needs.

    a. _____

    b. _____

    c. _____

    d. _____

Implementation

Health Promotion

52. Describe the purpose of the influenza and pneumococcal vaccines and explain for whom the vaccines are recommended.

    _____

    _____

53. Identify some healthy lifestyle behaviours that decrease the risk of cardiopulmonary disease.

    _____

    _____

Acute Care

54. Nursing interventions for the client with acute pulmonary illnesses are directed toward _____, _____ _____, and _____.

55. List four treatment modalities appropriate for a client with dyspnea.

    a. _____

    b. _____

    c. _____

    d. _____

Mobilization of Pulmonary Secretions

56. Nursing interventions that promote mobilization of pulmonary secretions include the following. Briefly explain each one.

    a. Dyspnea management:

    _____

    _____

b. Humidification:

    _____

    _____

c. Nebulization:

    _____

    _____

d. Chest physiotherapy (CPT):

    _____

    _____

57. Briefly describe the three activities involved in CPT.

    a. Postural drainage:

    _____

    _____

    b. Chest percussion:

    _____

    _____

    c. Vibration:

    _____

    _____

58. Briefly explain the following types of suctioning techniques.

    a. Oropharyngeal and nasopharyngeal:

    _____

    _____

    b. Orotracheal and nasotracheal:

    _____

    _____

    c. Tracheal:

    _____

    _____

59. Describe selected nursing interventions used to promote and maintain adequate oxygenation by completing the grid that follows. Include the purpose of the intervention.

Nursing Interventions	Purpose
Oropharyngeal and nasopharyngeal suctioning	
Tracheal suctioning	
Oral airway	
Tracheal airway	

60. Nursing interventions that maintain or promote lung expansion include the following noninvasive techniques. Briefly explain each.

   a. Positioning:

   _____

   _____

   b. Incentive spirometry:

   _____

   _____

61. Identify the three reasons for inserting chest tubes.

   a. _____

   b. _____

   c. _____

62. Define the following.

   a. Pneumothorax:

   _____

   _____

   b. Hemothorax:

   _____

   _____

63. List the two types of drainage systems used with chest tubes.

   a. _____

   b. _____

64. Identify five special considerations the nurse needs to address when dealing with chest tubes.

   a. _____

   b. _____

   c. _____

   d. _____

   e. _____

65. Promotion of lung expansion, mobilization of secretions, and maintenance of a patent airway assist the client in meeting oxygenation needs.

66. Identify the goal of oxygen therapy.

   _____

   _____

67. List five safety measures to institute when a client receives oxygen.

   a. _____

   b. _____

   c. _____

   d. _____

   e. _____

68. Describe the following methods of oxygen delivery and identify the usual flow rates.

a. Nasal cannula:

_____

_____

b. Face mask:

_____

_____

c. Venturi mask:

_____

_____

69. Identify the indications for a client to receive home oxygen therapy.

_____

_____

70. Identify the teaching required by the client for use of home oxygen therapy.

_____

_____

71. List the three goals of cardiopulmonary resuscitation (CPR).

a. _____

b. _____

c. _____

Restorative and Continuing Care

72. Cardiopulmonary rehabilitation is

_____

_____

73. Briefly explain the following breathing exercises used to improve ventilation and oxygenation.

a. Pursed-lip breathing:

_____

_____

b. Diaphragmatic breathing:

_____

_____

Evaluation

Client Care

74. The nurse evaluates the actual care provided to the client by the health care team based on the expected outcomes.

75. The client is the only person who can evaluate his or her degree of breathlessness.

76. The evaluation of _____ and _____ are done by comparing the client's _____ with the goals and _____ of the nursing care plan

Client Expectations

77. Evaluate the care from the client's perspective.

78. Working closely with the client will enable the nurse to redefine those client expectations that can be realistically met within the limitations of the client's condition and treatment.

Review Questions

Select the appropriate answer and cite the rationale for choosing that particular answer.

1. Ventilation, perfusion, and exchange of gases are the major purposes of
   a. Respiration
   b. Circulation
   c. Aerobic metabolism
   d. Anaerobic metabolism

Answer: _____   Rationale: _____

_____

_____

2. Afterload refers to
   a. The amount of blood ejected from the left ventricle each minute
   b. The amount of blood ejected from the left ventricle with each contraction
   c. The resistance to left ventricle ejection
   d. The amount of blood in the left ventricle at the end of diastole

Answer: _____   Rationale: _____

_____

_____

3. The movement of gases into and out of the lungs depends on the
   a. Fifty percent oxygen content in the atmospheric air
   b. Pressure gradient between the atmosphere and the alveoli

c. Use of accessory muscles of respiration during expiration

d. Amount of carbon dioxide dissolved in the fluid of the alveoli

Answer: _____   Rationale: _____

_____

_____

4. The client's ECG shows an abnormal rhythm that slows during inspiration and increases with expiration. The rate is 70 to 80 beats per minute. The P-wave, PR interval, and QRS complex are normal. This is referred to as
   a. Sinus tachycardia
   b. Sinus dysrhythmia
   c. Supraventricular tachycardia
   d. Premature ventricular contractions

Answer: _____   Rationale: _____

_____

_____

5. Mr. Isaac comes to the ER complaining of difficulty breathing. An objective finding associated with his dyspnea might include
   a. Statements about a sense of impending doom
   b. Complaints of shortness of breath
   c. Feelings of heaviness in the chest
   d. Use of accessory muscles of respiration

Answer: _____   Rationale: _____

_____

_____

6. The use of chest physiotherapy to mobilize pulmonary secretions involves the use of
   a. Hydration
   b. Percussion
   c. Nebulization
   d. Humidification

Answer: _____   Rationale: _____

_____

_____

Critical Thinking Model for the Nursing Care Plan for Ineffective Airway Clearance/Retained Secretions

Imagine that you are the student nurse in the Care Plan on page 901 of your text. Complete the *assessment phase* of the critical thinking model by writing your answers in the appropriate boxes of the model shown. Think about the following:

• What knowledge base was applied to Mr. Edwards?

• In what way might your previous experience apply in this case?

• What intellectual or professional standards were applied to Mr. Edwards?

• What critical thinking attitudes did you use in assessing Mr. Edwards?

• As you review your assessment, what key areas did you cover?

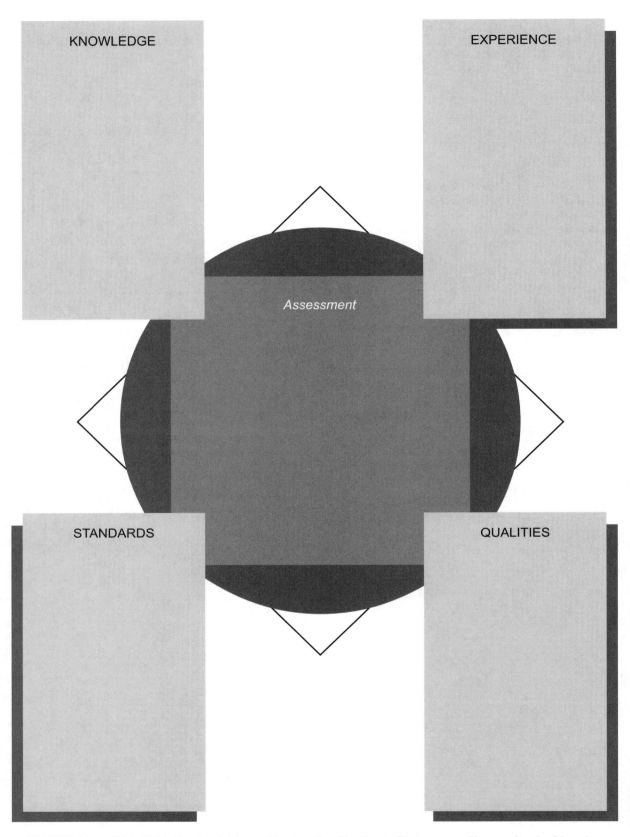

CHAPTER 39   Critical Thinking Model for the Nursing Care Plan for *Ineffective Airway Clearance/Retained Secretions*
See answers on page 536.

40

Fluid, Electrolyte, and Acid–Base Balances

Preliminary Reading

Chapter 40, pp. 933–986

Comprehensive Understanding

Scientific Knowledge Base

1. _____ is the largest single component of the body, 60% of the average adult's weight.

Distribution of Body Fluids

2. Body fluids are distributed in two distinct compartments. Briefly explain each one.

   a. Extracellular:

   _____
   _____

   b. Intracellular:

   _____
   _____

3. Extracellular fluids (ECF) are divided into two smaller compartments. Explain each.

   a. Interstitial:

   _____
   _____

   b. Intravascular:

   _____
   _____

Composition of Body Fluids

4. Define *electrolytes*.

   _____
   _____

5. Define the following terms related to the composition of body fluids.

   a. Cations:

   _____
   _____

   b. Anions:

   _____
   _____

   c. mmol/L:

   _____
   _____

   d. Solute:

   _____
   _____

   e. Solvent:

   _____
   _____

   f. Minerals:

   _____
   _____

Movement of Body Fluids

6. Fluids and electrolytes constantly shift between compartments to facilitate body processes.

7. List and briefly describe the four factors responsible for the movement of body fluids.

a. _____

b. _____

c. _____

d. _____

8. Define the following terms related to osmosis.

a. Osmotic pressure:

_____

_____

b. Isotonic:

_____

_____

c. Hypotonic:

_____

_____

d. Hypertonic:

_____

_____

9. Define *hydrostatic pressure*.

_____

_____

Regulation of Body Fluids

10. Body fluids are regulated by _____ _____, _____, and _____ _____. This balance is termed _____.

11. Briefly describe the physiological stimuli triggering the thirst mechanism.

_____

_____

12. For each hormone in the grid below, identify the stimuli for its release and its influence on fluid and electrolyte balance.

Hormone	Stimuli	Action
ADH		
Aldosterone		

13. Fluid output occurs through four organs. List and explain each one.

a. _____

b. _____

c. _____

d. _____

14. Define the following.

a. Insensible water loss:

_____

_____

b. Sensible water loss:

_____

_____

Regulation of Electrolytes

15. The major cations within the body fluids include _____, _____, _____ _____, and _____.

16. The major anions are _____, _____ ____, and _____.

17. Give the normal values, function, and regulatory mechanisms for the major body electrolytes in the following grid.

Electrolyte	Value	Function	Regulatory Mechanism
Sodium			
Potassium			
Calcium			
Magnesium			
Chloride			
Bicarbonate			
Phosphate			

Regulation of Acid–Base Balance

18. Identify and describe the acid–base regulatory mechanisms for each of the following buffering systems.

a. Chemical regulation:

_____

_____

b. Biological regulation:

_____

_____

c. Physiological regulation:

_____

_____

19. Describe the physiological mechanism through which the lungs regulate hydrogen ion concentration.

_____

_____

Disturbances in Electrolyte, Fluid, and Acid–Base Balances

20. For each electrolyte disturbance, identify the diagnostic laboratory finding, and list at least four characteristic signs and symptoms in the grid below.

Imbalance	Lab Finding	Signs and Symptoms
Hyponatremia		
Hypernatremia		
Hypokalemia		
Hyperkalemia		
Hypocalcemia		
Hypercalcemia		
Hypomagnesemia		
Hypermagnesemia		

21. The basic types of fluid imbalances are _____ _____ and _____.

22. Isotonic deficit and excess exist when

    _____

    _____

23. Osmolar imbalances are

    _____

    _____

24. Arterial blood gas (ABG) analysis is the best way to evaluate acid–base balance. Give the normal value for each.

   a. pH:

    _____

   b. $PaCO_2$:

    _____

c. PaO_2:

_____

d. Base excess:

_____

e. HCO_3^-:

25. Complete the grid below giving the causes and signs and symptoms of the listed fluid disturbances.

Fluid Disturbances	Causes	Signs and Symptoms
Fluid volume deficit (FVD)		
Fluid volume deficit (FVE)		
Hyperosmolar imbalance		
Hypo-osmolar imbalance		

26. Briefly explain the following components of the acid–base balance.

a. pH:

_____
_____

b. $PaCO_2$:

_____
_____

c. PaO_2:

_____
_____

d. Oxygen saturation:

_____
_____

e. Base excess:

_____
_____

f. Bicarbonate:

_____
_____

27. The four primary types of acid–base imbalances are listed in the following grid. For each acid–base imbalance, identify the diagnostic laboratory finding and list the characteristic signs and symptoms.

Acid–Base Imbalance	Lab Findings	Signs and Symptoms
Respiratory acidosis		
Respiratory alkalosis		
Metabolic acidosis		
Metabolic alkalosis		

Knowledge Base of Nursing Practice

28. List the five major risk factors that can affect fluid and electrolyte imbalances. Give two examples of each.

a. _____
   _____

b. _____
   _____

c. _____
   _____

d. _____
   _____

e. _____
   _____

Nursing Process

Assessment

29. Briefly describe the fluid changes that are associated with aging and development.

a. Infants:
   _____
   _____

b. Children:
   _____
   _____

c. Adolescents:
   _____
   _____

d. Older adults:
   _____
   _____

30. Explain how the following acute illnesses affect fluid, electrolyte, and acid–base balances.

a. Surgery:
   _____
   _____
   _____

b. Burns:
   _____
   _____
   _____

c. Respiratory disorders:
   _____
   _____

d. Head injury:

_____

_____

_____

31. Describe how the following chronic illnesses affect fluid, electrolyte, and acid–base imbalances.

a. Cancer:

_____

_____

_____

b. Cardiovascular disease:

_____

_____

_____

c. Renal disorders:

_____

_____

_____

d. Gastrointestinal disturbances:

_____

_____

_____

e. HIV/AIDS:

_____

_____

_____

32. Briefly explain how the following affect fluid, electrolyte, and acid–base imbalances.

a. Diet:

_____

_____

_____

b. Lifestyle factors:

_____

_____

_____

c. Medication:

_____

_____

_____

33. Indicate the possible fluid, electrolyte, or acid–base imbalances associated with each physical finding.

a. Weight loss of 5% to 10%:

_____

_____

b. Irritability:

_____

_____

c. Lethargy:

_____

_____

d. Periorbital edema:

_____

_____

e. Sticky, dry mucous membranes:

_____

_____

f. Distended neck veins:

_____

_____

g. Dysrhythmias:

_____

_____

h. Weak pulse:

_____

_____

i. Low blood pressure:

_____

_____

j. Third heart sound:

_____

_____

k. Increased respiratory rate:

_____

_____

l. Crackles:

_____

_____

m. Anorexia:

_____

_____

n. Abdominal cramps:

_____

_____

o. Poor skin turgor:

_____

_____

p. Oliguria or anuria:

_____

_____

q. Increased specific gravity:

_____

_____

r. Muscle cramps, tetany:

_____

_____

s. Hypertonicity of muscles on palpation:

_____

_____

t. Decreased or absent deep tendon reflexes:

_____

_____

u. Increased temperature:

_____

_____

v. Distended abdomen:

_____

_____

w. Cold, clammy skin:

_____

_____

x. Edema (dependent body parts):

_____

_____

34. Recording intake and output (I&O) is essential for obtaining an accurate database. Accurate I&O measurements can identify both clients at risk for and clients who are experiencing fluid, electrolyte, and acid–base disturbances.

35. Intake includes _____,
_____, _____,
and _____.

36. Output includes _____, _____,
_____, _____ and
_____.

Nursing Diagnosis

37. List five potential or actual nursing diagnoses for a client with fluid, electrolyte, or acid–base imbalances.

a. _____

b. _____

c. _____

d. _____

e. _____

Planning

38. List three goals that are appropriate for a client with a fluid, electrolyte, or acid–base imbalance.

a. _____

b. _____

c. _____

Implementation

Health Promotion

39. Identify some common risk factors for imbalances for which the caregiver may implement appropriate preventive measures.

_____

_____

_____

Acute Care

40. When implementing specific measures to increase or decrease fluid, two interventions are necessary. Explain each one.

a. Daily weights:

_____

_____

b. I&O:

_____

_____

41. List and briefly describe the enteral replacement of fluids.

    a. _____

    b. _____

42. Briefly explain the need for a restricted fluid intake and how the nurse would implement the restriction.

    _____
    _____
    _____

43. List the three methods of parenteral replacement.

    a. _____
    b. _____
    c. _____

44. Vascular assist devices are

    _____
    _____

45. Total parenteral nutrition (TPN) is

    _____
    _____

46. Identify the primary goal of IV fluid administration.

    _____
    _____

47. Define the following types of electrolyte solutions.

    a. Isotonic:

    _____
    _____

    b. Hypotonic:

    _____
    _____

    c. Hypertonic:

    _____

48. List two major purposes of infusion pumps.

    a. _____
    b. _____

49. List three groups of clients for whom venipunctures may be difficult.

    a. _____
    b. _____
    c. _____

50. List four factors that may affect IV flow rates.

    a. _____
    b. _____
    c. _____
    d. _____

51. Indicate the sequence to be followed when changing the gown of a client with an IV line.

    a. _____
    b. _____
    c. _____
    d. _____
    e. _____
    f. _____

52. Complete the grid below describing complications of IV therapy.

Complication	Assessment Finding	Nursing Action
Infiltration		
Phlebitis		
Fluid volume excess (FVE)		
Bleeding		

53. Briefly summarize the procedure for discontinuing intravenous infusions.

_____

_____

b. _____

_____

c. _____

_____

54. List three objectives for blood transfusion.

a. _____

_____

55. Complete the grid below describing the major blood groups.

	A	B	O	AB
Antigens present				
Antibodies present				

56. Define *autotransfusion*.

_____

_____

57. Identify the five nursing interventions associated with blood transfusions and give the rationale for each.

a. _____

_____

b. _____

_____

c. _____

_____

d. _____

_____

e. _____
_____

58. Define *transfusion reaction* and identify its cause.
_____
_____
_____

59. Identify types of transfusion reactions and their causes.

a. _____
_____

b. _____
_____

c. _____
_____

d. _____
_____

e. _____
_____

f. _____
_____

60. List the steps the nurse should follow if a transfusion reaction is suspected.

a. _____
b. _____
c. _____
d. _____
e. _____
f. _____
g. _____
h. _____

Restorative Care

61. Older adults and clients with chronic illnesses require special considerations to prevent complications from developing. Briefly summarize the following.

a. Home intravenous therapy:
_____
_____
_____

b. Nutritional support:
_____
_____

c. Medication safety:
_____
_____
_____

Evaluation

Client Care

62. The nurse evaluates the actual care delivered by the health care team based on the expected outcomes.

63. The nurse will perform evaluative measures and determine if changes have occurred since the last client assessment. The client's level of progress determines whether the nurse needs to continue or revise the care plan.

Client Expectations

64. Nurses routinely review with their client their success in meeting expectations of care.

65. Often the client's level of satisfaction with care also depends on the nurse's success in involving friends and family.

Review Questions

Select the appropriate answer and cite the rationale for choosing that particular answer.

1. The body fluids comprising the interstitial fluid and blood plasma are
   a. Intracellular
   b. Extracellular
   c. Hypotonic
   d. Hypertonic

Answer: _____   Rationale: _____
_____
_____

2. Which of the following statements is true with regard to the lungs' regulation of acid–base balance?
   a. The lungs serve a minor role in the physiological buffering of H ions.
   b. It takes several days for the lungs to restore pH to a normal level.

c. The lungs correct imbalances by altering the rate and depth of respiration.
d. The lungs maintain normal pH by either retaining or excreting bicarbonate.

Answer: _____   Rationale: _____

_____

_____

3. Mrs. Singh's arterial blood gas results are as follows: pH: 7.32; $PaCO_2$: 52; PaO_2: 78; HCO_3^-: 24. Mrs. Singh has
a. Respiratory acidosis
b. Respiratory alkalosis
c. Metabolic acidosis
d. Metabolic alkalosis

Answer: _____   Rationale: _____

_____

_____

4. Mr. Frank is an 82-year-old client who has had a 3-day history of vomiting and diarrhea. Which symptom would you expect to find on a physical examination?
a. Neck vein distension
b. Crackles in the lungs
c. Tachycardia
d. Hypertension

Answer: _____   Rationale: _____

_____

_____

5. Which of the following is most likely to result in respiratory alkalosis?
a. Fad dieting
b. Hyperventilation
c. Chronic alcoholism
d. Steroid use

Answer: _____   Rationale: _____

_____

_____

Critical Thinking Model for Planning Fluid, Electrolyte, and Acid–Base Balances

Imagine that you are the student nurse in the Care Plan on page 953 of your text. Complete the *planning phase* of the critical thinking model by writing your answers in the appropriate boxes of the model shown. Think about the following:

• When developing a plan of care, what intellectual and professional standards did you apply?

• In developing Mrs. Topping's plan of care, what knowledge did you apply?

• In what way might your previous experience assist you in developing a plan of care for Mrs. Topping?

• What critical thinking attitudes might have been applied to developing Mrs. Topping's care?

• How will you accomplish your goals?

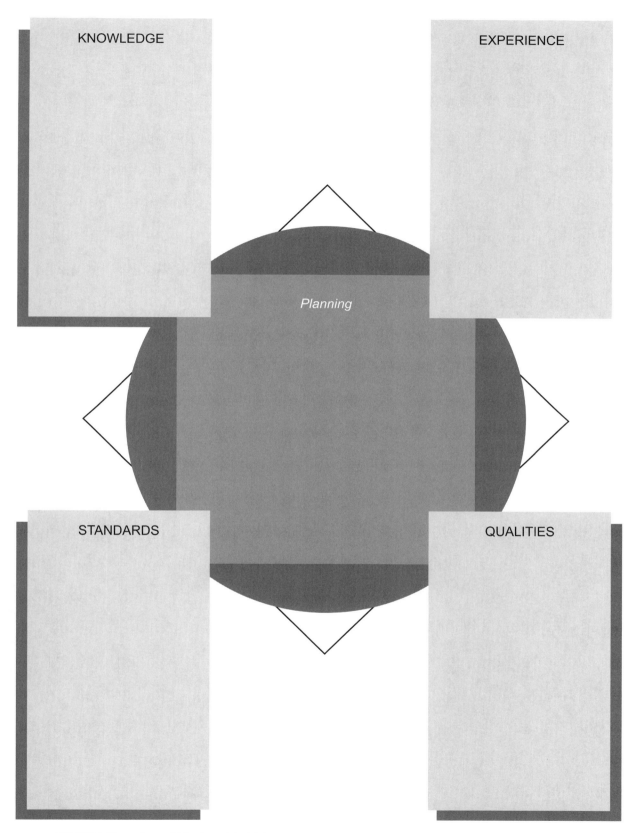

KNOWLEDGE

EXPERIENCE

Planning

STANDARDS

QUALITIES

CHAPTER 40   Critical Thinking Model for Nursing Care Plan for *Fluid, Electrolyte, and Acid–Base Balances*
See answers on page 537.

41

Sleep

Preliminary Reading

Chapter 41, pp. 987–1008

Comprehensive Understanding

Scientific Knowledge Base

Physiology of Sleep

1. Define *sleep*.

   _____

   _____

2. Define the following terms related to sleep.
   a. Circadian rhythm:

   _____

   _____

   b. Biological clocks:

   _____

   _____

3. Sleep involves a sequence of physiological states maintained by highly integrated central nervous system activity that is associated with changes in the _____,

   _____, _____, _____,

   and _____ systems.

4. The control and regulation of sleep may depend on the interrelationship between two cerebral mechanisms that intermittently activate and suppress the brain's higher centres to control sleep and wakefulness.

5. Summarize the function of the reticular activating system (RAS).

   _____

   _____

6. The area of the brain called the *bulbar synchronizing region* (BSR) is responsible for

   _____

   _____

   _____

7. Explain the two stages of sleep.
   a. NREM:

   _____

   _____

   b. REM:

   _____

   _____

8. Describe the characteristics of the following cycles of sleep.
   a. Stage 1:

   _____

   b. Stage 2:

   _____

   c. Stage 3:

   _____

   d. Stage 4:

   _____

   e. REM:

   _____

Functions of Sleep

9. Explain briefly the functions of sleep.

   _____

   _____

Physical Illness

10. Explain how the following conditions affect sleep.

    a. Discomfort:

    _____

    b. Respiratory disease:

    _____

    c. Hypertension:

    _____

    d. Hypothyroidism:

    _____

    e. Hyperthyroidism:

    _____

    f. Nocturia:

    _____

    g. Restless leg syndrome:

    _____

Sleep Disorders

11. Briefly describe the following categories of sleep disorders.

    a. Hypersomnias:

    _____

    b. Parasomnias:

    _____

12. Define *insomnia*.

    _____
    _____

13. List two conditions that are associated with insomnia.

    a. _____
    b. _____

14. Define *sleep apnea*.

    _____
    _____

15. Define the following types of apnea.

    a. Central sleep apnea:

    _____
    _____

    b. Obstructive sleep apnea:

    _____
    _____

16. Briefly explain excessive daytime sleepiness (EDS).

    _____
    _____

17. Define *narcolepsy*.

    _____
    _____

18. Define *cataplexy*.

    _____
    _____

19. Identify the developmental stage in which narcolepsy symptoms first develop.

    _____
    _____

20. Identify the treatment modalities for a client with narcolepsy.

    _____
    _____

21. Sleep deprivation is

    _____
    _____

22. Explain the following parasomnias.

    a. Somnambulism:

    _____
    _____

    b. Nocturnal enuresis:

    _____
    _____

    c. Bruxism:

    _____
    _____

Nursing Knowledge Base

Sleep and Rest

23. Define *rest*.

    _____
    _____

Normal Sleep Requirements and Patterns

24. Complete the grid that follows listing the normal sleep patterns and rituals for the various developmental stages.

Developmental Stage	Sleep Patterns	Usual Rituals
Neonates		
Infants		
Toddlers		
Preschoolers		
School-age children		
Adolescents		
Young adults		
Middle adults		
Older adults		

Factors Affecting Sleep

25. A number of factors affect the quantity and quality of sleep.

26. Sleepiness and sleep deprivation are common side effects of medications. Describe how each of the following affects sleep and give an example.

a. Drugs and substances:

_____

_____

b. Lifestyle:

_____

_____

27. List three alterations in routine that can disrupt sleep patterns.

    a. _____

    b. _____

    c. _____

28. Explain how emotional stress affects sleep.

    _____

    _____

29. List and briefly describe three environmental factors that affect sleep.

    a. _____

    b. _____

    c. _____

30. Explain how exercise promotes sleep.

    _____

    _____

31. List and briefly describe five foods that affect sleep and why.

    a. _____

    b. _____

    c. _____

    d. _____

    e. _____

Nursing Process

Assessment

32. Sleep and restfulness are subjective experiences.

33. Assessment is aimed at understanding the characteristics of a sleep problem and the client's sleep habits.

34. Identify three sources for sleep assessment.

    a. _____

    b. _____

    c. _____

35. List seven components of a sleep history.

    a. _____

    b. _____

    c. _____

    d. _____

    e. _____

    f. _____

    g. _____

36. List and briefly describe the six areas to assess with a client when asking about the nature of a sleeping problem.

    a. _____
       _____

    b. _____
       _____

    c. _____
       _____

    d. _____
       _____

    e. _____
       _____

    f. _____
       _____

37. Identify the information recorded in a sleep–wake log.

    _____

    _____

38. Briefly explain how the following factors interfere with sleep.

    a. Physical and psychological illness:

       _____

       _____

    b. Current life events:

       _____

       _____

    c. Bedtime routines:

       _____

       _____

    d. Bedtime environment:

       _____

       _____

39. List four behaviours a client may manifest with sleep deprivation.

    a. _____

    b. _____

    c. _____

    d. _____

Nursing Diagnosis

40. If a sleep pattern disturbance is identified, the nurse specifies the condition.

41. Assessment should also identify the related factor or probable cause of the sleep disturbance.

Planning

42. It is important for the plan of care to include strategies that are appropriate for the client's environment and lifestyle.

43. List four goals appropriate for a client needing rest or sleep.

    a. _____
    b. _____
    c. _____
    d. _____

Implementation

44. Nursing interventions designed to improve the quality of a person's sleep are largely focused on health promotion.

Health Promotion

45. Many factors affect the ability to gain adequate rest and sleep. Briefly give examples of each of the following.

    a. Environmental controls:
    _____
    _____

    b. Promoting bedtime routines:
    _____
    _____

    c. Promoting safety:
    _____
    _____

    d. Promoting comfort:
    _____
    _____

    e. Periods of rest and sleep:
    _____
    _____

    f. Stress reduction:
    _____
    _____

    g. Bedtime snacks:
    _____

    h. Pharmacological approaches:
    _____
    _____

Acute Care

46. For each of the following situations, give two examples of nursing measures that will promote sleep.

    a. Environmental controls:
        1. _____
        2. _____

    b. Promoting comfort:
        1. _____
        2. _____

    c. Establishing periods of rest and sleep:
        1. _____
        2. _____

    d. Promoting safety:
        1. _____
        2. _____

    e. Stress reduction:
        1. _____
        2. _____

Restorative or Continuing Care

47. Give an example of the following interventions that are implemented in the restorative environment.

    a. Promoting comfort:
    _____

    b. Controlling physiological disturbances:
    _____

    c. Pharmacological approaches:
    _____

48. Briefly describe the effect of benzodiazepines in promoting sleep.
    _____
    _____

49. Identify three types of clients who should not use benzodiazepines and explain why.

    a. _____

    b. _____

    c. _____

50. The regular use of sleeping medication can lead to

    _____

    _____

Evaluation

Client Care

51. The client is the only person who knows if sleep problems are improved and which interventions or therapies are successful.

Client Expectations

52. Identify some subtle behaviours a client may exhibit that indicate sleep satisfaction.

    _____

    _____

Review Questions

Select the appropriate answer and cite the rationale for choosing that particular answer.

1. The 24-hour day–night cycle is known as the
   a. Circadian rhythm
   b. Infradium rhythm
   c. Ultradian rhythm
   d. Non-REM rhythm

   Answer: _____   Rationale: _____

   _____

   _____

2. Which of the following substances will promote normal sleep patterns?
   a. L-tryptophan
   b. Beta-blockers
   c. Alcohol
   d. Narcotics

   Answer: _____   Rationale: _____

   _____

   _____

3. All of the following are symptoms of sleep deprivation, except
   a. Hyperactivity
   b. Irritability
   c. Rise in body temperature
   d. Decreased motivation

   Answer: _____   Rationale: _____

   _____

   _____

4. Mrs. Phan complains of difficulty falling asleep, awakening earlier than desired, and not feeling rested. She attributes these problems to leg pain that is secondary to her arthritis. What would be the appropriate nursing diagnosis for her?
   a. *Sleep pattern disturbances related to arthritis*
   b. *Fatigue related to leg pain*
   c. *Knowledge deficit related to sleep hygiene measures*
   d. *Sleep pattern disturbances related to chronic leg pain*

   Answer: _____   Rationale: _____

   _____

   _____

5. A nursing care plan for a client with sleep problems has been implemented. All of the following would be expected outcomes except
   a. Client reports no episodes of awakening during the night.
   b. Client falls asleep within 1 hour of going to bed.
   c. Client reports satisfaction with amount of sleep.
   d. Client rates sleep as an 8 or above on the visual analogue scale.

   Answer: _____   Rationale: _____

   _____

   _____

Critical Thinking Model for Nursing Care Plan for Disturbed Sleep Pattern

Imagine that you are the nurse in the Care Plan on pages 1000–1001 of your text. Complete the *evaluation phase* of the critical thinking model by writing your answers in the appropriate boxes of the model shown. Think about the following:

- What knowledge did you apply in evaluating Julie's care?

- In what way might your previous experience influence your evaluation of Julie's care?

- During evaluation, what intellectual and professional standards were applied to Julie's care?

- In what way do critical thinking attitudes play a role in how you approach the evaluation of Julie's care plan?

- How might you evaluate Julie's care plan?

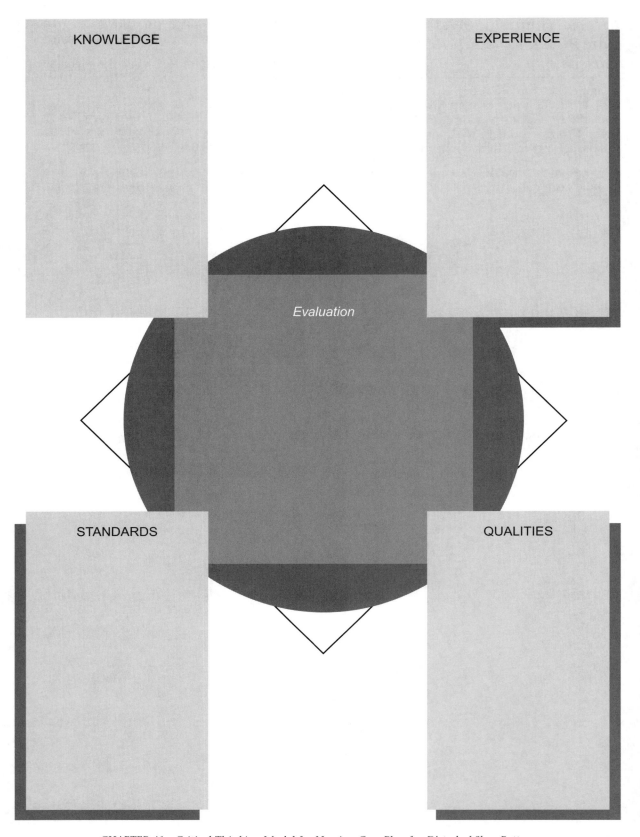

KNOWLEDGE

EXPERIENCE

Evaluation

STANDARDS

QUALITIES

CHAPTER 41   Critical Thinking Model for Nursing Care Plan for *Disturbed Sleep Pattern*
See answers on page 538.

42

Pain and Comfort

Preliminary Reading

Chapter 42, pp. 1009–1042

Comprehensive Understanding

1. Pain is subjective; no two people experience pain in the same way, and no two painful events create identical responses or feelings in a person.

2. Pain and pain management options are viewed within the context of comfort; providing comfort is central to nursing.

3. The relief from pain is considered a basic human right and is incorporated into the Canadian Pain Society's *Patient Pain Manifesto*.

Scientific Knowledge Base

Nature of Pain

4. Define *pain*.

   _____

   _____

Physiology of Pain

5. Explain the four processes of nociceptive pain.

   a. Transduction:

   _____

   _____

   b. Transmission:

   _____

   _____

   c. Perception:

   _____

   _____

   d. Modulation:

   _____

   _____

6. Explain the two types of neuroregulators.

   a. Neurotransmitters:

   _____

   _____

   b. Neuromodulators:

   _____

   _____

7. Identify the neurophysiological function of the following neuroregulators.

   a. Substance P:

   _____

   b. Prostaglandins:

   _____

   c. Serotonin:

   _____

   d. Endorphins:

   _____

   e. Bradykinin:

   _____

8. Explain the gate-control theory of pain.

   _____

   _____

   _____

9. List some physiological responses to pain.

   a. Sympathetic stimulation:

   1. _____

   2. _____

   3. _____

4. _____

5. _____

b. Parasympathetic stimulation:

1. _____

2. _____

3. _____

4. _____

5. _____

10. Identify four behavioural changes that characterize a client experiencing pain.

a. _____

b. _____

c. _____

d. _____

11. List four characteristics of acute pain.

a. _____

b. _____

c. _____

d. _____

12. Define *chronic pain*.

_____

_____

_____

Nursing Knowledge Base

Knowledge, Attitudes, and Beliefs

13. The medical model of illness describes pain as

_____

_____

_____

14. Identify common biases and misconceptions about pain.

_____

_____

_____

Factors Influencing Pain

15. Explain the developmental differences of the following clients' reaction to pain.

a. Young children:

_____

_____

b. Toddlers and preschoolers:

_____

_____

c. Older adults:

_____

_____

16. Identify five misconceptions about pain in older clients.

a. _____

b. _____

c. _____

d. _____

e. _____

17. Fatigue heightens the perception of pain. Explain.

_____

_____

_____

18. Explain how a client's neurological function can influence pain.

_____

_____

19. Give an example how each of the following influences pain.

a. Attention:

_____

_____

b. Previous experience:

_____

_____

c. Family and social support:

_____

_____

d. Spiritual factors:

_____

_____

20. Explain how the following psychological factors affect pain.

a. Anxiety:

_____

_____

b. Coping style:

_____

_____

c. Meaning of pain:

_____

_____

21. Explain how cultural factors affect pain.

_____

_____

_____

Nursing Process and Pain

22. Pain management extends beyond pain relief, encompassing the client's _____ _____ and ability to _____, _____, and _____ _____.

Assessment

23. For clients with an acute episode of pain, the nurse assesses and responds to the _____, _____, and _____ of the pain.

24. Assessment of chronic pain should focus on _____, _____, and _____ dimensions of the pain and on its history and context.

25. Explain what is meant by the pain assessment and management approach "ABCDE."

    A: _____

    B: _____

    C: _____

    D: _____

    E: _____

26. Identify examples of non-verbal expressions of pain.

_____

_____

_____

27. Cognitively impaired clients might require simple assessment approaches involving close observation of behaviour changes, especially movement.

28. Briefly explain the common characteristics of pain.

    a. Onset and duration:

    _____

    _____

b. Location:

_____

c. Intensity:

_____

_____

29. Describe the following descriptive scales for measuring the severity of pain.

    a. Numerical rating scale (NRS):

    _____

    _____

    b. Verbal descriptor scale (VDS):

    _____

    _____

    c. Visual analogue scale (VAS):

    _____

    _____

    d. FACES scale:

    _____

    _____

30. Identify some terms a client can use to describe the quality of his or her pain.

_____

_____

_____

31. Identify some measures a client may use to relieve pain.

_____

_____

_____

32. Identify some contributing symptoms that may make pain worsen.

_____

_____

_____

33. Summarize how pain affects the psychological well-being of the client.

_____

_____

_____

34. Give examples of the following behavioural indicators of pain.

    a. Vocalizations:

    _____

b. Facial expressions:

_____

c. Body movement:

_____

d. Social interaction:

_____

35. Explain how pain can influence activities of daily living in regard to the following.

a. Sleep:

_____

_____

b. Hygiene:

_____

_____

c. Sexual relations:

_____

_____

d. Employment:

_____

_____

e. Social activities:

_____

_____

Nursing Diagnosis

36. The nursing diagnosis focuses on the nature of the pain so that the nurse can identify the best interventions for relieving pain and minimizing its effect on the client's lifestyle and function.

37. List five potential or actual nursing diagnoses related to a client in pain.

a. _____

b. _____

c. _____

d. _____

e. _____

Planning

38. An intervention that works for one client will not work for all clients.

39. When developing a plan of care, the nurse selects priorities based on the client's level of pain and its effect on the client's condition.

40. List the client outcomes appropriate for the client experiencing pain.

a. _____

b. _____

c. _____

d. _____

e. _____

Implementation

Health Promotion

41. Teaching clients about the pain experience reduces anxiety and helps clients achieve a sense of control.

42. Describe how you would teach a child about a painful procedure.

_____

_____

_____

43. The Agency for Health Care Policy and Research (AHCPR) guidelines for acute pain management cite nonpharmacological interventions appropriate for clients who meet certain criteria. List those criteria.

a. _____

b. _____

c. _____

d. _____

e. _____

44. Briefly explain how relaxation lessens pain.

_____

_____

45. Briefly explain how the nurse would lead a client through guided imagery.

_____

_____

46. Briefly explain how the nurse would guide a client through progressive relaxation exercises.

_____

_____

47. Define *distraction*, and list one disadvantage and advantage of using distraction.

_____

_____

_____

48. Describe the effects of using music as a distraction to decrease pain.

_____

_____

_____

49. Define the following pain-relief measures and the rationale for their use.

a. Biofeedback:

_____

_____

b. Cutaneous stimulation:

_____

_____

c. Herbals:

_____

_____

d. Reducing pain perception:

_____

_____

50. What is TENS, and how is it believed to reduce pain?

_____

_____

Acute Care

51. Analgesics are the most common method of pain relief.

52. Identify the three types of analgesics and explain the conditions for which they are generally prescribed.

a. _____

b. _____

c. _____

53. One way to maximize pain relief while minimizing drug toxicity is to administer the medication on a(n) _____ basis, rather than on a(n) _____ basis.

54. Describe four major principles for analgesic administration.

a. _____

b. _____

c. _____

d. _____

55. Explain the benefits of patient-controlled analgesia (PCA).

_____

_____

56. Describe what a local anaesthetic is, how it may be applied, and possible side effects.

_____

_____

_____

57. Describe what a regional anaesthetic is and list three types.

a. _____

_____

b. _____

_____

c. _____

_____

58. Explain an advantage of epidural analgesia and how it is administered.

_____

_____

_____

59. Describe six goals of nursing care for a client with epidural infusions. Explain one intervention for each goal.

a. _____

_____

b. _____

_____

c. _____

_____

d. _____

_____

e. _____

_____

f. _____

_____

60. Explain the following surgical interventions for pain.

a. Dorsal rhizotomy:

_____

_____

b. Chordotomy:

_____

_____

61. Identify the three-step approach to cancer pain management recommended by the World Health Organization (1990).

    a. _____

    b. _____

    c. _____

62. Identify clients who are candidates for continuous infusions.

    a. _____

    b. _____

    c. _____

    d. _____

63. List four guidelines for safe administration of morphine sulfate via ambulatory infusion pumps.

    a. _____

    b. _____

    c. _____

    d. _____

Restorative and Continuing Care

64. Explain hospice programs.

    _____

    _____

Evaluation

Client Care

65. If a client continues to have discomfort after an intervention, a different approach may be needed. For example, if an analgesic provides only partial relief, the nurse may add relaxation exercises or guided-imagery exercises.

66. Pain assessment and responses to intervention should be accurately and thoroughly documented so that they can be communicated to others caring for the client.

Client Perceptions

67. The client, if able, is the best judge of whether pain-relief measures work.

68. The family often is another valuable resource, particularly in the case of the client with cancer who may not be able to express

discomfort during the latter stages of terminal illness.

Review Questions

Select the appropriate answer and cite the rationale for choosing that particular answer.

1. Pain is a protective mechanism warning of tissue injury and is largely a(n)
   a. Symptom of a severe illness or disease
   b. Subjective experience
   c. Objective experience
   d. Acute symptom of short duration

   Answer: _____   Rationale: _____

   _____

   _____

2. A substance that can cause analgesia when it attaches to opiate receptors in the brain is
   a. Substance P
   b. Serotonin
   c. Prostaglandin
   d. Endorphin

   Answer: _____   Rationale: _____

   _____

   _____

3. To adequately assess the quality of a client's pain, which question would be appropriate?
   a. "Tell me what your pain feels like."
   b. "Is your pain a crushing sensation?"
   c. "How long have you had this pain?"
   d. "Is it a sharp pain or a dull pain?"

   Answer: _____   Rationale: _____

   _____

   _____

4. The use of client distraction in pain control is based on the principle that
   a. Small C fibres transmit impulses via the spinothalamic tract.
   b. The reticular formation can send inhibitory signals to gating mechanisms.
   c. Large A fibres compete with pain impulses to close gates to painful stimuli.

d. Transmission of pain impulses from the spinal cord to the cerebral cortex can be inhibited.

Answer: _____ Rationale: _____

_____

_____

5. Teaching a child about painful procedures is best achieved by
   a. Early warnings of the anticipated pain
   b. Storytelling about the upcoming procedure
   c. Relevant play directed toward procedure activities
   d. Avoiding explanations until the pain is experienced

Answer: _____ Rationale: _____

_____

_____

Critical Thinking Model for Nursing Care Plan for Acute Pain

Imagine that you are the student nurse in the Care Plan on page 1027 of your text. Complete the *assessment phase* of the critical thinking model by writing your answers in the appropriate boxes of the model shown. Think about the following:

- What knowledge base was applied to Mrs. Mays?

- In what way might previous experience assist you in this case?

- What intellectual or professional standards were applied to the care of Mrs. Mays?

- What critical thinking attitudes did you use in assessing Mrs. Mays?

- As you review your assessment, what key areas did you cover?

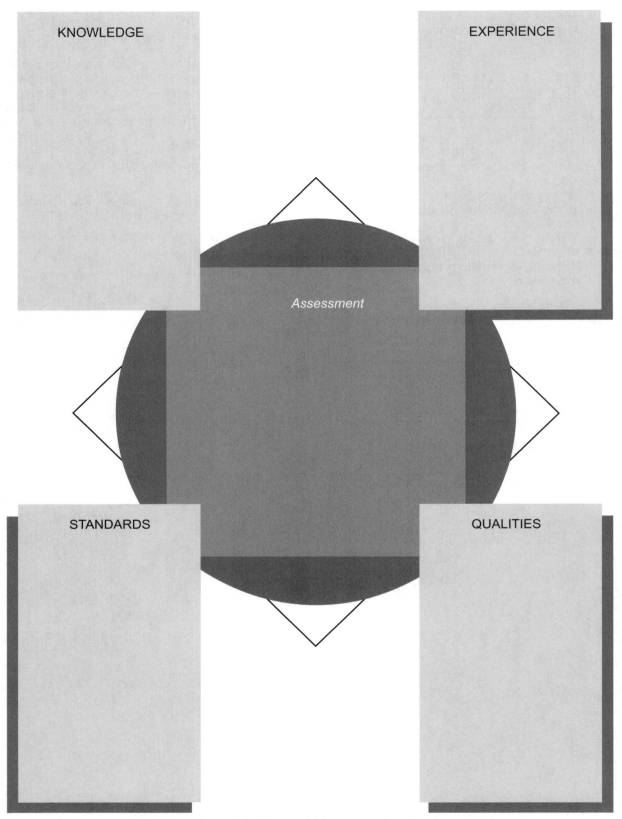

KNOWLEDGE

EXPERIENCE

Assessment

STANDARDS

QUALITIES

CHAPTER 42   Critical Thinking Model for Nursing Care Plan for *Acute Pain*
See answers on page 539.

43

Nutrition

Preliminary Reading

Chapter 43, pp. 1043–1096

Comprehensive Understanding

Scientific Knowledge Base

Nutrients: The Biochemical Units of Nutrition

1. The body requires fuel to provide energy for activities, building and repairing tissues, and regulating organs and systems.

2. Define the following terms.
    a. Basal metabolic rate (BMR):

    _____
    _____

    b. Resting energy expenditure (REE):

    _____
    _____

    c. Nutrients:

    _____
    _____

    d. Nutrient density:

    _____
    _____

3. List the six categories of nutrients.
    a. _____
    b. _____
    c. _____
    d. _____
    e. _____
    f. _____

Carbohydrates

4. Each gram of carbohydrate produces _____ ____ kilocalories (kcal).

5. Identify the three classifications of carbohydrates.
    a. _____
    b. _____
    c. _____

Proteins

6. Proteins are essential for _____ of body tissue in _____, _____, and _____.

7. The simplest form of protein is the _____.

8. Explain the two forms of protein.
    a. Essential amino acids:

    _____
    _____

    b. Non-essential amino acids:

    _____
    _____

9. Define the following terms.
    a. Complete protein:

    _____
    _____

    b. Incomplete protein:

    _____
    _____

    c. Complementary proteins:

    _____
    _____

10. Protein is the only major nutrient that contains _____ and is the only source of _____ for the body.

11. *Nitrogen balance* is

_____

_____

Fats

12. Fats (lipids) are the most calorically dense nutrient, providing _____ kilocalories per gram.

13. Describe the following composition of fats.

    a. Triglycerides:

    _____

    _____

    b. Fatty acids:

    _____

    _____

14. Define the following types of fatty acids and give an example of each.

    a. Saturated:

    _____

    _____

    b. Unsaturated:

    _____

    _____

    c. Monounsaturated:

    _____

    _____

    d. Polyunsaturated:

    _____

    _____

    e. Trans:

    _____

    _____

15. Define cholesterol and identify two sources of cholesterol.

    a. _____

    b. _____

Water

16. Water composes _____ of total body weight.

17. _____ have the greatest percentage of total body weight as water, and _____ _____ people have the least.

18. Fluid needs are met by ingesting _____ and _____, and by water produced during _____.

19. Identify the role of water in the body.

_____

_____

Vitamins

20. Vitamins are

_____

_____

_____

21. Identify the fat-soluble vitamins:

    a. _____

    b. _____

    c. _____

    d. _____

22. Identify the water-soluble vitamins:

    a. _____

    b. _____

23. Define *hypervitaminosis*.

_____

_____

_____

Minerals

24. Minerals are

_____

_____

_____

25. Minerals are classified as _____ when the daily requirement is 100 mg or more, and _____ or _____ when less than 100 mg is needed daily.

Anatomy and Physiology of the Digestive System

26. Digestion of food consists of the mechanical breakdown and chemical reactions by which food is reduced to its simplest form.

27. Enzymes are

_____

_____

28. The following activities of digestion are interdependent. Explain each one.

a. Mechanical:

_____

_____

b. Chemical:

_____

_____

c. Hormonal:

_____

_____

29. The major portion of digestion occurs in the

_____

_____

30. Define the following terms.

a. Peristalsis:

_____

_____

b. Dysphagia:

_____

_____

c. Chyme:

_____

_____

31. The primary absorption site of nutrients is the

_____

_____

32. The main source of water absorption is via the _____.

33. In addition to water, electrolytes and minerals are absorbed, and bacteria in the colon synthesize vitamins _____ and some _____.

34. *Metabolism* refers to

_____

_____

35. Describe the two types of metabolism.

a. Anabolism:

_____

_____

b. Catabolism:

_____

_____

36. Nutrient metabolism consists of three main processes. Explain each one.

a. Glycogenolysis:

_____

_____

b. Glycogenesis:

_____

_____

c. Gluconeogenesis:

_____

_____

37. Glycogen is synthesized from _____.

38. The body's major form of reserved energy is _____, which is stored as _____.

39. Feces contain

_____

_____

Dietary Guidelines

40. Explain dietary reference intakes (DRIs).

_____

_____

41. Define the four components to the DRIs.

a. _____

b. _____

c. _____

d. _____

42. Using the space below, diagram and label Canada's Food Guide.

43. List five dietary guidelines identified in *Eating Well with Canada's Food Guide*.

 a. _____
 _____

 b. _____
 _____

 c. _____
 _____

 d. _____
 _____

 e. _____
 _____

44. List the nutritional recommendations identified in *Eating Well with Canada's Food Guide*.

 a. _____
 _____

 b. _____
 _____

 c. _____
 _____

 d. _____
 _____

 e. _____
 _____

 f. _____
 _____

 g. _____
 _____

 h. _____
 _____

45. List the parts of a food label.

    a. _____

    b. _____

    c. _____

    d. _____

    e. _____

    f. _____

Nursing Knowledge Base

Nutrition During Human Growth and Development

Infants Through School-Age Children

46. An energy intake of approximately _____ _____ kcal/kg is needed in the first half of infancy, and _____ kcal/kg is needed in the second half.

47. A full-term newborn is able to digest and absorb _____, _____, and _____.

48. Infants need _____ mL/kg per day of fluid.

49. List at least four benefits for breastfeeding an infant.

    a. _____

    b. _____

    c. _____

    d. _____

50. Explain why the following should not be used in infant formula.

    a. Cow's milk:

    _____

    _____

    b. Honey:

    _____

    _____

51. The addition of solid foods to an infant's diet should be governed by the infant's

    a. _____

    b. _____

    c. _____

    d. _____

    e. _____

    f. _____

52. When should dental visits begin?

53. What practice puts children at risk for developing early childhood tooth decay? Why?

    _____

    _____

54. What is the role of parents in ensuring the dental health of their young child?

    _____

    _____

55. The toddler needs _____ kilocalories, but an increased amount of _____ in relation to body weight.

56. Identify examples of foods that have been implicated in the choking deaths of toddlers and preschoolers.

    _____

    _____

57. School-age children's diets should be assessed for

    _____

    _____

58. Explain some reasons for the increase in childhood obesity.

    _____

    _____

Adolescents

59. Identify the common nutritional deficiencies in the following adolescent population groups.

    a. Girls:

    _____

    _____

    b. Boys:

    _____

    _____

    c. Those who eat fast food:

    _____

    _____

    d. Pregnant women:

    _____

    _____

    e. Athletes:

    _____

    _____

60. Identify the diagnostic criteria for the following eating disorders.

a. Anorexia nervosa:

_____

_____

_____

b. Bulimia nervosa:

_____

_____

_____

Young and Middle-Aged Adults

61. Obesity may become a problem because of

_____

_____

62. Adult women who use oral contraceptives need extra

_____

63. The energy requirements of pregnancy are related to _____ and _____.

64. During pregnancy, supplementation is usually recommended along with dietary modification to increase intake of the following:

a. _____

b. _____

c. _____

d. _____

e. _____

65. During lactation, there is an increased need for vitamins _____ and _____.

Older Adults

66. List four factors that influence the nutritional status of the older adult.

a. _____

b. _____

c. _____

d. _____

Alternative Food Patterns

67. Briefly describe the vegetarian diet.

_____

_____

68. What knowledge is necessary to implement a healthy vegetarian diet?

_____

_____

_____

Nursing Process and Nutrition

69. Close daily contact with clients and their families enables nurses to make observations about their physical status, food intake, weight changes, and responses to therapy.

Assessment

70. Define the following terms.

a. Nutritional screening:

_____

_____

b. Body mass index (BMI):

_____

_____

c. Ideal body weight (IBW):

_____

_____

d. Anthropometry:

_____

_____

71. Describe how to obtain a waist circumference measurement.

_____

_____

_____

72. Identify the common laboratory tests used to study the nutritional status of a client.

_____

_____

73. List twelve components of a dietary history and provide a sample question for each.

a. _____

_____

b. _____

_____

c. _____

_____

d. _____

_____

e. _____

_____

f. _____

_____

g. _____

_____

h. _____

_____

i. _____

_____

j. _____

_____

k. _____

_____

l. _____

_____

74. For each assessment area, list at least two signs of good and poor nutrition.

a. General appearance

1. _____
2. _____

b. General vitality

1. _____
2. _____

c. Weight

1. _____
2. _____

d. Hair

1. _____
2. _____

e. Skin

1. _____
2. _____

f. Mouth, oral membranes

1. _____
2. _____

g. Gastrointestinal function

1.
2. _____

h. Cardiovascular function

1. _____
2. _____

i. Nervous system function

1. _____
2. _____

j. Muscles

1. _____
2. _____

75. Define the following terms:

a. Aspiration

_____

_____

b. Dysphagia

_____

_____

76. Which clients are at risk for aspiration?

_____

_____

77. Identify how the nurse checks swallow adequacy.

_____

_____

78. Describe the steps involved in an in-depth assessment for aspiration risk.

_____

_____

_____

79. Identify the warning signs of dysphagia.

_____

_____

Nursing Diagnosis

80. List three potential or actual nursing diagnoses for altered nutritional status.

a. _____
b. _____
c. _____

Planning

81. Nurses frequently collaborate with dietitians to ensure nutrition plans are appropriate and to learn how to obtain accurate data, for example, how to conduct calorie counts. A good care plan requires the accurate exchange of information between disciplines.

82. Provide an example of a goal and associated outcomes appropriate for a client with nutritional problems.

    Goal: _____
    _____

    Outcomes: _____
    _____

    a. _____
    b. _____
    c. _____
    d. _____

Implementation

Health Promotion

83. Clients can prevent _____ by incorporating knowledge of nutrition into their lifestyle.

84. Summarize menu planning and identify the factors that should be considered.

    _____
    _____
    _____

85. Describe the relationship between income and healthy eating.

    _____
    _____
    _____

86. List two examples of interventions to counter the threat to nutrition and health from lack of purchasing power.

    a. Individual level:

    _____
    _____

    b. Collective level:

    _____
    _____

87. Client education about food safety and reducing the risk of food-borne illnesses includes the following instructions:

    a. _____

b. _____
c. _____
d. _____
e. _____
f. _____
g. _____
h. _____
i. _____
j. _____

Acute Care

88. List three factors that can cause anorexia (loss of appetite) in acute care settings.

    a. _____
    b. _____
    c. _____

89. Identify factors that put clients at nutritional risk during hospitalizations.

    _____
    _____
    _____

90. Describe the following therapeutic diets.

    a. Clear Liquid:

    _____
    _____

    b. Thickened Liquid:

    _____
    _____

    c. Full Liquid:

    _____
    _____

    d. Pureed:

    _____
    _____

    e. Mechanical Soft:

    _____
    _____

    f. Soft or Low Residue:

    _____
    _____

    g. High Fibre:

    _____
    _____

h. Low Sodium:

_____

_____

i. Low Cholesterol:

_____

_____

j. Diabetic:

_____

_____

k. Regular:

_____

_____

91. List five ways in which you can promote appetite.

a. _____

b. _____

c. _____

d. _____

e. _____

92. List eight nursing interventions to assist dysphagic clients with feeding.

a. _____

b. _____

c. _____

d. _____

e. _____

f. _____

g. _____

h. _____

93. List six nursing measures to help clients retain comfort and a sense of independence in relation to their food intake.

a. _____

b. _____

c. _____

d. _____

e. _____

f. _____

Restorative and Continuing Care

94. Restorative care includes _____ _____ and _____ care in _____ and _____ settings.

Evaluation

95. Multidisciplinary collaboration remains essential in the provision of nutritional support.

Client Care

96. The effectiveness of nutritional interventions delivered by the health care team is based on meeting the client's _____ _____ and _____.

97. The client's ability to incorporate dietary changes into _____ _____ will ensure that outcome measures are successfully met.

Client Expectations

98. Clients expect competent and accurate care. The _____ must be altered if the outcomes are not being met.

Review Questions

Select the appropriate answer and cite the rationale for choosing that particular answer.

1. Which nutrient is the body's most preferred energy source?
   a. Protein
   b. Fat
   c. Carbohydrate
   d. Vitamin

   Answer: _____   Rationale: _____

   _____

   _____

2. Positive nitrogen balance would occur in which condition?
   a. Infection
   b. Starvation
   c. Burn injury
   d. Wound healing

   Answer: _____   Rationale: _____

   _____

   _____

3. Mrs. Schultz is talking with you about the dietary needs of her 23-month-old daughter, Anita. Which of the following responses would be appropriate?
   a. "Use skim milk to cut down on the fat in Anita's diet."
   b. "Anita should be drinking at least 720 mL of milk per day."

c. "Anita needs fewer calories in relation to her body weight now than she did as an infant."

d. "Anita needs less protein in her diet now because she isn't growing as fast."

Answer: _____   Rationale: _____

_____

_____

4. All of the following clients are at risk for alteration in nutrition except
   a. Client J, who is 86 years old, lives alone, and has poorly fitting dentures
   b. Client K, who has been NPO for seven days following bowel surgery and is receiving intravenous fluids
   c. Client L, whose weight is 10% above his ideal body weight
   d. Client M, a 17-year-old girl who weighs 40 kg and frequently complains about her baby fat

Answer: _____   Rationale: _____

_____

_____

5. To help counter childhood obesity, you should recommend which of the following for 9–11-year-olds?
   a. Consume 2–3 servings of fruit and vegetables daily
   b. Consume 2–3 servings of milk products daily
   c. Eliminate all fat from the daily diet
   d. Reduce the hours spent in front of the television

Answer: _____   Rationale: _____

_____

_____

6. The current diet of Aboriginal peoples is high in which of the following?
   a. Calcium
   b. Fibre
   c. Fat and sugar
   d. Fruit and vegetables

Answer: _____   Rationale: _____

_____

_____

Critical Thinking Model for Nursing Care Plan for Imbalanced Nutrition: Less Than Body Requirements

Imagine that you are Belinda, the nurse in the Care Plan on page 1066 of your text. Complete the *planning phase* of the critical thinking model by writing your answers in the appropriate boxes of the model shown. Think about the following:

• In developing Mrs. Cooper's plan of care, what knowledge did Belinda apply?

• In what ways might Belinda's previous experience assist in developing Mrs. Cooper's plan of care?

• When developing a plan of care for Mrs. Cooper, what intellectual and professional standards were applied?

• What critical thinking attitudes might have been applied in developing Mrs. Cooper's plan of care?

• How will Belinda accomplish these goals?

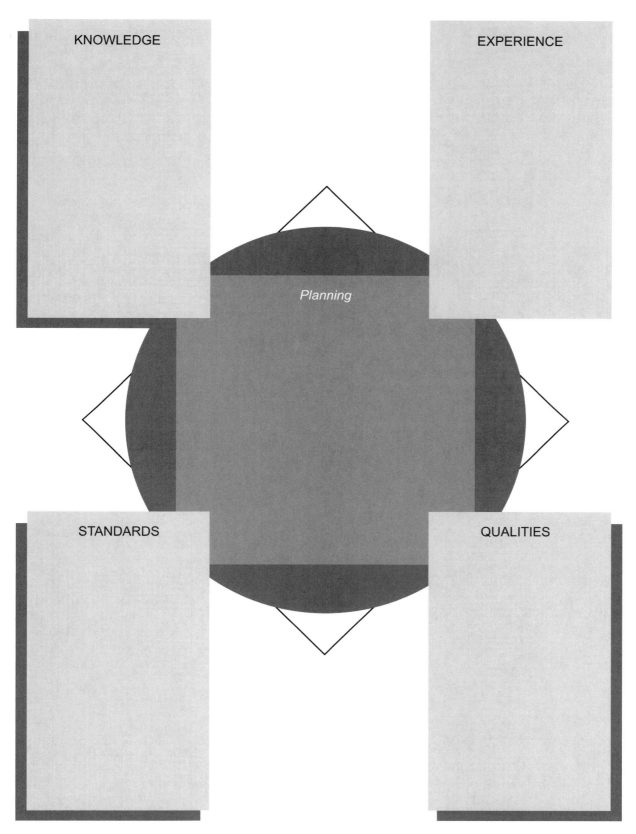

KNOWLEDGE

EXPERIENCE

Planning

STANDARDS

QUALITIES

CHAPTER 43   Critical Thinking Model for Nursing Care Plan for *Imbalanced Nutrition: Less Than Body Requirements*
See answers on page 540.

44

Urinary Elimination

Preliminary Reading

Chapter 44, pp. 1097–1140

Comprehensive Understanding

Scientific Knowledge Base

1. Summarize the function of each of the following organs in the urinary system.

   a. Kidneys:

   _____
   _____
   _____

   b. Ureters:

   _____
   _____
   _____

   c. Bladder:

   _____
   _____
   _____

   d. Urethra:

   _____
   _____
   _____

2. Define the following terms related to urine elimination.

   a. Nephron:

   _____
   _____

   b. Proteinuria:

   _____
   _____

   c. Erythropoietin:

   _____
   _____

   d. Renin:

   _____
   _____

   e. Micturition:

   _____
   _____

   f. Urethral meatus:

   _____
   _____

3. The ability of the urethra to maintain adequate closure is critical to continence.

4. Briefly describe how the following contribute to urethral closure.

   a. Smooth muscle:

   _____
   _____

   b. Striated muscle:

   _____
   _____

   c. Rhabdosphincter (urethral sphincter, external sphincter):

   _____
   _____

Act of Urination

5. Number the steps describing the normal act of micturition in sequential order.

    _____ The detrusor muscle contracts.

    _____ Urine volume stretches the bladder walls, sending impulses to the micturition centre in the spinal cord.

    _____ The urethral sphincter relaxes.

    _____ Impulses travel from the pontine micturition centre.

    _____ The bladder empties.

Factors Influencing Urination

6. Problems related to the act of urination may be of cognitive, functional, or physical origin, and may result in incontinence, retention, or infection.

7. Disease processes that primarily affect renal function (changes in urine volume or quality) are generally categorized as follows. Briefly explain each.

    a. Prerenal:

    _____

    _____

    b. Renal:

    _____

    _____

    c. Postrenal:

    _____

    _____

8. Define *oliguria*.

    _____

    _____

9. Define *anuria*.

    _____

    _____

10. List the characteristic signs of the uremic syndrome.

    _____

    _____

11. Briefly describe the two methods of dialysis.

    a. Peritoneal:

    _____

    _____

    b. Hemodialysis:

    _____

    _____

12. Identify some indications for dialysis.

    _____

    _____

13. Discuss how each of the following can impact urinary elimination.

    a. Cerebral vascular accident:

    _____

    _____

    b. Diabetes mellitus:

    _____

    _____

    c. Parkinson's disease:

    _____

    _____

    d. Alzheimer's disease:

    _____

    _____

    e. Rheumatoid arthritis:

    _____

    _____

14. Explain how the following affect the balance of urine excreted.

    a. Alcohol:

    _____

    _____

    b. Caffeine drinks:

    _____

    _____

    c. Peripheral edema:

    _____

    _____

    d. Febrile conditions:

    _____

    _____

15. List three types of medications that affect urination, and describe their major effect.

    a. _____

    b. _____

    c. _____

16. Explain how pelvic floor muscle tone affects urinary elimination.

   _____

   _____

17. Explain what a cystoscopy is and how it may affect urination.

   _____

   _____

18. Briefly explain how the stress of surgery affects urine output.

   _____

   _____

19. Briefly explain how anaesthetics and narcotic analgesics affect urine output.

   _____

   _____

Common Alterations in Urinary Elimination

20. Most clients with urinary problems have disturbances in the act of micturition that involve a failure to store urine, a failure to empty urine, or both. List the three most common alterations in urinary elimination.

   a. _____

   b. _____

   c. _____

21. Although many microorganisms may cause urinary tract infections (UTIs), the most frequent causative pathogen is _____.

22. Describe two host defence mechanisms specific to each of the following.

   a. Females:

   _____

   _____

   b. Males:

   _____

   _____

   c. Both females and males:

   _____

   _____

23. List six signs or symptoms of UTIs.

   a. _____

   b. _____

   c. _____

   d. _____

   e. _____

   f.

24. Identify the most common cause of UTIs.

   _____

25. List four risk factors for UTI in women.

   a. _____

   b. _____

   c. _____

   d. _____

26. Define the following terms related to UTIs.

   a. Bacteriuria:

   _____

   _____

   b. Dysuria:

   _____

   _____

   c. Hematuria:

   _____

   _____

   d. Pyelonephritis:

   _____

   _____

   e. Cystitis:

   _____

   _____

27. Explain why residual urine is a risk factor for UTIs.

   _____

   _____

28. Define *urinary incontinence*.

   _____

   _____

29. Briefly describe the major types of urinary incontinence.

   a. Transient:

   _____

   _____

   b. Urge:

   _____

   _____

   c. Stress:

   _____

   _____

d. Mixed:

_____

_____

e. Functional:

_____

_____

f. Overflow:

_____

_____

g. Reflex:

_____

_____

h. Total:

_____

_____

30. Explain the term *overactive bladder*.

_____

_____

31. Define *urinary retention*.

_____

_____

32. List five signs of urinary retention.
a. _____
b. _____
c. _____
d. _____
e. _____

33. Identify three indications for urinary diversions.
a. _____
b. _____
c. _____

34. Briefly describe the following urinary diversions.

a. Ileal loop or conduit:

_____

_____

b. Ureterostomy:

_____

_____

c. Nephrostomy:

_____

_____

Nursing Knowledge Base

35. You need to know concepts other than anatomy and physiology, such as infection control, hygiene measures, growth and development, and psychosocial influences.

36. Hospital-acquired UTIs are often related to _____, _____, or _____.

37. Briefly summarize the developmental changes that may influence urination.

_____

_____

_____

38. Identify the psychosocial and cultural factors that may influence urination.

_____

_____

Nursing Process and Alterations in Urinary Function

Assessment

39. List three factors to be explored when completing a health history related to urinary elimination.
a. _____
b. _____
c. _____

40. List five topics that should be included in a urinary diary.
a. _____
b. _____
c. _____
d. _____
e. _____

41. Describe the following symptoms of urinary alterations.

a. Incontinence:

_____

b. Urgency:

_____

c. Dysuria:

_____

d. Frequency:

_____

e. Hesitancy:

_____

f. Polyuria:

_____

g. Oliguria:

_____

h. Nocturia:

_____

i. Dribbling:

_____

j. Hematuria:

_____

k. Retention:

_____

l. Elevated postvoid residual urine:

_____

42. Briefly explain the four structures, organs, or both that you would assess to determine the presence and severity of urinary problems.

a. _____

b. _____

c. _____

d. _____

43. Assessment of urine involves _____ _____and_____ _____.

44. Describe the following characteristics of urine.

a. Colour:

_____

b. Clarity:

_____

c. Odour:

_____

45. Describe the following types of urine specimens collected for testing.

a. Random:

_____

_____

b. Clean-voided or midstream:

_____

_____

c. Sterile:

_____

d. Timed:

_____

_____

46. Common urine tests include the following. Briefly explain each.

a. Urinalysis:

_____

_____

b. Specific gravity:

_____

_____

c. Urine culture:

_____

_____

47. Briefly explain the following types of diagnostic examinations and give the nursing implications for each.

a. Abdominal roentgenogram:

_____

_____

b. Intravenous pyelogram (IVP):

_____

_____

c. Renal scan:

_____

_____

d. Computerized axial tomography (CT) scan:

_____

_____

e. Ultrasound:

_____

_____

48. List the three types of invasive diagnostic examinations and the nursing implications.

a. _____

_____

b. _____

_____

c. _____

_____

Nursing Diagnosis

49. List six potential or actual nursing diagnoses related to urinary elimination.

    a. _____

    b. _____

    c. _____

    d. _____

    e. _____

    f. _____

Planning

50. List two examples of goals appropriate for a client with a urinary elimination problem.

    _____

    _____

    _____

Implementation

Health Promotion

51. Maintaining regular patterns of urinary elimination can help prevent many urination problems. You should reinforce the importance of voiding regularly every _____ _____ to _____ hours during the day.

52. List three techniques that may be used to stimulate the micturition reflex.

    a. _____

    b. _____

    c. _____

53. List several food substances that can be irritating to the bladder mucosa.

    _____

    _____

54. Urine is normally acidic and tends to inhibit the growth of microorganisms. List four types of foods that increase urine acidity.

    a. _____

    b. _____

    c. _____

    d. _____

Acute Care

55. Briefly explain how you can help the hospitalized client maintain normal elimination habits.

    _____

    _____

    _____

56. List and explain three types of medications that can be used to treat incontinence or retention.

    a. _____

    b. _____

    c. _____

57. Briefly describe the following types of catheters.

    a. Straight:

    _____

    _____

    b. Foley:

    _____

    _____

    c. Coudé:

    _____

    _____

58. List three indications for each of the following.

    a. Short-term catheterization:

    _____

    _____

    b. Long-term catheterization:

    _____

    _____

    c. Intermittent catheterization:

    _____

    _____

59. Explain the following nursing measures taken to maintain client comfort, prevent infection, and maintain an unobstructed flow of urine in catheterized clients.

    a. Fluid intake:

    _____

    _____

    b. Perineal hygiene:

    _____

    _____

    c. Catheter care:

    _____

    _____

60. Briefly describe catheter irrigations and instillations.

    _____

    _____

    _____

61. Name two principles to follow when removing an in-dwelling catheter.

    a. _____

    b. _____

62. Briefly explain the two alternatives for urinary catheterization and give the nursing implications for each.

    a. Suprapubic catheterization:

       _____

       _____

    b. Condom catheterization:

       _____

       _____

63. Name two precautions that should be taken to ensure client safety and comfort when using a condom catheter.

    a. _____

    b. _____

64. List the nursing measures used to maintain skin integrity when urine comes in contact with the skin.

    a. _____

    b. _____

    c. _____

    d. _____

65. List comfort measures for a client with the following sources of discomfort.

    a. Inflamed tissues near urethral meatus:

       _____

       _____

    b. Painful distension:

       _____

       _____

Conservative Therapies to Restore Bladder Control and Promote Continence

66. List measures the nurse can teach the incontinent client to gain control over elimination.

    a. _____

    b. _____

    c. _____

    d. _____

    e. _____

    f. _____

    g. _____

    h. _____

    i.

    j. _____

    k. _____

67. Conservative therapies should be the first line of treatment because they are _____, have _____, and _____.

68. Describe three lifestyle modifications that can improve symptoms of UI.

    a. _____

    b. _____

    c. _____

69. Define *pelvic floor muscle exercises* (PFMEs or Kegel exercises) and list the types of incontinence for which they are generally indicated.

    _____

    _____

    _____

70. Describe a regimen of bladder training and the clients most likely to benefit.

    _____

    _____

    _____

71. Describe the behavioural therapies most appropriate for clients with cognitive impairment, physical impairment, or both.

    a. _____

    b. _____

Evaluation

Client Care

72. The client is the best source of evaluation of outcomes and responses to nursing care; however, the nurse also evaluates interventions through comparisons with baseline data.

73. You should evaluate for changes in the _____ _____, _____ _____, and _____.

Client Expectations

74. You need to confirm whether the client's expectations have been met to his or her full satisfaction.

75. You can also assist the client in redefining unrealistic goals when an impairment is not likely to be altered as completely as the client might like.

Review Questions

Select the appropriate answer and cite the rationale for choosing that particular answer.

1. All of the following factors will influence the production of urine except
   a. Poor pelvic floor muscle tone
   b. Acute renal disease
   c. Febrile conditions
   d. Diuretic medications

Answer: _____   Rationale: _____

_____

_____

2. Mrs. Rantz complains of a small amount of leaking urine when she coughs or laughs. This is known as
   a. Transient incontinence
   b. Stress incontinence
   c. Urge incontinence
   d. Reflex incontinence

Answer: _____   Rationale: _____

_____

_____

3. Ms. Worobetz has a urinary tract infection. Which of the following symptoms would you expect her to exhibit?
   a. Proteinuria
   b. Dysuria
   c. Oliguria
   d. Polyuria

Answer: _____   Rationale: _____

_____

_____

4. The nurse is working with a client who is having an intravenous pyelogram. Which of the following complaints by the client is an abnormal response?
   a. Shortness of breath and audible wheezing
   b. Feeling dizzy and warm with obvious facial flushing

   c. Thirst and feeling "worn out"
   d. Frequent, loose stools

Answer: _____   Rationale: _____

_____

_____

5. A postsurgical client who has recently had her in-dwelling catheter removed complains of feeling the urge to void every 20 to 30 minutes, but is only voiding small amounts. Which of the following behavioural therapies would be most appropriate?
   a. Habit retraining
   b. Prompted voiding
   c. Pelvic floor muscle exercise
   d. Bladder training

Answer: _____   Rationale: _____

_____

_____

Critical Thinking Model for Nursing Care Plan for Functional Urinary Incontinence

Imagine that you are Kay, the home care nurse in the Care Plan on page 1091 of your text. Complete the *assessment phase* of the critical thinking model by writing your answers in the appropriate boxes of the model shown. Think about the following:

- What knowledge base was applied to the care of Mrs. Grayson?

- In what way might Kay's previous experience assist in this case?

- What intellectual or professional standards were applied to Mrs. Grayson?

- What critical thinking attitudes did you utilize in assessing Mrs. Grayson?

- As you review the assessment, what key areas did Kay cover?

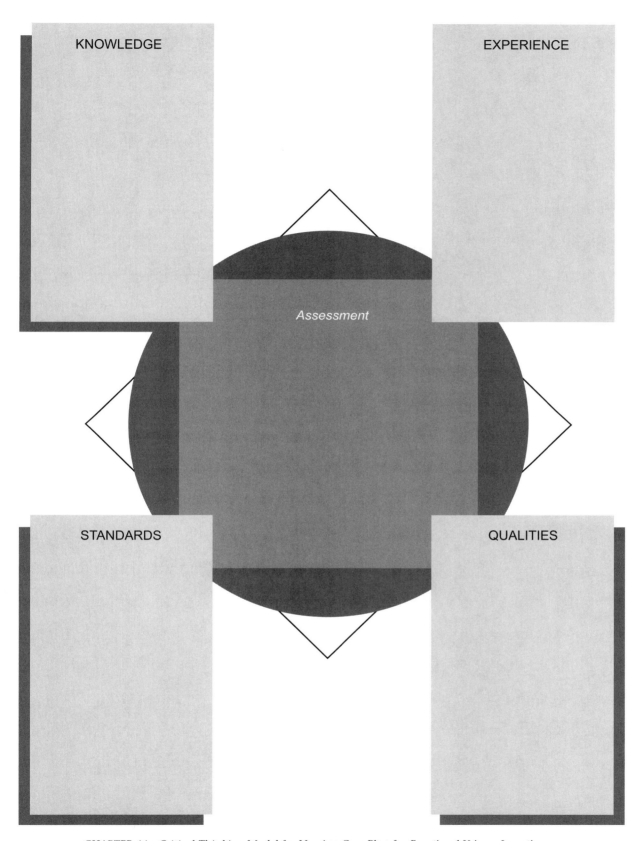

KNOWLEDGE

EXPERIENCE

Assessment

STANDARDS

QUALITIES

CHAPTER 44   Critical Thinking Model for Nursing Care Plan for *Functional Urinary Incontinence*
See answers on page 541.

45

Bowel Elimination

Preliminary Reading

Chapter 45, pp. 1141–1184

Comprehensive Understanding

Scientific Knowledge Base

1. The volume of fluids absorbed by the GI tract is high, making fluid and electrolyte balance a key function of the GI system.

2. Summarize the functions of the following.

   a. Mouth:

   _____

   _____

   b. Esophagus:

   _____

   _____

   c. Stomach:

   _____

   _____

   d. Small intestine:

   _____

   _____

   e. Large intestine:

   _____

   _____

3. Define the following terms and identify the portion of the GI tract to which they relate.

   a. Masticate:

   _____

   _____

   b. Bolus:

   _____

   _____

   c. Peristalsis:

   _____

   _____

   d. Chyme:

   _____

   _____

   e. Flatus:

   _____

   _____

   f. Feces:

   _____

   _____

4. Indicate the correct sequence of mechanisms involved in normal defecation.

   _____ Abdominal muscles contract, increasing intrarectal pressure.

   _____ The external sphincter relaxes.

   _____ The internal sphincter relaxes and awareness of the need to defecate occurs.

   _____ Movement in the left colon occurs, moving stool toward the anus.

5. Describe the Valsalva manoeuvre and the risk it poses to certain clients.

   _____

   _____

Nursing Knowledge Base

Factors Affecting Bowel Elimination

6. Briefly describe the normal elimination pattern of an infant.

   _____

   _____

7. List six changes that occur in the GI system of the older adult that impair normal digestion and elimination.

   a. _____

   b. _____

   c. _____

   d. _____

   e. _____

   f. _____

8. Identify the mechanisms that cause high-fibre diets to promote elimination.

   _____

   _____

9. List five types of foods that are considered high in fibre (bulk).

   a. _____

   b. _____

   c. _____

   d. _____

   e. _____

10. Define *lactose intolerance*.

   _____

   _____

11. Summarize how an inadequate intake of fluids can affect the character of feces.

   _____

   _____

12. Physical activity _____ peristalsis; immobilization _____ peristalsis.

13. Weakened abdominal and pelvic floor muscles impair the ability to _____ and to _____.

14. List two diseases of the GI tract that may be associated with stress.

   a. _____

   b. _____

15. List four personal elimination habits that influence bowel function.

   a. _____

   b. _____

   c. _____

   d. _____

16. Describe how the squatting position facilitates defecation.

   _____

   _____

17. List conditions that may result in painful defecation.

   a. _____

   b. _____

   c. _____

   d. _____

18. Identify the common problems related to defecation that occur during pregnancy and explain why they occur.

   _____

   _____

   _____

19. Summarize the effects of anaesthetic agents and peristalsis on defecation.

   _____

   _____

20. Describe the effect on elimination of each of the following medications.

   a. Mineral oil:

   _____

   _____

   b. Dicyclomine HCl (Bentyl):

   _____

   _____

   c. Narcotics:

   _____

   _____

   d. Anticholinergics:

   _____

   _____

   e. Antibiotics:

   _____

   _____

f. Histamines:

_____

_____

g. Nonsteroidal anti-inflammatory drugs:

_____

_____

21. List three types of diagnostic tests for visualization of GI structures.

a. _____

b. _____

c. _____

Common Bowel Elimination Problems

22. List five factors that place a client at risk for
elimination problems.

a. _____

b. _____

c. _____

d. _____

e. _____

23. Define *constipation*.

_____

_____

24. List and briefly describe four causes of
constipation.

a. _____

b. _____

c. _____

d. _____

25. List three groups of clients in whom
constipation could pose a significant health
hazard.

a. _____

b. _____

c. _____

26. Define *fecal impaction*.

_____

_____

27. List four signs and symptoms of fecal
impaction.

a. _____

b. _____

c. _____

d. _____

28. Define *diarrhea*.

_____

29. Name the two major complications associated with diarrhea.

a. _____

b. _____

30. List five conditions and the physiological
effects that cause diarrhea.

a. _____

b. _____

c. _____

d. _____

e. _____

31. Define *fecal incontinence*.

_____

_____

32. *Flatulence* results from _____
_____. It is a common cause
of _____, _____, and
_____.

33. Define *hemorrhoids*.

_____

_____

34. List four conditions that cause hemorrhoids.

a. _____

b. _____

c. _____

d. _____

Bowel Diversions

35. Define the following.

a. Stoma:

_____

_____

b. Ileostomy:

_____

_____

c. Colostomy:

_____

_____

36. The location of the ostomy determines the
consistency of the stool.

37. Briefly explain each of the following types
of colostomy construction.

a. Loop colostomy:

_____

_____

b. End colostomy:

_____

_____

c. Double-barrel colostomy:

_____

_____

38. Briefly describe the following surgical procedures that provide continence for selected colectomy clients.

a. Ileoanal pouch anastomosis:

_____

_____

b. Kock continent ileostomy:

_____

_____

39. Identify a major psychological concern of a client with an ostomy.

_____

_____

Nursing Process and Bowel Elimination

Assessment

40. List 16 factors affecting elimination that need to be included in a health history for clients with altered elimination status.

a. _____

b. _____

c. _____

d. _____

e. _____

f. _____

g. _____

h. _____

i. _____

j. _____

k. _____

l. _____

m. _____

n. _____

o. _____

p. _____

41. Summarize the following steps for assessing the abdomen.

a. Inspection:

_____

_____

b. Auscultation:

_____

_____

c. Palpation:

_____

_____

d. Percussion:

_____

_____

42. Summarize the assessment of the rectum.

_____

_____

_____

43. Briefly describe the appropriate technique for collecting a fecal specimen.

_____

_____

44. Define *fecal occult blood test (FOBT)*.

_____

_____

45. Describe the normal fecal characteristics.

a. Colour:

_____

_____

b. Odour:

_____

_____

c. Consistency:

_____

_____

d. Frequency:

_____

_____

e. Amount:

_____

_____

f. Shape:

_____

_____

g. Constituents:

_____

_____

46. Indicate the possible cause for each of the following fecal characteristics.

a. White or clay colour:

_____

_____

b. Black and tarry (melena):

_____

_____

c. Liquid consistency:

_____

_____

d. Narrow, pencil-shaped:

_____

_____

Nursing Diagnosis

47. List five potential or actual nursing diagnoses for a client with alterations in bowel elimination.

a. _____
b. _____
c. _____
d. _____
e. _____

Planning

48. List an example of a goal and five associated outcomes appropriate for clients with elimination problems.

a. _____
b. _____
c. _____
d. _____
e. _____

Implementation

Health Promotion

49. Explain how the following can assist the client to evacuate his or her bowels.

a. Sitting position:

_____

b. Positioning on the bedpan:

_____

_____

50. Explain the proper technique for positioning a client on a bedpan.

_____

_____

Acute Care

51. Identify the primary action of the following.

a. Cathartics:

_____

_____

b. Laxatives:

_____

_____

c. Antidiarrheals:

_____

_____

52. The primary reason for an enema is:

_____

_____

53. Briefly describe the following types of enemas.

a. Tap water:

_____

_____

b. Normal saline:

_____

_____

c. Soapsuds:

_____

_____

d. Hypertonic solution:

_____

_____

e. Oil-retention:

_____

_____

f. Carminative:

_____

_____

54. Explain the physician's order, "Give enemas until clear."

_____

_____

55. List three complications of digital removal of stool.

a. _____

b. _____

c. _____

56. List four reasons to insert a nasogastric (NG) tube for decompression.

a. _____

b. _____

c. _____

d. _____

57. Explain how the Salem sump tube works.

_____

_____

58. Explain how you would provide comfort to a client with an NG tube.

_____

_____

59. Explain how an NG tube can cause distention and how this can be prevented.

_____

_____

Continuing and Restorative Care

Care of Ostomies

60. List eight factors to consider when selecting a pouching system for a client.

a. _____

b. _____

c. _____

d. _____

e. _____

f. _____

g. _____

h. _____

61. Summarize the nutritional considerations for clients with ostomies.

_____

_____

62. Summarize the goals of a bowel-training program.

_____

_____

63. Briefly explain bowel training.

_____

_____

64. Describe two nursing interventions that promote comfort for clients who experience the following:

a. Hemorrhoids:

1. _____

2. _____

b. Risks to skin integrity:

1. _____

2. _____

Evaluation

Client Care

65. The effectiveness of care depends on success in meeting the goals and expected outcomes of care.

66. The client is the only one who is able to determine if the bowel elimination problems have been relieved and which therapies were the most effective.

Client Expectations

67. The client will relate a feeling of comfort and freedom from pain as elimination needs are met within the limits of the client's condition and treatment.

Review Questions

Select the appropriate answer and cite the rationale for choosing that particular answer.

1. Most nutrients and electrolytes are absorbed in the
   a. Esophagus
   b. Small intestine
   c. Colon
   d. Stomach

Answer: _____   Rationale: _____

_____

_____

2. Regarding diagnostic examinations involving visualization of the lower GI structures, all of the following are true except
   a. The client must drink fluids immediately before the test.

b. The client will likely receive a prescribed bowel preparation before the test.
c. The client is not allowed to eat or drink before the test.
d. Changes in elimination may occur following the procedure until normal eating patterns resume.

Answer: _____ Rationale: _____
_____
_____

3. Mrs. Ahmed is concerned about her breastfed infant's stool, stating that it is yellow instead of brown. The nurse explains that
a. A change to formula may be necessary.
b. Her infant is dehydrated and she should increase his fluid intake.
c. The stool is normal for an infant.
d. It will be necessary to send a stool specimen to the lab.

Answer: _____ Rationale: _____
_____
_____

4. After positioning a client on the bedpan, you should
a. Leave the head of the bed flat.
b. Raise the head of the bed 30 degrees.
c. Raise the head of the bed to a 90-degree angle.
d. Raise the bed to the highest working level.

Answer: _____ Rationale: _____
_____
_____

5. The physician has ordered a cleansing enema for 7-year-old Michael. The nurse calculates that the maximum volume to be given should be
a. 100 to 150 mL
b. 150 to 250 mL
c. 300 to 500 mL
d. 600 to 700 mL

Answer: _____ Rationale: _____
_____
_____

Critical Thinking Model for Nursing Care Plan for Constipation

Imagine that you are Javier, the nurse in the Care Plan on page 1137 of your text. Complete the *planning phase* of the critical thinking model by writing your answers in the appropriate boxes of the model shown. Think about the following:

- In developing Larry's plan of care, what knowledge did Javier apply?
- In what way might Javier's previous experience assist in developing a plan of care for Larry?
- When developing a plan of care, what intellectual and professional standards were applied?
- What critical thinking attitudes might have been applied in developing a plan for Larry?
- How will Javier accomplish the goals?

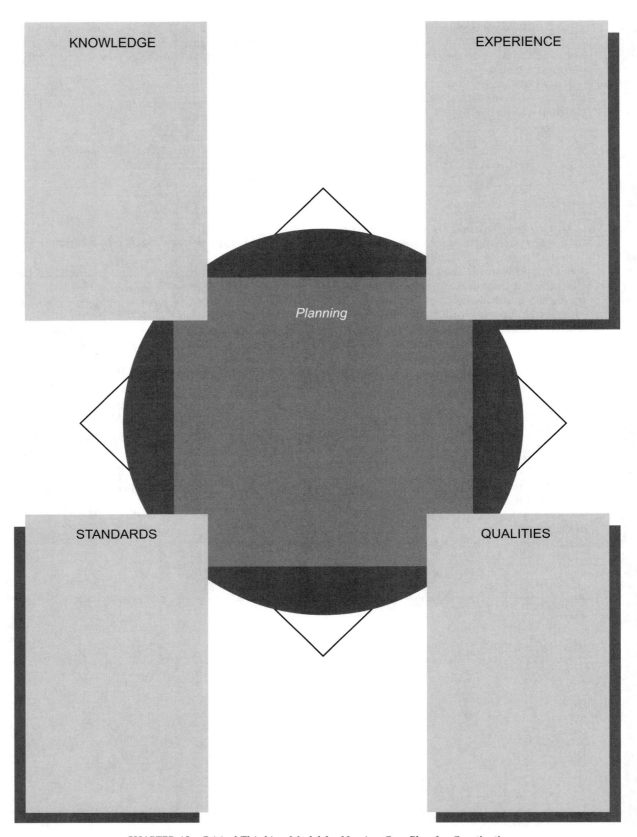

KNOWLEDGE

EXPERIENCE

Planning

STANDARDS

QUALITIES

CHAPTER 45 Critical Thinking Model for Nursing Care Plan for *Constipation*
See answers on page 542.

46

Mobility and Immobility

Preliminary Reading

Chapter 46, pp. 1185–1238

Comprehensive Understanding

1. *Mobility* refers to

_____

_____

Scientific Knowledge Base

Physiology and Principles of Body Mechanics

2. Define the following.

   a. Body mechanics:

   _____

   _____

   b. Body alignment or posture:

   _____

   _____

3. Balance is required for _____,
   for _____, and for _____.

4. The ability to balance can be compromised
   by many situations, such as

   _____

   _____

Gravity and Friction

5. Define *friction*.

   _____

   _____

6. List two techniques that minimize friction.

   a. _____

   b. _____

Regulation of Movement

7. List three systems responsible for coordinating body movements.

   a. _____

   b. _____

   c. _____

Pathological Influences on Mobility

8. Briefly explain how the following pathological conditions affect mobility.

   a. Postural abnormalities:

   _____

   _____

   b. Impaired muscle development:

   _____

   _____

   c. Damage to the central nervous system:

   _____

   _____

   d. Direct trauma to the musculoskeletal system:

   _____

   _____

9. Describe *pathological fractures*.

   _____

   _____

Nursing Knowledge Base

Mobility-Immobility

10. Define *bed rest*.

_____

_____

11. *Impaired physical mobility* is defined as

_____

_____

Systemic Effects of Immobility

12. When there is an alteration in mobility, each body system is at risk. Identify at least two hazards of immobility for each area.

   a. Metabolic changes:

      1. _____

      2. _____

   b. Respiratory changes:

      1. _____

      2. _____

   c. Cardiovascular changes:

      1. _____

      2. _____

   d. Musculoskeletal changes:

      1. _____

      2. _____

   e. Urinary elimination changes:

      1. _____

      2. _____

   f. Integumentary changes:

      1. _____

      2. _____

   g. Psychosocial effects:

      1. _____

      2. _____

Developmental Changes

13. Identify the descriptive characteristics of body alignment and mobility related to the following developmental stages.

   a. Infants:

_____

   b. Toddlers:

_____

   c. Preschoolers:

_____

   d. Adolescents:

_____

   e. Adults:

_____

   f. Older adults:

_____

Nursing Process for Impaired Body Alignment and Mobility

Assessment

14. Briefly describe the four major areas for assessment of client mobility.

   a. Range of motion:

_____

_____

   b. Gait:

_____

_____

   c. Exercise and activity tolerance:

_____

_____

   d. Body alignment:

_____

_____

15. Briefly describe the physiological hazards of immobility in relation to the following systems.

   a. Metabolic:

_____

_____

   b. Respiratory:

_____

_____

   c. Cardiovascular:

_____

_____

   d. Musculoskeletal:

_____

_____

e. Integumentary:

_____

_____

f. Elimination:

_____

_____

16. Briefly describe the hazards of immobility in hospitalized older adults.

a. Musculoskeletal:

_____

_____

b. Elimination:

_____

_____

c. Nutrition:

_____

_____

d. Psychosocial:

_____

_____

Nursing Diagnosis

17. List six actual or potential nursing diagnoses related to an immobilized or partially immobilized client.

a. _____

b. _____

c. _____

d. _____

e. _____

f. _____

Planning

18. The nurse plans therapies according to the severity of risks to the client, and the plan is individualized according to the client's _____, _____, and _____.

Implementation

Health Promotion

19. Many health care agencies have a "no-lift" policy, whereby manual lifting of the whole or a large part of the weight of the client by a health care worker is prohibited except in exceptional or life-threatening situations. Therefore, you should not attempt to lift a client without assistance unless the client is a _____ _____ or a _____.

20. List alternatives to manual lifting.

a. _____

b. _____

c. _____

21. Briefly explain the benefits of exercise.

_____

_____

Acute Care

22. Identify two nursing interventions to meet each of the following goals for the immobilized client.

a. Maintain optimal nutritional (metabolic) state:

1. _____
2. _____

b. Promote expansion of the chest and lungs:

1. _____
2. _____

c. Prevent stasis of pulmonary secretions:

1. _____
2. _____

d. Maintain a patent airway:

1. _____
2. _____

e. Reduce orthostatic hypotension:

1. _____
2. _____

f. Reduce cardiac workload:

1. _____
2. _____

g. Prevent thrombus formation:

1. _____
2. _____

h. Maintain muscle strength and joint mobility:

1. _____
2. _____

i. Maintain normal elimination patterns:

1. _____

2. _____

j. Prevent pressure ulcers:

1. _____

2. _____

k. Maintain usual psychosocial state:

1. _____

2. _____

23. Identify two nursing interventions for the immobilized child.

a. _____

b. _____

Positioning Devices and Techniques

24. List some general guidelines to apply in any transfer procedure.

_____

_____

25. List four areas the nurse needs to consider in determining if assistance is required when moving a client in bed.

a. _____

b. _____

c. _____

d. _____

Restorative Care

26. The goal of restorative care for the immobile client is to

_____

_____

27. Instrumental activities of daily living (IADLs) are

_____

_____

Joint Mobility

28. Indicate the type of joint and range-of-motion exercises for the body parts listed in the table below.

Body Part	Type of Joint	Type of Movement
Neck		
Shoulder		
Elbow		
Forearm		
Wrist		

(Continued)

Body Part	Type of Joint	Type of Movement
Fingers and thumb		
Hip		
Knee		
Ankle and foot		
Toes		

Walking

29. Identify the steps you should take to prepare to assist a client to walk.

_____

_____

30. Describe how you would assist clients with hemiplegia or hemiparesis in walking.

_____

_____

31. The nurse, in collaboration with others, promotes activity and exercise by teaching the use of assistive devices most appropriate for a client's condition. Briefly explain the appropriate use of the following.

a. Canes:

_____

_____

b. Crutches:

_____

_____

c. Walkers:

_____

_____

32. Explain the following crutch gaits.

a. Four-point:

_____

_____

b. Three-point:

_____

_____

c. Two-point:

_____

_____

d. Swing-through:

_____

_____

33. Explain how you would instruct the client in each of the following.

a. Crutch walking on stairs:

_____

_____

b. Sitting in the chair with crutches:

_____

_____

Evaluation

Client Care

34. To evaluate outcomes, the nurse measures the effectiveness of all interventions. The actual outcomes are compared with the outcomes selected during planning.

35. The optimal outcomes are the client's ability to maintain or improve body alignment and joint mobility.

Client Expectations

36. Client expectations evaluate care from the client's perspective.

Review Questions

Select the appropriate answer and cite the rationale for choosing that particular answer.

1. The nurse would expect all of the following physiological effects of exercise on the body systems except
   a. Decreased cardiac output
   b. Increased respiratory rate and depth
   c. Increased muscle tone, size, and strength
   d. Change in metabolic rate

   Answer: _____   Rationale: _____
   _____
   _____

2. Which of the following is a potential hazard for which you should assess when the client is in the prone position?
   a. Unprotected pressure points at the sacrum and heels
   b. Internal rotation of the shoulder
   c. Increased cervical flexion
   d. Plantar flexion

   Answer: _____   Rationale: _____
   _____
   _____

3. Which of the following is a physiological effect of prolonged bed rest?
   a. A decrease in urinary excretion of nitrogen
   b. An increase in cardiac output
   c. A decrease in lean body mass
   d. A decrease in lung expansion

   Answer: _____   Rationale: _____
   _____
   _____

4. All of the following measures are used to assess for deep vein thrombosis except
   a. Measuring the circumference of each leg daily, placing the tape measure at the midpoint of the knee
   b. Observing the dorsal aspect of lower extremities for redness, warmth, and tenderness
   c. Asking the client about the presence of calf pain
   d. Checking for a positive Homans' sign, if not contraindicated

   Answer: _____   Rationale: _____
   _____
   _____

5. Which of the following is *not* true of the two-point gait with crutches?
   a. The client requires at least partial weight bearing on each foot.
   b. The client is required to bear all of the weight on one foot.
   c. The client moves one crutch at the same time as the opposing leg.
   d. Crutch movements are similar to arm motion during normal walking.

   Answer: _____   Rationale: _____
   _____
   _____

6. Which of the following is an appropriate intervention to maintain the respiratory system of the immobilized client?
   a. Turn the client every 4 hours.
   b. Maintain a maximum fluid intake of 1500 mL per day.
   c. Apply and maintain an abdominal binder.
   d. Encourage the use of an incentive spirometer.

Answer: _____   Rationale: _____
_____
_____

Critical Thinking Model for Nursing Care Plan for Impaired Physical Mobility

Imagine that you are the student nurse in the Care Plan on pages 1181–1182 of your text. Complete the *evaluation phase* of the critical thinking model by writing your answers in the appropriate boxes of the model shown. Think about the following:

- What knowledge did you apply in evaluating Ms. Adams's care?

- In what way might your previous experience influence your evaluation of Ms. Adams?

- During evaluation, what intellectual and professional standards were applied to Ms. Adams's care?

- In what ways do critical thinking attitudes play a role in how you approach evaluation of Ms. Adams's care?

- How might you adjust Ms. Adams's care?

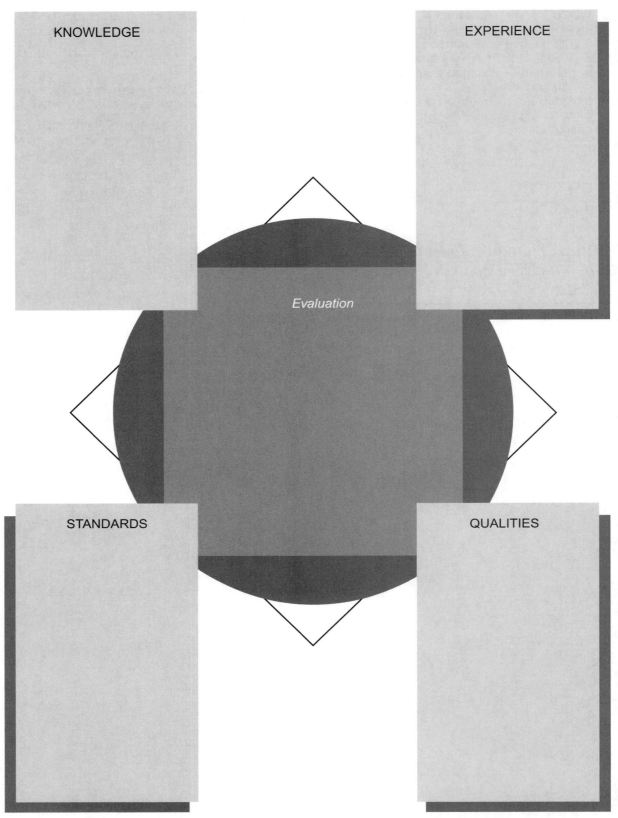

CHAPTER 46   Critical Thinking Model for Nursing Care Plan for *Impaired Physical Mobility*
See answers on page 543.

47

Skin Integrity and Wound Care

Preliminary Reading

Chapter 47, pp. 1239–1289

Comprehensive Understanding

Scientific Knowledge Base

Skin

1. Describe the function of each of the following layers of skin.

   a. Epidermis:

   _____

   _____

   b. Dermis:

   _____

   _____

   c. Subcutaneous tissue:

   _____

   _____

Pressure Ulcers

2. Define *pressure ulcer*.

   _____

   _____

3. Identify the pressure factors that contribute to pressure ulcer development.

   a. _____

   _____

   b. _____

   _____

   c. _____

   _____

4. Define the following.

   a. Erythema:

   _____

   _____

   b. Blanching:

   _____

   _____

5. Explain the difference between normal reactive hyperemia and abnormal reactive hyperemia. Indicate which of the two is a sign of deep tissue damage.

   _____

   _____

Nursing Knowledge Base

Prediction and Prevention of Pressure Ulcers

6. You should assess the skin for signs of pressure ulcers at least _____; however, high-risk clients will need more frequent skin assessments.

7. Briefly explain how the following factors contribute to an increased risk for pressure ulcers.

   a. Impaired mobility:

   _____

   _____

   b. Altered level of consciousness:

   _____

   _____

c. Impaired sensory perception:

_____
_____

d. Friction:

_____
_____

e. Shear:

_____
_____

f. Moisture:

_____
_____

g. Nutrition:

_____
_____

h. Tissue perfusion:

_____
_____

i. Infection

_____
_____

j. Pain

_____
_____

k. Advanced age:

_____
_____

8. Identify the factors that may affect the client's perception of the wound.

_____
_____

Nursing Process

Assessment

Risk Assessment

9. Explain what factors should be considered in each of the four areas when assessing skin integrity:

a. Sensation:

_____
_____

b. Mobility:

_____
_____

c. Continence:

_____
_____

d. Presence of a wound:

_____
_____

Braden Scale

10. List the six categories of the Braden Scale used to predict for pressure ulcer risk.

a. _____
b. _____
c. _____
d. _____
e. _____
f. _____

Classification of Pressure Ulcers

11. A pressure ulcer is classified in stages according to its severity. Briefly describe the staging system devised by the National Pressure Ulcer Advisory Panel.

a. Suspected Deep Tissue Injury:

_____
_____

b. Stage I:

_____
_____

c. Stage II:

_____
_____

d. Stage III:

_____
_____

e. Stage IV:

_____
_____

f. Unstageable:

_____
_____

Wound Classification

12. Describe the physiological process involved with wound healing.
    a. Primary intention:

    _____

    _____

    _____

    b. Secondary intention:

    _____

    _____

    _____

    c. Tertiary intention:

    _____

    _____

    _____

13. Explain the three components involved in the healing of a partial-thickness wound.
    a. _____

    _____

    b. _____

    _____

    c. _____

    _____

14. Explain the three phases involved in the healing of a full-thickness wound.
    a. Inflammatory phase:

    _____

    _____

    b. Proliferative phase:

    _____

    _____

    c. Remodelling:

    _____

    _____

Process of Wound Healing

15. Depending on the nature of the wound, wounds heal by either primary intention or secondary intention. Explain.
    a. Primary intention:

    _____

    _____

    b. Secondary intention:

    _____

Wound Repair

16. Explain the three phases of full-thickness wound repair.
    a. Inflammatory phase:

    _____

    _____

    b. Proliferative phase:

    _____

    _____

    c. Remodelling phase:

    _____

    _____

17. Briefly describe the etiology of and two main treatment points to consider for each type of wound listed below.
    a. Skin tear

    _____

    _____

    _____

    b. Malignant or fungating wound

    _____

    _____

    _____

    c. Venous ulcer

    _____

    _____

    _____

    d. Arterial ulcer

    _____

    _____

    e. Diabetic ulcer

    _____

    _____

    _____

    f. Acute or surgical wound

    _____

    _____

    _____

18. Describe the four major types of wound drainage (*exudate*).

    a. _____

    b. _____

    c. _____

    d. _____

19. What is the purpose of obtaining a wound culture?

    _____

    _____

20. Describe the method of obtaining a wound culture.

    _____

    _____

    _____

Complications of Wound Healing

21. Briefly explain the following complications of wound healing.

    a. Hemorrhage:

       _____

       _____

       _____

    b. Infection:

       _____

       _____

       _____

    c. Dehiscence:

       _____

       _____

       _____

    d. Evisceration:

       _____

       _____

       _____

    e. Fistulas:

       _____

       _____

       _____

22. What are the characteristics of wound infection?

    a. _____

    b. _____

    c. _____

    d. _____

    e. _____

Nursing Diagnosis

23. List three nursing diagnoses related to impaired skin integrity.

    a. _____

    b. _____

    c. _____

Planning

24. List six possible goals for the client at risk for pressure ulcers.

    a. _____

    b. _____

    c. _____

    d. _____

    e. _____

    f. _____

Collaborative Care

25. List information that should be provided when a client is discharged or moves to another care setting.

    a. _____

    b. _____

    c. _____

    d. _____

    e. _____

    f. _____

    g. _____

    h. _____

    i. _____

Implementation: Preventing Skin Breakdown

26. Briefly explain the following nursing interventions for the prevention of pressure ulcers.

    a. Topical skin care:

       _____

       _____

    b. Positioning:

       _____

       _____

    c. Support surfaces (therapeutic beds and mattresses):

       _____

       _____

d. Nutrition:

_____

_____

e. Education:

_____

_____

f. Management of pressure ulcers:

_____

_____

Wound Management

27. Prevention of wound infection includes wound cleansing and removal of nonviable tissue (debridement).

28. List and explain three principles to follow when cleansing a wound or the area around a drain.

a. _____

b. _____

c. _____

29. _____ is a common method of delivering the wound cleansing solution to the wound and removing debris.

30. Irrigation of an open wound requires _____ _____ technique.

31. Describe the following methods of debridement.

a. Mechanical:

_____

_____

b. Autolytic:

_____

_____

c. Surgical:

_____

_____

Dressings

32. List the purposes for dressings.

a. _____

b. _____

c. _____

d. _____

e. _____

f. _____

g. _____

33. List the clinical guidelines to use when selecting the appropriate dressing.

a.

b. _____

c. _____

d. _____

e. _____

f. _____

34. Briefly describe the following types of dressings and their uses.

a. Woven gauze:

_____

_____

b. Self-adhesive, transparent film:

_____

_____

c. Hydrocolloid:

_____

_____

d. Hydrogel:

_____

_____

e. Calcium alginate:

_____

_____

f. Composite:

_____

_____

g. Foam:

_____

_____

h. Hypertonic sodium:

_____

_____

i. Soft silicone:

_____

_____

j. Silver:

_____

_____

k. Cadexomer iodine:

_____

_____

l. Negative pressure wound therapy (NPWT):

_____

_____

35. To prepare for a dressing change, you must know _____, _____ _____, and _____.

36. Dressings over closed wounds should be removed or changed when they _____ _____ or the client _____.

37. List the activities you would perform to prepare a client for a dressing change.

a. _____

b. _____

c. _____

d. _____

e. _____

38. The first step in packing a wound is to assess the _____, _____, and _____ _____ of the wound.

39. Summarize the principles of packing a wound.

_____

_____

_____

40. A dressing may be secured by _____, ___ _____, _____, or _____ _____.

Surgical or Traumatic Wound Considerations

41. Summarize the nursing responsibilities for suture care.

_____

_____

42. The most important principle in suture removal is to

_____

_____

Drainage Evacuation

43. Explain the purpose for drainage evacuation.

_____

_____

Bandages and Binders

44. Explain how bandages and binders applied over or around dressings provide extra protection and therapeutic benefits.

a. _____

b. _____

c. _____

45. List the nursing responsibilities when applying a bandage or binder.

a. _____

b. _____

c. _____

d. _____

46. Describe the abdominal binder.

_____

_____

Evaluation

47. Nursing interventions for wound care and reducing the risk of pressure ulcers are evaluated by determining the client's response to nursing therapies and by determining whether each goal was achieved.

48. The optimal outcomes are to _____, _____, and _____ _____.

Review Questions

Select the appropriate answer and cite the rationale for choosing that particular answer.

1. Ischemia is defined as
   a. Increased tissue buildup during the healing process
   b. A reduction of blood flow to the tissues
   c. Decreased fluid to the tissues
   d. Increased irritability of nerves

Answer: _____   Rationale: _____

_____

_____

2. Mr. Prada is in a Fowler's position to improve his oxygenation status. You note that he frequently slides down in the bed and needs to be repositioned. Mr. Prada is at risk for developing a pressure ulcer on his coccyx because of
   a. Friction
   b. Shearing force
   c. Maceration
   d. Impaired peripheral circulation

Answer: _____   Rationale: _____

_____

_____

3. Which of the following is not a subscale on the Braden Scale for predicting pressure ulcer risk?
   a. Age
   b. Sensory perception
   c. Moisture
   d. Activity

Answer: _____ Rationale: _____

_____

_____

4. Which of the following clients has a nutritional risk for pressure ulcer development?
   a. Client A has a serum albumin level of 37 g/L.
   b. Client B has a lymphocyte count of 2000/mm^3.
   c. Client C has a body mass index of 17.
   d. Client D has a body weight that is 5% greater than his ideal weight.

Answer: _____ Rationale: _____

_____

_____

5. Mrs. Tootoosis is an immobilized client. Which of the following will *not* increase her risk of developing a pressure ulcer?
   a. She has unrelieved pressure to her hip of greater than 32 mm Hg.
   b. After being turned to her side, she displays normal reactive hyperemia on her coccyx that lasts for 5 minutes.
   c. She has low-intensity pressure over a long period to her heels as a result of elastic stockings.
   d. She is positioned so that she has an unequal distribution of body weight.

Answer: _____ Rationale: _____

_____

_____

6. Mr. Wong has a stage II ulcer of his right heel. What would be the most appropriate treatment for this ulcer?
   a. Apply a thick layer of enzymatic ointment to the ulcer and the surrounding skin.
   b. Apply a calcium alginate dressing and change when strikethrough is noted.
   c. Apply a heat lamp to the area for 20 minutes twice daily.
   d. Apply a hydrocolloid dressing and change it as necessary.

Answer: _____ Rationale: _____

_____

_____

Critical Thinking Model for Impaired Skin Integrity

Imagine that you are the student nurse in the Critical Thinking Exercise on page 1264 of your text. Complete the *assessment phase* of the critical thinking model by writing your answers in the appropriate boxes of the model shown. Think about the following:

- What knowledge base was applied to Mrs. Stein?
- In what way might your previous experience assist you in this case?
- What intellectual or professional standards were applied to Mrs. Stein?
- What critical thinking attitudes did you use in assessing Mrs. Stein?
- As you review your assessment, what key areas did you cover?

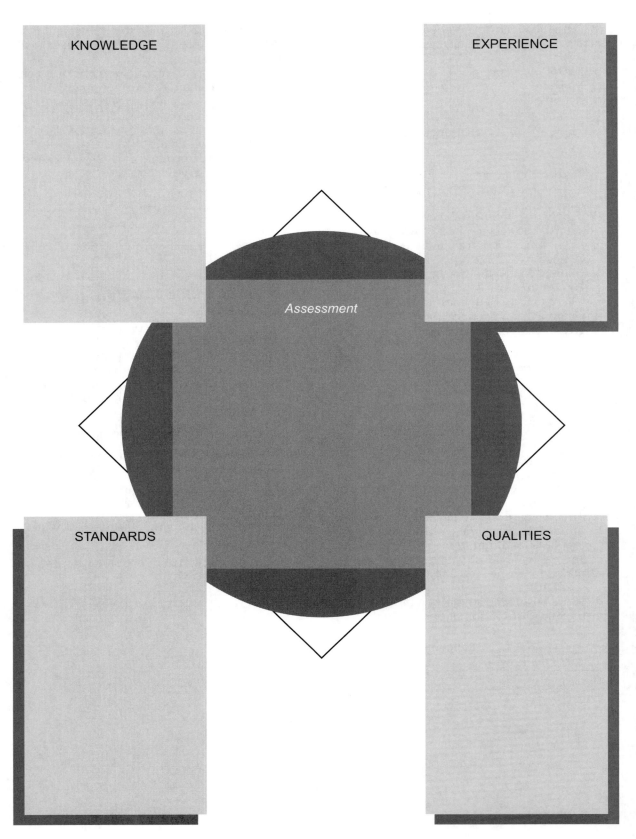

CHAPTER 47   Critical Thinking Model for *Impaired Skin Integrity*
See answers on page 544.

48

Sensory Alterations

Preliminary Reading

Chapter 48, pp. 1290–1311

Comprehensive Understanding

1. Define *stereognosis*.

   _____
   _____

Scientific Knowledge Base

Normal Sensation

2. List and briefly explain the three functional components necessary for any sensory experience.

   a. _____
   b. _____
   c. _____

Sensory Alterations

3. The types of sensory alterations commonly seen by the nurse are _____, _____, and _____,

4. Define *sensory deficit*.

   _____
   _____

5. For each of the following, describe a disease or condition that may cause it.

   a. Visual deficit:

   _____
   _____

   b. Hearing deficit:

   _____
   _____

   c. Balance deficit:

   _____
   _____

   d. Taste deficit:

   _____
   _____

   e. Neurological deficit:

   _____
   _____

6. List the three major types of sensory deprivation and give an example of each.

   a. _____
   b. _____
   c. _____

7. Define *sensory overload*.

   _____
   _____

8. Identify the behavioural changes that are associated with sensory overload.

   _____
   _____

Nursing Knowledge Base

Factors Affecting Sensory Function

9. Explain how and why the following factors affect sensory function.

   a. Age:

   _____
   _____

b. Quality of stimuli:

_____

_____

c. Quantity of stimuli:

_____

_____

d. Social interaction:

_____

_____

e. Family factors:

_____

_____

f. Environmental factors:

_____

_____

Nursing Process

Assessment

10. The nurse collects a history that assesses the client's current sensory status and the degree to which a sensory deficit affects the client's
_____, _____, _____
_____, _____, and
_____.

11. When assessing the client's mental status, you need to evaluate each of the following. Give an example of each.

a. Physical appearance and behaviour:

_____

_____

b. Cognitive ability:

_____

_____

c. Emotional status:

_____

_____

12. Complete the grid that follows by describing at least one assessment technique for the identified sensory function and the behaviours for an adult and child that would indicate a sensory deficit.

Sense	Assessment Technique	Child Behaviour	Adult Behaviour
Vision			
Hearing			
Touch			
Smell			
Taste			
Position sense			

13. Give an example of an assessment for the following that might assist you in deciding if the client has a sensory alteration.

   a. Ability to perform self-care:

_____
_____

   b. Health promotion habits:

_____
_____

   c. Hazards:

_____
_____

14. Define the following types of aphasia.

   a. Expressive:

_____
_____

   b. Receptive:

_____
_____

   c. Global:

_____
_____

Nursing Diagnosis

15. List six actual or potential nursing diagnoses that might apply to a client with sensory alterations.

   a. _____
   b. _____
   c. _____
   d. _____
   e. _____
   f. _____

Planning

16. List an example of a goal and four associated outcomes appropriate for a client with a sensory alteration.

   a. _____
   b. _____
   c. _____
   d. _____
   e. _____

Implementation

Health Promotion

17. List the three recommended vision screening interventions.

   a. _____
   b. _____
   c. _____

18. The most common visual problem is

_____
_____

19. Explain how hearing loss can be caused by exposure to excessive noise.

_____
_____

20. Identify the common injuries due to trauma that result in hearing or vision loss in both adults and children.

   a. Adults:

_____
_____

   b. Children:

_____
_____

21. Explain the measures to take to ensure that assistive devices being used help maintain sensory function at the highest level.

_____
_____
_____

22. Briefly explain how the nurse can promote meaningful stimulation for clients with sensory alterations in the following areas.

   a. Vision:

_____
_____

   b. Hearing:

_____
_____

   c. Taste and smell:

_____
_____

   d. Touch:

_____
_____

23. List three methods of establishing a safe environment with regard to the following adaptations.

    a. Visual loss:

        1. _____

        2. _____

        3. _____

    b. Reduced hearing:

        1. _____

        2. _____

        3. _____

    c. Reduced olfaction:

        1. _____

        2. _____

        3. _____

    d. Reduced tactile sensation:

        1. _____

        2. _____

        3. _____

24. Describe ten communication methods that are appropriate for clients with a hearing impairment.

    a. _____

    b. _____

    c. _____

    d. _____

    e. _____

    f. _____

    g. _____

    h. _____

    i. _____

    j. _____

Acute Care

25. When clients enter acute care settings for therapeutic management of sensory deficits or as a result of traumatic injury, the following approaches are used to maximize sensory function. Briefly explain each.

    a. Orientation to the environment:

        _____

        _____

    b. Communication:

        _____

        _____

    c. Controlling sensory stimuli:

        _____

        _____

    d. Safety measures:

        _____

        _____

Restorative and Continuing Care

26. After a client experiences a sensory loss, it becomes important to understand the implications of the loss and to make the adjustments needed to continue a normal lifestyle. Briefly explain each.

    a. Understanding sensory loss:

        _____

        _____

    b. Socialization:

        _____

        _____

    c. Promoting self-care:

        _____

        _____

Evaluation

Client Care

27. The client is the only one who will know if his or her sensory abilities are improved and which specific interventions or therapies are most successful in facilitating a change in performance.

Client Expectations

28. Client expectations are one of the evaluative criteria used by the nurse. What questions might you ask to determine if client expectations have been met?

    _____

    _____

Review Questions

Select the appropriate answer and cite the rationale for choosing that particular answer.

1. All of the following are true of age-related factors that influence sensory function except
   a. Refractive errors are the most common types of visual disorders in children.
   b. Visual changes in adulthood include presbyopia.
   c. Older adults hear high-pitched sounds best.
   d. Neonates are unable to discriminate sensory stimuli.

Answer: _____ Rationale: _____
_____
_____

2. Mr. McDonald, a 62-year-old farmer, has been hospitalized for 2 weeks for thrombophlebitis. He has no visitors, and the nurse notices that he appears bored, restless, and anxious. The type of alteration occurring because of sensory deprivation is
   a. Affective
   b. Cognitive
   c. Perceptual
   d. Receptual

Answer: _____ Rationale: _____
_____
_____

3. Which of the following would not provide meaningful stimuli for a client?
   a. A clock or calendar with large numbers
   b. A television that is kept on all day at a low volume
   c. Family pictures and personal possessions
   d. Interesting magazines and books

Answer: _____ Rationale: _____
_____
_____

4. Clients with existing sensory loss must be protected from injury. What determines the safety precautions taken?
   a. The existing dangers in the environment
   b. The financial means to make needed safety changes
   c. The nature of the client's actual or potential sensory loss
   d. The availability of a support system to enable the client to exist in his or her present environment

Answer: _____ Rationale: _____
_____
_____

5. A client who is unable to name common objects or express simple ideas in words or writing suffers from
   a. Expressive aphasia
   b. Receptive aphasia
   c. Global aphasia
   d. Intellectual disability

Answer: _____ Rationale: _____
_____
_____

Critical Thinking Model for Nursing Care Plan for Disturbed Sensory Perception

Imagine that you are the community health nurse in the Care Plan on page 1277 of your text. Complete the *planning phase* of the critical thinking model by writing your answers in the appropriate boxes of the model shown. Think about the following:

- In developing Judy's plan of care, what knowledge did you apply?
- In what way might your previous experience assist in developing a plan of care?
- When developing a plan of care, what intellectual and professional standards were applied?
- What critical thinking attitudes might have been applied in developing Judy's plan?
- How will you accomplish the goals?

KNOWLEDGE

EXPERIENCE

Planning

STANDARDS

QUALITIES

CHAPTER 48   Critical Thinking Model for Nursing Care Plan for *Disturbed Sensory Perception*
See answers on page 545.

49

Care of Surgical Clients

Preliminary Reading

Chapter 49, pp. 1312–1356

Comprehensive Understanding

History of Surgical Nursing

1. Summarize the historical changes that have occurred in surgical nursing.

_____

_____

_____

_____

Ambulatory Surgery

2. List the benefits of ambulatory surgery.

a. _____

b. _____

c. _____

d. _____

Scientific Knowledge Base

Classification of Surgery

3. Define the following surgical procedure classifications.

a. Palliative:

_____

_____

b. Ablative:

_____

_____

c. Emergency:

_____

_____

d. Minor:

_____

_____

e. Urgent:

_____

_____

f. Major:

_____

_____

g. Reconstructive:

_____

_____

h. Constructive:

_____

_____

i. Elective:

_____

_____

j. Procurement for transplant:

_____

_____

k. Diagnostic:

_____

_____

l. Cosmetic

_____

_____

The Nursing Process in the Preoperative Surgical Phase

Assessment

4. Identify the data you should collect from the client's medical history.

_____

_____

5. Briefly explain the following factors that increase the client's risk in surgery.

   a. Age:

   _____

   _____

   b. Nutrition:

   _____

   _____

   c. Obesity:

   _____

   _____

   d. Immunocompetence:

   _____

   _____

   e. Fluid and electrolyte imbalances:

   _____

   _____

   f. Pregnancy:

   _____

   _____

6. Briefly explain the rationale for assessing the following.

   a. Previous surgeries:

   _____

   _____

   b. Perceptions and understanding of surgery:

   _____

   _____

   c. Medication history:

   _____

   _____

   d. Allergies:

   _____

   _____

   e. Smoking habits:

   _____

   _____

   f. Alcohol ingestion and substance use and abuse:

   _____

   _____

   g. Family support:

   _____

   _____

   h. Occupation:

   _____

   _____

   i   Pain:

   _____

   _____

7. Briefly explain each of the following factors that need to be assessed in order to understand the impact of surgery on a client's and family's emotional health.

   a. Body image:

   _____

   _____

   b. Coping resources:

   _____

   _____

8. Cultural differences influence the surgical experience. Give an example.

   _____

   _____

9. Briefly describe the findings on which you should focus related to the physical examination of the following body systems.

   a. General survey:

   _____

   _____

   b. Head and neck:

   _____

   _____

   c. Integument:

   _____

   _____

d. Thorax and lungs:

_____

_____

e. Heart and vascular system:

_____

_____

f. Abdomen:

_____

_____

g. Neurological status:

_____

_____

10. Describe the following routine screening tests for surgical clients.

a. CBC:

_____

_____

b. Serum electrolytes:

_____

_____

c. Coagulation studies:

_____

_____

d. Serum creatinine:

_____

_____

e. BUN:

_____

_____

f. Glucose:

_____

_____

Nursing Diagnosis

11. List ten potential or actual nursing diagnoses appropriate for the preoperative client.

a. _____

b. _____

c. _____

d. _____

e. _____

f. _____

g. _____

h. _____

i. _____

j. _____

Planning

12. Give examples of associated outcomes related to the goal of a perioperative client being able to verbalize the significance of postoperative exercises.

a. _____

b. _____

c. _____

d. _____

Implementation

13. Surgery cannot be performed until a client understands the following:

a. _____

b. _____

c. _____

d. _____

e. _____

14. Preparatory information helps clients anticipate the steps of a procedure and thus helps them form realistic images of the surgical experience. When events occur as predicted, clients are better able to cope and attend to the experiences.

15. Describe the criteria that may demonstrate the client's understanding of the surgical procedure.

a. _____

_____

b. _____

_____

c. _____

_____

d. _____

_____

e. _____

_____

f. _____

_____

g. _____
_____

h. _____
_____

Acute Care

Physical Preparation

16. Briefly describe the following preoperative preparations.

   a. Maintenance of normal fluid and electrolyte balances:
   _____
   _____

   b. Reduction of risk of surgical wound infection:
   _____
   _____

   c. Prevention of bowel and bladder incontinence:
   _____
   _____

   d. Promotion of rest and comfort:
   _____
   _____

Preparation on the Day of Surgery

17. List nine responsibilities of a nurse caring for a client the day of surgery.

   a. _____
   b. _____
   c. _____
   d. _____
   e. _____
   f. _____
   g. _____
   h. _____
   i. _____

18. The signs and symptoms of a latex reaction are
_____
_____
_____

19. Describe methods to eliminate wrong site and wrong procedure surgery.
_____
_____
_____

Transport to the Operating Room

20. After the client leaves the nursing division, the nurse prepares the bed and room for the client's return if the client is returning to the same nursing division. List ten pieces of equipment that should be present in the postoperative bedside unit.

   a. _____
   b. _____
   c. _____
   d. _____
   e. _____
   f. _____
   g. _____
   h. _____
   i. _____
   j. _____

Intraoperative Surgical Phase

21. In the holding area, two nursing responsibilities are
_____
_____

The Nursing Process in the Intraoperative Surgical Phase

Implementation

Acute Care

Introduction of Anaesthesia

22. General anaesthesia involves
_____
_____
_____
_____

23. Regional anaesthesia results in
_____
_____
_____
_____

24. Local anaesthesia involves

_____

_____

_____

25. Describe conscious sedation and identify its advantages.

_____

_____

_____

Positioning the Client for Surgery

26. Identify factors to consider when positioning the client for surgery.

_____

_____

_____

27. During the intraoperative phase, the nursing staff continues the preoperative plan.

28. Documentation of intraoperative care provides useful data for the nurse who cares for the client postoperatively.

Postoperative Surgical Phase

Immediate Postoperative Recovery

29. Describe the assessment data that you should obtain in the postanaesthesia care unit (PACU).

_____

_____

Discharge From the Postanaesthesia Care Unit

30. Identify the criteria for discharge from the PACU.

a. _____

b. _____

c. _____

d. _____

e. _____

f. _____

g. _____

h. _____

Recovery in Ambulatory Surgery

31. Describe the two phases of postanaesthesia recovery.

a. Phase I:

_____

_____

b. Phase II:

_____

Postanaesthesia Recovery Score for Ambulatory Patients (PARSAP)

32. Describe what this tool is and what minimum score is required for discharge.

_____

_____

The Nursing Process in Postoperative Care

Assessment

33. Explain the frequency of assessments needed during the postoperative period.

_____

_____

34. List four major causes of airway obstruction in the postoperative client.

a. _____

b. _____

c. _____

d. _____

35. List four areas to assess in order to determine a postoperative client's circulatory status.

a. _____

b. _____

c. _____

d. _____

36. Describe the characteristic findings associated with postoperative hemorrhage.

a. Blood pressure

_____

_____

b. Heart rate and character of pulse

_____

_____

c. Respiratory rate

_____

_____

d. Skin

_____

_____

e. Level of consciousness

_____

_____

37. Explain why clients awakening from surgery often complain of feeling cold.

_____

_____

_____

38. Define *malignant hyperthermia*.

_____

_____

39. List three areas you should assess to determine fluid and electrolyte alterations.

a. _____

b. _____

c. _____

40. List the areas of assessment that help to determine a postoperative client's neurological status.

a. _____

b. _____

c. _____

d. _____

41. The nurse assesses the condition of the skin, noting _____, _____, _____, and _____.

42. Describe how the nurse would assess the amount of drainage from a wound.

_____

_____

43. Depending on the surgery, a client may not regain voluntary control over urinary function for hours after anaesthesia.

44. Distension may occur in the client who develops a _____.

45. Normally during the immediate recovery phase, faint or absent bowel sounds are auscultated in all four quadrants. _____ loud gurgles per minute over each quadrant indicate that peristalsis has returned.

46. Pain can be perceived before full consciousness is regained. Acute incisional pain causes clients to become _____ and may be responsible for temporary changes in _____.

47. Assessment of the client's discomfort and evaluation of pain relief therapies are essential nursing functions.

Nursing Diagnosis

48. Identify two actual or potential nursing diagnoses that are appropriate for a postoperative client.

a. _____

b. _____

Planning

49. List the typical postoperative plans prescribed by surgeons and seen, for example, on clinical pathways.

a. _____

b. _____

c. _____

d. _____

e. _____

f. _____

g. _____

h. _____

i. _____

j. _____

50. Give five goals of care and associated outcomes for a postoperative client.

a. _____

b. _____

c. _____

d. _____

e. _____

Implementation

Health Promotion

51. To prevent respiratory complications, begin pulmonary interventions early. Describe measures that will promote the following.

a. Airway patency:

_____

_____

_____

b. Expansion of the lungs:

_____

_____

_____

c. Removal of pulmonary secretions:

_____

_____

_____

52. Briefly describe measures to promote normal venous return and circulatory blood flow.

a. _____

b. _____

c. _____

d. _____

e. _____

f. _____

53. List three nonpharmacological pain-relief measures.

a. _____

b. _____

c. _____

Evaluation

Client Care

54. The nurse evaluates the effectiveness of care provided to the surgical client on the basis of expected outcomes following nursing interventions.

55. Describe how you should evaluate the ambulatory surgical client.

_____

_____

_____

Review Questions

Select the appropriate answer and cite the rationale for choosing that particular answer.

1. Mrs. Yong-Hing, a 45-year-old client with diabetes, is having a hysterectomy in the morning. Because of her history, the nurse would expect
   a. An increased risk of hemorrhaging
   b. Fluid imbalances

c. Altered elimination of anaesthetic agents
d. Impaired wound healing

Answer: _____   Rationale: _____

_____

_____

2. The purposes of the health history for the client who is to have surgery include all of the following except
   a. Identifying the client's perception about surgery
   b. Obtaining information about the client's past experience with surgery
   c. Deciding whether surgery is indicated
   d. Understanding the impact surgery has on the client's and family's emotional health

Answer: _____   Rationale: _____

_____

_____

3. All of the following clients are at risk for developing serious fluid and electrolyte imbalances during and after surgery, except
   a. Client E, who is 81 years old and having emergency surgery for a bowel obstruction following 4 days of vomiting and diarrhea
   b. Client F, who is 1 year old and having a cleft palate repair
   c. Client G, who is 55 years old and has a history of chronic respiratory disease
   d. Client H, who is 79 years old and has a history of congestive heart failure

Answer: _____   Rationale: _____

_____

_____

4. The primary purpose of postoperative leg exercises is to
   a. Promote venous return
   b. Promote lymphatic drainage
   c. Assess range of motion
   d. Exercise fatigued muscles

Answer: _____   Rationale: _____

_____

_____

5. The PACU nurse notices that the client is shivering. This is most commonly caused by
   a. The use of a reflective blanket on the operating room table
   b. Side effects of certain anaesthetic agents

c. Intravenous narcotics used for pain management
d. Malignant hypothermia

Answer: _____   Rationale: _____

_____

_____

Critical Thinking Model for Nursing Care Plan for Deficient Knowledge Regarding Preoperative and Postoperative Care Requirements

Imagine that you are Joe, the nurse in the Care Plan on page 1303 of your text. Complete the *evaluation phase* of the critical thinking model by writing your answers in the appropriate boxes of the model shown. Think about the following:

- During evaluation, what knowledge and professional standards were applied to Mrs. Campana's care?

- In what way might Joe's previous experience influence his evaluation of Mrs. Campana's care?

- In what way do critical thinking attitudes play a role in how you approach evaluation of Mrs. Campana's care?

- How might Joe adjust Mrs. Campana's care?

- What knowledge did Joe apply in evaluating Mrs. Campana's care?

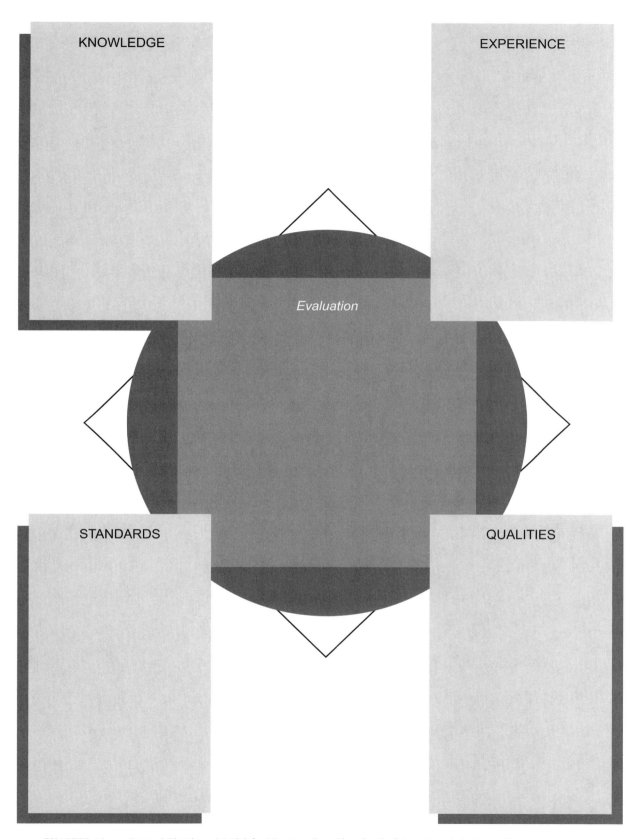

KNOWLEDGE

EXPERIENCE

Evaluation

STANDARDS

QUALITIES

CHAPTER 49   Critical Thinking Model for Nursing Care Plan for *Deficient Knowledge Regarding Preoperative and Postoperative Care Requirements*
See answers on page 546.

Skills Performance Checklists

Skill 31–1 Measuring Body Temperature

	S	U	NP	Comments
1. Assess for temperature alterations and factors that influence body temperature.	___	___	___	_____
2. Determine any activity that may interfere with accuracy of temperature measurement.	___	___	___	_____
3. Determine appropriate site and measurement device to be used.	___	___	___	_____
4. Explain to client how temperature will be taken and importance of maintaining proper position.	___	___	___	_____
5. Perform hand hygiene.	___	___	___	_____
6. Obtain temperature reading:				
A. *Oral temperature measurement with electronic thermometer*				
(1) Apply disposable gloves (optional).	___	___	___	_____
(2) Remove thermometer pack from charging unit. Attach oral probe (blue tip) to thermometer unit. Grasp top of probe stem, being careful not to apply pressure on the ejection button.	___	___	___	_____
(3) Slide disposable plastic probe cover over thermometer probe until it locks in place.	___	___	___	_____
(4) Have client sit or lie in bed. Ask client to open mouth, then place thermometer probe under tongue in posterior sublingual pocket lateral to centre of lower jaw.	___	___	___	_____
(5) Ask client to hold thermometer probe with lips closed.	___	___	___	_____
(6) Leave thermometer probe in place until audible signal occurs and temperature appears on digital display. Remove thermometer probe from client's mouth.	___	___	___	_____
(7) Push ejection button on thermometer stem to discard plastic probe cover into appropriate receptacle.	___	___	___	_____
(8) Return thermometer stem to storage well of recording unit.	___	___	___	_____
(9) If gloves were worn, remove and dispose of them in appropriate receptacle. Perform hand hygiene.	___	___	___	_____
(10) Return thermometer to charger.	___	___	___	_____
B. *Rectal temperature measurement with electronic thermometer*				
(1) Provide privacy and assist client to Sims' position. Drape client.	___	___	___	_____
(2) Apply disposable gloves.	___	___	___	_____
(3) Remove thermometer pack from charging unit. Attach rectal probe (red tip) to thermometer unit. Grasp top of probe stem.	___	___	___	_____
(4) Slide disposable plastic probe cover over thermometer probe until it locks in place.	___	___	___	_____
(5) Lubricate 2.5 to 3.5 cm of probe for an adult.	___	___	___	_____
(6) Separate buttocks to expose anus. Ask client to breathe slowly and relax.	___	___	___	_____
(7) Gently insert thermometer 3.5 cm for adult.	___	___	___	_____
(8) If resistance is felt, withdraw thermometer immediately. Never force thermometer.	___	___	___	_____
(9) Leave thermometer probe in place until audible signal occurs and temperature appears on digital display. Remove thermometer probe from client's anus.	___	___	___	_____
(10) Push ejection button on thermometer stem to discard plastic probe cover. Wipe probe with alcohol swab.	___	___	___	_____
(11) Return thermometer stem to storage well of recording unit.	___	___	___	_____
(12) Wipe client's anal area with soft tissue and discard tissue. Assist client to a comfortable position.	___	___	___	_____
(13) Remove and dispose of gloves. Perform hand hygiene.	___	___	___	_____
(14) Return thermometer to charger.	___	___	___	_____

Continued

	S	U	NP	Comments

C. *Axillary temperature measurement with electronic thermometer*

(1) Provide privacy.   ___ ___ ___ _____

(2) Assist client to supine or sitting position.   ___ ___ ___ _____

(3) Move client's clothing or gown away from his or her shoulder and arm.   ___ ___ ___ _____

(4) Remove thermometer pack from charging unit. Be sure oral probe (blue tip) is attached to thermometer unit. Grasp top of probe stem.   ___ ___ ___ _____

(5) Slide disposable plastic probe cover over thermometer probe until it locks in place.   ___ ___ ___ _____

(6) Raise client's arm away from torso and inspect for skin lesions and excessive perspiration. Insert probe into centre of client's axilla, lower arm over probe, and place arm across chest.   ___ ___ ___ _____

(7) Hold probe in place until audible signal occurs and temperature appears on digital display.   ___ ___ ___ _____

(8) Remove probe from axilla.   ___ ___ ___ _____

(9) Push ejection button on probe to discard plastic probe cover.   ___ ___ ___ _____

(10) Return probe to storage well of recording unit.   ___ ___ ___ _____

(11) Assist client to a comfortable position.   ___ ___ ___ _____

(12) Perform hand hygiene.   ___ ___ ___ _____

(13) Return thermometer to charger.   ___ ___ ___ _____

D. *Tympanic membrane temperature with electronic thermometer*

(1) Assist client to a comfortable position with head turned toward the side, away from you.   ___ ___ ___ _____

(2) Note if there is obvious cerumen in the ear canal.   ___ ___ ___ _____

(3) Remove handheld thermometer unit from charging base, being careful not to apply pressure on the ejection button.   ___ ___ ___ _____

(4) Slide disposable speculum cover over tip until it locks into place.   ___ ___ ___ _____

(5) Insert speculum into ear canal following manufacturer's instructions for tympanic probe positioning:

    a. Pull ear pinna backward, up, and out for adult.   ___ ___ ___ _____

    b. Move thermometer in a figure-eight pattern.   ___ ___ ___ _____

    c. Fit probe gently in ear canal and do not move it.   ___ ___ ___ _____

    d. Point probe toward client's nose.   ___ ___ ___ _____

(6) Depress scan button on handheld unit. Leave thermometer probe in place until audible signal occurs and client's temperature appears on digital display.   ___ ___ ___ _____

(7) Carefully remove speculum from client's auditory canal.   ___ ___ ___ _____

(8) Push ejection button on handheld unit to discard plastic probe cover.   ___ ___ ___ _____

(9) If second reading is required, replace probe cover and wait 2 to 3 minutes.   ___ ___ ___ _____

(10) Return handheld unit to charging base.   ___ ___ ___ _____

(11) Assist client to a comfortable position.   ___ ___ ___ _____

7. Perform hand hygiene.   ___ ___ ___ _____

8. Discuss findings with client as needed.   ___ ___ ___ _____

9. If temperature is being assessed for the first time, establish temperature as baseline if within normal range.   ___ ___ ___ _____

10. Compare temperature reading with previous baseline and normal temperature range for client's age group.   ___ ___ ___ _____

11. Record temperature and report abnormal findings.   ___ ___ ___ _____

STUDENT: _____ DATE: _____

INSTRUCTOR: _____ DATE: _____

Skill 31–2 Assessing the Radial and Apical Pulses

	S	U	NP	Comments
1. Determine need to assess radial or apical pulse.	___	___	___	_____
2. Assess for factors that influence pulse rate.	___	___	___	_____
3. Determine previous baseline apical rate (if available) from client's record.	___	___	___	_____
4. Explain that pulse or heart rate is to be assessed. Encourage client to relax and not speak.	___	___	___	_____
5. Perform hand hygiene.	___	___	___	_____
6. Provide privacy.	___	___	___	_____
7. Obtain pulse measurement.				
A. *Radial pulse*				
(1) Assist client to supine or sitting position.	___	___	___	_____
(2) If client is supine, place client's forearm straight alongside the body or across lower chest or upper abdomen with wrist extended straight. If client is sitting, bend client's elbow 90 degrees and support his or her lower arm on a chair or on your arm. Slightly flex client's wrist, with palm down.	___	___	___	_____
(3) Place tips of first two fingers of hand over groove along radial or thumb side of client's inner wrist.	___	___	___	_____
(4) Lightly compress against client's radius, obliterate pulse initially, then relax pressure.	___	___	___	_____
(5) Determine strength of pulse.	___	___	___	_____
(6) After pulse can be felt regularly, look at watch's second hand and begin to count rate.	___	___	___	_____
(7) If pulse is regular, count rate for 30 seconds and multiply total by 2.	___	___	___	_____
(8) If pulse is irregular, count rate for 60 seconds. Assess frequency and pattern of irregularity.	___	___	___	_____
B. *Apical pulse*				
(1) Assist client to supine or sitting position. Expose client's sternum and left side of chest.	___	___	___	_____
(2) Locate anatomical landmarks to identify the point of maximal impulse.	___	___	___	_____
(3) Place diaphragm of stethoscope in palm of your hand for 5 to 10 seconds.	___	___	___	_____
(4) Place diaphragm of stethoscope over point of maximal impulse at the fifth intercostal space at the left midclavicular line and auscultate for normal S_1 and S_2 heart sounds.	___	___	___	_____
(5) When S_1 and S_2 are heard with regularity, look at watch's second hand and begin to count rate.	___	___	___	_____
(6) If apical rate is regular, count for 30 seconds and multiply by 2.	___	___	___	_____
(7) If rate is irregular or client is receiving cardiovascular medication, count for 60 seconds.	___	___	___	_____
(8) Note regularity of any dysrhythmia.	___	___	___	_____
(9) Replace client's gown and bed linen; assist client to a comfortable position.	___	___	___	_____
(10) Clean earpieces and diaphragm of stethoscope with alcohol swab as needed.	___	___	___	_____
8. Perform hand hygiene.	___	___	___	_____
9. Discuss findings with client as needed.	___	___	___	_____
10. Compare readings with client's previous baseline and/or acceptable range of heart rate for client's age group.	___	___	___	_____
11. Compare peripheral pulse rate with apical rate and note discrepancy.	___	___	___	_____
12. Compare radial pulse equality and note discrepancy.	___	___	___	_____
13. Correlate pulse rate with data obtained from blood pressure and related signs and symptoms.	___	___	___	_____

STUDENT: _____ DATE: _____

INSTRUCTOR: _____ DATE: _____

Skill 31–3 Assessing Respirations

	S	U	NP	Comments
1. Determine need to assess client's respirations.	___	___	___	_____
2. Assess pertinent laboratory values.	___	___	___	_____
3. Determine previous baseline respiratory rate (if available) from client's record.	___	___	___	_____
4. Perform hand hygiene. Provide privacy.	___	___	___	_____
5. Assist client to a comfortable position, preferably sitting or lying with the head of the bed elevated 45 to 60 degrees. Be sure client's chest is visible. If necessary, move client's bed linen or gown.	___	___	___	_____
6. Place client's arm in relaxed position across the abdomen or lower chest, or place your hand directly over client's upper abdomen.	___	___	___	_____
7. Observe complete respiratory cycle (one inspiration and one expiration).	___	___	___	_____
8. After cycle is observed, look at watch's second hand and begin to count rate.				
9. If rhythm is regular, count number of respirations in 30 seconds and multiply by 2. If rhythm is irregular, less than 12, or greater than 20, count respirations for 60 seconds.	___	___	___	_____
10. Note depth of respirations.	___	___	___	_____
11. Note rhythm of ventilatory cycle.	___	___	___	_____
12. Replace client's bed linen and gown.	___	___	___	_____
13. Perform hand hygiene.	___	___	___	_____
14. Discuss findings with client as needed.	___	___	___	_____
15. If respirations are being assessed for the first time, establish rate, rhythm, and depth as baseline if within normal range.	___	___	___	_____
16. Compare respirations with client's previous baseline and normal rate, rhythm, and depth.	___	___	___	_____
17. Record respiratory rate and character and any use of oxygen and report abnormal findings.	___	___	___	_____

STUDENT: _____   DATE: _____

INSTRUCTOR: _____   DATE: _____

Skill 31–4 Measuring Oxygen Saturation (Pulse Oximetry)

	S	U	NP	Comments
1. Determine need to measure client's oxygen saturation.	___	___	___	_____
2. Assess for factors that influence measurement of SpO_2.	___	___	___	_____
3. Review client's record for prescriber's order.	___	___	___	_____
4. Determine previous baseline SpO_2 (if available) from client's record.	___	___	___	_____
5. Perform hand hygiene.	___	___	___	_____
6. Explain purpose and method of procedure to client.	___	___	___	_____
7. Assess site for sensor probe placement.	___	___	___	_____
8. Assist client to a comfortable position. If client's finger is chosen as monitoring site, support client's lower arm.	___	___	___	_____
9. Instruct client to breathe normally.				
10. Use acetone to remove any fingernail polish from digit to be assessed.	___	___	___	_____
11. Attach sensor probe to monitoring site. Tell client that clip-on probe will feel like a clothespin on the finger and will not hurt.	___	___	___	_____
12. Turn on oximeter by activating power. Observe pulse waveform/ intensity display and audible beep. Correlate oximeter pulse rate with client's radial pulse.	___	___	___	_____
13. Leave probe in place until oximeter readout reaches constant value and pulse display reaches full strength during each cardiac cycle. Read SpO_2 on digital display.				
14. Verify SpO_2 alarm limits and alarm volume for continuous monitoring. Verify that alarms are on. Assess skin integrity under sensor probe and relocate sensor probe at least every 4 hours.	___	___	___	_____
15. Assist client in returning to a comfortable position.	___	___	___	_____
16. Perform hand hygiene.	___	___	___	_____
17. Discuss findings with client as needed.	___	___	___	_____
18. Remove probe and turn oximeter power off after intermittent measurements. Store probe in appropriate location.	___	___	___	_____
19. Compare SpO_2 reading with client baseline and acceptable values.	___	___	___	_____
20. Correlate SpO_2 reading with SaO_2 reading obtained from arterial blood gas measurements, if available.	___	___	___	_____
21. Correlate SpO_2 reading with data obtained from respiratory assessment.	___	___	___	_____

STUDENT: _____ DATE: _____

INSTRUCTOR: _____ DATE: _____

Skill 31–5 Measuring Blood Pressure

	S	U	NP	Comments
1. Determine need to assess client's blood pressure (BP).	___	___	___	_____
2. Determine best site for BP assessment.	___	___	___	_____
3. Select appropriate cuff size.	___	___	___	_____
4. Determine previous baseline BP (if available) from client's record.	___	___	___	_____
5. Encourage client to avoid exercise and smoking for 30 minutes and ingestion of caffeine for 60 minutes before assessment of BP.	___	___	___	_____
6. Perform hand hygiene. Assist client to sitting or lying position. Make sure room is warm, quiet, and relaxing.	___	___	___	_____
7. Explain to client that BP is to be assessed and have client rest at least 5 minutes before measurement is taken. Ask client not to speak while BP is being measured.	___	___	___	_____
8. With client sitting or lying, position client's forearm or thigh and provide support if needed.	___	___	___	_____
9. Expose extremity by removing constricting clothing.	___	___	___	_____
10. Palpate brachial artery or popliteal artery. Position cuff 2.5 cm above site of pulsation.	___	___	___	_____
11. Centre bladder of cuff above artery. With cuff fully deflated, wrap cuff evenly and snugly around extremity.	___	___	___	_____
12. To determine BP (two-step method), palpate artery distal to cuff with fingertips of one hand while inflating cuff rapidly to pressure 30 mm Hg above point at which pulse disappears. Slowly deflate cuff and note point when pulse reappears. Deflate cuff fully and wait 30 seconds.	___	___	___	_____
13. Place stethoscope earpieces in ears.	___	___	___	_____
14. Relocate brachial or popliteal artery and place bell or diaphragm chestpiece of stethoscope over it.	___	___	___	_____
15. Close valve of pressure bulb clockwise until tight. Inflate cuff to 30 mm Hg above palpated systolic pressure.	___	___	___	_____
16. Slowly release valve and allow mercury to fall at rate of 2 mm Hg/second.	___	___	___	_____
17. Note point on manometer when first clear sound is heard.	___	___	___	_____
18. Continue to deflate cuff, noting point at which muffled or dampened sound appears.	___	___	___	_____
19. Continue to deflate cuff gradually, noting point at which sound disappears in adults. Listen for 10 to 20 mm Hg after the last sound, then allow remaining air to escape quickly.	___	___	___	_____
20. Remove cuff from client's extremity unless measurement must be repeated. If this is the first assessment of the client, repeat procedure on other extremity.	___	___	___	_____
21. Assist client in returning to a comfortable position and cover upper arm if previously clothed.	___	___	___	_____
22. Perform hand hygiene.	___	___	___	_____
23. Discuss findings with client as needed.	___	___	___	_____
24. Compare reading with previous baseline and/or acceptable BP for client's age group.	___	___	___	_____
25. Compare BP in both of client's arms or legs.	___	___	___	_____
26. Correlate BP with data obtained from pulse assessment and related cardiovascular signs and symptoms.	___	___	___	_____
27. Inform client of value of and need for periodic reassessment of BP.	___	___	___	_____

STUDENT: _____   DATE: _____

INSTRUCTOR: _____   DATE: _____

Skill 32–1 Critical Components of Indirect Percussion Techniques

	S	U	NP	Comments
1. Trim the fingernail short on the plexor finger.	___	___	___	_____
2. Place pleximeter finger (finger being struck) on the skin surface over the area to be percussed.	___	___	___	_____
3. Place pleximeter firmly.	___	___	___	_____
4. Do not move pleximeter.	___	___	___	_____
5. Limit contact of pleximeter to one small area on the skin; preferably only the distal interphalangeal joint (DIP) touches the skin surface.	___	___	___	_____
6. Strike a sharp, perpendicular blow to the DIP joint of the stationary pleximeter with the plexor finger (striking finger).	___	___	___	_____
7. Use brisk arclike wrist action with relaxed wrist.	___	___	___	_____
8. Limit movement to wrist action, avoiding movement at elbow.	___	___	___	_____
9. Limit percussion to one or two sharp blows.	___	___	___	_____
10. Select the appropriate force of blow to achieve a clear percussion note.	___	___	___	_____
11. Use the lightest blow possible to achieve a clear percussion note.	___	___	___	_____

Adapted from Skillen, D. L. (2004). *A primer on physical examination techniques* [WebCT]. Edmonton, AB: Faculty of Nursing, University of Alberta.

STUDENT: _____ DATE: _____

INSTRUCTOR: _____ DATE: _____

Skill 32–2 Assessing the Face

	S	U	NP	Comments
INSPECTION				
Skin, face, lips				
1. Inspect skin, face, and lips.	____	____	____	_____
PALPATION				
Temporal arteries				
1. Palpate temporal arteries with fingertips or pads.	____	____	____	_____
Temporomandibular joint				
1. Position index fingertips in front of each tragus.	____	____	____	_____
2. Instruct client to open and close jaw with fingertips in position.	____	____	____	_____
Cranial nerve (CN) V (trigeminal) motor function				
1. Instruct client to clench teeth.	____	____	____	_____
2. Palpate temporal and masseter muscles with fingertips or pads.	____	____	____	_____
3. Note strength and symmetry of contraction.	____	____	____	_____
Sensory function				
1. Demonstrate how sharp, dull, and light touch feels before beginning tests.	____	____	____	_____
2. Instruct client to close eyes and indicate when touched.	____	____	____	_____
3. Test side to side, varying rhythm, touching ophthalmic, maxillary, and mandibular regions lightly with cotton ball.	____	____	____	_____
4. Repeat with splintered tongue blade. Use dull touch to check client's reliability at least once.	____	____	____	_____
5. Compare sides.	____	____	____	_____
CN VII (facial) motor function				
1. Instruct client to				
A. Show upper and lower teeth	____	____	____	_____
B. Puff out cheeks	____	____	____	_____
C. Smile	____	____	____	_____
2. Observe for symmetry.	____	____	____	_____
3. Instruct client to				
A. Frown	____	____	____	_____
B. Raise eyebrows	____	____	____	_____
C. Close eyes tight and resist opening by examiner	____	____	____	_____
4. Attempt to open client's closed eyes, exerting pressure on bony orbit, avoiding pressure on eye.	____	____	____	_____
5. Observe for symmetry and strength of motion.	____	____	____	_____

From Skillen, D. L., & Day, R. A. (Eds.). (2004). *A syllabus for adult health assessment* (pp. 31, 34–35). Edmonton, AB: Faculty of Nursing, University of Alberta.

STUDENT: _____ DATE: _____

INSTRUCTOR: _____ DATE: _____

Skill 32–3 Inspecting the External Structures of the Eyes

	S	U	NP	Comments

INSPECTION

Eyebrows, lids, lashes

1. Inspect eyebrows, lids, lashes.

Cornea

1. Use tangential lighting, with penlight, to inspect cornea.

Lens, iris, pupils

1. Inspect
   - Lens from anterior view
   - Iris of each eye
   - Size, shape, equality of pupils

Sclera, conjunctiva

1. Instruct client to look up while gently retracting lower lid to inspect sclera and conjunctiva.
2. Instruct client to look down and side to side while gently retracting upper lid to view sclera and possibly lacrimal gland.

Lacrimal sacs/glands

1. Inspect lacrimal sac puncta/gland regions bilaterally.

PUPILLARY REACTION CN II, III (optic, oculomotor)

Test each eye separately.

1. Instruct client to look past examiner.

Pupillary reaction to light; direct, consensual reactions

2. Shine a bright light from temporal region on each pupil in turn.
3. Inspect for direct and consensual reactions.

NEAR REACTION (accommodation)

Test each eye separately.

Dilatation

1. Instruct client to look into distance with each eye.
2. Observe pupil for dilatation.

Constriction

3. Instruct client to look at examiner's finger held 10 cm from client's eye.
4. Observe for pupillary constriction while client focuses on finger.
5. Repeat for other eye.

CONVERGENCE CN III, IV (oculomotor, trochlear)

1. Instruct client to follow finger.

Convergence

2. From directly in front of client, move finger to within 5 to 8 cm from bridge of client's nose.
3. Observe convergence.

CORNEAL REFLEX

Test each eye separately.

Continued

340

	S	U	NP	Comments

CN V, VII (trigeminal, facial)

1. Ask client if wearing contact lenses.
2. Instruct client to look up and away from examiner.
3. Approach from side with fine wisp of cotton.
4. Touch cornea, avoiding eyelashes and sclera.

Bilateral blink

5. Observe for bilateral blink.

From Skillen, D. L., & Day, R. A. (Eds.). (2004). *A syllabus for adult health assessment* (pp. 29–31). Edmonton, AB: Faculty of Nursing, University of Alberta.

STUDENT: _____   DATE: _____

INSTRUCTOR: _____   DATE: _____

Skill 32–4 Assessing Visual Fields and Extraocular Movements

	S	U	NP	Comments

VISUAL FIELDS BY CONFRONTATION

1. Position self 60 cm away from client with eyes level.

CN II (optic); visual fields

2. Instruct client to cover one eye and to look at examiner's eye directly opposite.
3. Cover own eye opposite to client's covered eye.
4. Instruct client to indicate when wiggling finger seen.
5. Test temporal, inferotemporal, and superotemporal fields of vision by placing wiggling finger somewhat behind client and slowly moving it within client's visual field.
6. Test nasal, superior, and inferior fields of vision in turn by maintaining wiggling finger equidistant between client and self. Test eight different positions for each eye.
7. Slowly move wiggling finger within visual fields.
8. Compare client's visual field against own.

Extraocular muscles and movements

1. Inspect extraocular muscle function by performing
   A. Cardinal directions test **AND**
   B. Cover test **OR**
   C. Corneal reflection test

CN III, IV, VI (oculomotor, trochlear, abducens)

   A. Cardinal directions (extraocular movements)
      (1) Ask client if wearing contact lenses.
      (2) Position self so client can focus.
      (3) Instruct client to follow finger or pen (consider age) without moving head.
      (4) Move finger slowly avoiding straight up and down midline position to client's (R) in line with shoulder, upward to (R) of midline, downward to (R) of midline, to client's (L) in line with shoulder, upward to (L) of midline, downward to (L) of midline.

Parallel tracking, nystagmus, lid lag

      (5) Avoid fixation of extreme lateral points.
      (6) Observe for parallel tracking (conjugate movements), nystagmus, and lid lag.
   B. Cover test
      (1) Keep eyes level with those of client.
      (2) Instruct client to look at examiner.
      (3) Hold opaque cover over one eye for 5 to 10 seconds before removing it quickly, without warning and without touching.
      (4) Observe eye that was covered.
      (5) Repeat with other eye.
   C. Corneal reflections
      (1) Stand at least 0.6 m away from client.
      (2) Shine penlight from midline of examiner directly onto bridge of client's nose; ask client to look directly at light.
      (3) Observe site on each cornea from which light is reflected.

From Skillen, D. L., & Day, R. A. (Eds). (2004). *A syllabus for adult health assessment* (p. 32). Edmonton, AB: Faculty of Nursing, University of Alberta.

STUDENT: _____   DATE: _____

INSTRUCTOR: _____   DATE: _____

Skill 32–5 Assessing the Internal Structures of the Eyes

	S	U	NP	Comments

FUNDUS: INSPECTION BY OPHTHALMOSCOPE

Both eyes

	S	U	NP	Comments
1. Instruct client to look slightly up and over examiner's shoulder at specific point on wall.	___	___	___	_____
2. Turn lens disc of ophthalmoscope to 0 diopters.	___	___	___	_____
3. Maintain index finger on lens disc for refocusing during examination.	___	___	___	_____
4. Use (R) hand, (R) eye for client's (R) eye.	___	___	___	_____
5. Use (L) hand, (L) eye for client's (L) eye.	___	___	___	_____
6. Shine small light beam on pupil from about 40 cm away from client and 15 degrees lateral to midline.	___	___	___	_____
7. Place hand on client's forehead above eye being examined with thumb extended.	___	___	___	_____

Red reflex

	S	U	NP	Comments
8. Observe for red reflex.	___	___	___	_____
9. Move in toward client while maintaining focus on pupil and until eyelashes almost touch.	___	___	___	_____

Disc, cups, arterioles

	S	U	NP	Comments
10. Inspect disc, cup, arterioles, veins, crossings, adjusting lens disc if necessary.	___	___	___	_____

Veins, crossings

	S	U	NP	Comments
11. Move head and ophthalmoscope as one unit and follow vessels peripherally in four directions.	___	___	___	_____

Macula

	S	U	NP	Comments
12. Instruct client to briefly look directly at the light.	___	___	___	_____
13. Inspect macula and fovea.	___	___	___	_____

From Skillen D. L., & Day, R. A. (Eds.). (2004). *A syllabus for adult health assessment* (p. 33). Edmonton, AB: Faculty of Nursing, University of Alberta.

Skill 32–6 Inspecting and Palpating the Ears

	S	U	NP	Comments

INSPECTION

Ears fully exposed

Auricle, mastoid surface

1. Inspect auricle and mastoid bilaterally, adjusting hair where necessary for clear vision. ___ ___ ___ _____

Alignment

1. Inspect alignment of ears from anterior and lateral views (angle of attachment, horizontal, vertical). ___ ___ ___ _____

PALPATION

1. Inquire about tenderness during palpation. ___ ___ ___ _____

Mastoid surface

2. Palpate both mastoid surfaces of temporal bones with pads of fingers. ___ ___ ___ _____

Auricle

3. Pull up on each auricle. ___ ___ ___ _____

Tragus

4. Press on each tragus with fingertip. ___ ___ ___ _____

From Skillen, D. L., & Day, R. A. (Eds.). (2004). *A syllabus for adult health assessment* (p. 28). Edmonton, AB: Faculty of Nursing, University of Alberta.

STUDENT: _____ DATE: _____

INSTRUCTOR: _____ DATE: _____

Skill 32–7 Assessing Hearing Acuity

	S	U	NP	Comments

CN VIII (ACOUSTIC):

Test hearing; gross hearing; cranial nerve VIII. Assess each ear separately.
1. Mask hearing in one ear by moving fingertip in client's auditory canal. ___ ___ ___ _____
2. Stand 0.3 to 0.6 m from client (ensuring that client cannot lip-read). ___ ___ ___ _____
3. Exhale fully and direct whisper toward ear being tested. ___ ___ ___ _____
4. Start with three low-whispered, two-syllable, equally accented numbers or words. *Only if* client does not identify first numbers or words in low whispers, gradually increase intensity of whispering (while changing numbers or words) to spoken voice.

WEBER TEST

1. Select tuning fork of 512 or 1024 Hz.
2. Activate tuning fork using
   A. Thumb and finger **OR** ___ ___ ___ _____
   B. Reflex hammer **OR** ___ ___ ___ _____
   C. Other part of hand ___ ___ ___ _____
3. Hold base of vibrating tuning fork. ___ ___ ___ _____
4. Press end of base of vibrating tuning fork firmly on ___ ___ ___ _____
   A. Midline of skull **OR** ___ ___ ___ _____
   B. Midline of forehead ___ ___ ___ _____
5. Ask client, "Where do you hear the sound?" ___ ___ ___ _____

RINNÉ TEST

1. Select tuning fork of 512 or 1024Hz. ___ ___ ___ _____
2. Activate tuning fork using ___ ___ ___ _____
   A. Thumb and finger **OR** ___ ___ ___ _____
   B. Reflex hammer **OR** ___ ___ ___ _____
   C. Other part of hand ___ ___ ___ _____
3. Hold base of vibrating tuning fork and place end on mastoid surface level with ear canal. ___ ___ ___ _____
4. Request client to indicate when sound is no longer heard. ___ ___ ___ _____
5. Following client response, place vibrating tuning fork about 2.54 cm from auditory meatus of same ear with "U" facing forward (anteriorly).
6. Ask client if sound is heard. ___ ___ ___ _____

From Skillen D. L., & Day, R. A. (Eds.). (2004). *A syllabus for adult health assessment* (p. 28–29). Edmonton, AB: Faculty of Nursing, University of Alberta.

STUDENT: _____   DATE: _____

INSTRUCTOR: _____   DATE: _____

Skill 32–8 Otoscopy

	S	U	NP	Comments

INSPECTION BY OTOSCOPY

Otoscopic examination (each ear, tender ear last)

	S	U	NP	Comments
1. Select largest ear speculum that fits in canal.	___	___	___	_____
2. Brace hand against head when holding otoscope.	___	___	___	_____
3. Lift auricle upward, backward, and slightly out from head *before inserting* speculum.	___	___	___	_____
4. Instruct client to tilt head slightly toward other shoulder.	___	___	___	_____
5. Insert speculum gently and not deeply.	___	___	___	_____

Auditory canal

	S	U	NP	Comments
6. Inspect auditory canal.	___	___	___	_____

Tympanic membrane, cone of light, umbo, handle of the malleus, short process

	S	U	NP	Comments
7. Inspect tympanic membrane, handle of malleus, umbo, cone of light, short process (structures and vascularity).	___	___	___	_____
8. Adjust position of speculum in order to visualize drum entirely.	___	___	___	_____
9. Remove speculum before releasing auricle.	___	___	___	_____

From Skillen, D. L., & Day, R. A. (Eds.). (2004). *A syllabus for adult health assessment* (p. 29). Edmonton, AB: Faculty of Nursing, University of Alberta.

STUDENT: _____   DATE: _____

INSTRUCTOR: _____   DATE: _____

Skill 32–9 Assessing the Nose and Paranasal Sinuses

	S	U	NP	Comments
INSPECTION				
Nose				
1. Inspect nose from anterior view and profile.	___	___	___	_____
Frontal and maxillary sinuses				
2. Inspect frontal and maxillary sinus regions.	___	___	___	_____
PALPATION				
Nose				
1. Palpate entire length of nose with finger pads.	___	___	___	_____
2. Inquire of tenderness.	___	___	___	_____
Frontal, maxillary sinuses				
3. Palpate maxillary sinuses simultaneously by pressing upward on maxillae with thumbs and ask about tenderness.	___	___	___	_____
4. Palpate frontal sinuses by pressing upward, inferior to the supraorbital ridge, from medial border of eyebrow to mideyebrow, using thumbs, and ask about tenderness	___	___	___	_____
Test for patency				
1. Occlude each nostril in turn.	___	___	___	_____
2. Instruct client to breathe with mouth closed.	___	___	___	_____
3. Listen to complete inspiration for each nostril.	___	___	___	_____
Test of smell (cranial nerve): CN I				
1. Instruct client to close eyes.	___	___	___	_____
2. Occlude one nostril (naris).	___	___	___	_____
3. Hold pungent odour for client identification at opposite nostril. Ask client what odour is.	___	___	___	_____
4. Change pungent odour and repeat on other side.	___	___	___	_____
INSPECTION WITH NASAL SPECULUM				
Nose				
1. Instruct to tilt head back slightly.	___	___	___	_____
2. Insert nasal speculum posteriorly in horizontal plane into vestibule of nares.	___	___	___	_____
3. Stabilize speculum with index finger.	___	___	___	_____
4. Avoid touching septum.	___	___	___	_____
Mucous membrane, septum, inferior and middle turbinates				
5. Inspect mucous membrane, septum, and inferior turbinates moving speculum slowly upward.	___	___	___	_____
6. Inspect middle turbinates and mucous membranes.	___	___	___	_____
7. Offer client a tissue if needed.	___	___	___	_____

From Skillen, D. L., & Day, R. A. (Eds.). (2004). *A syllabus for adult health assessment (pp. 33–34)*. Edmonton, AB: Faculty of Nursing, University of Alberta.

STUDENT: _____ DATE: _____

INSTRUCTOR: _____ DATE: _____

Skill 32–10 Assessing the Mouth and Pharynx

	S	U	NP	Comments

INSPECTION

Mouth

1. Ask client to remove dentures. ___ ___ ___ _____
2. Instruct client to sip some water. ___ ___ ___ _____

Gums, teeth, tongue, floor of mouth, uvula, palates, tonsils, tonsillar pillars, posterior pharynx

3. Use penlight and tongue blade to inspect ___ ___ ___ _____
   - Buccal mucosa bilaterally
   - Upper and lower gums
   - Upper and lower teeth
   - Dorsal and ventral surfaces and sides of tongue
   - Floor of mouth
   - Uvula, soft and hard palates
   - Tonsils, tonsillar pillars
   - Posterior pharyngeal wall
4. If lesion present, palpate with gloved hand. ___ ___ ___ _____

Cranial nerve (CN) IX, X (glossopharyngeal, vagus); motor and sensory

1. Depress tongue with tongue blade and instruct client to say "ah." ___ ___ ___ _____
2. Watch uvula and soft palate rise during "ah." ___ ___ ___ _____

Uvula, soft palate, gag reflex

3. Touch each side of posterior pharyngeal wall to elicit gag reflex (ability to swallow is tested during examination of the thyroid). ___ ___ ___ _____

CN XII (hypoglossal)

1. Observe tongue at rest on floor of mouth. ___ ___ ___ _____

Motor function

2. Instruct client to protrude tongue and observe. ___ ___ ___ _____

Symmetry and strength

3. Instruct client to ___ ___ ___ _____
   A. Wag tongue laterally ___ ___ ___ _____
   B. Stick tongue into each cheek ___ ___ ___ _____
4. Palpate for strength in each cheek ___ ___ ___ _____

From Skillen, D. L., & Day, R. A. (Eds.). (2004). *A syllabus for adult health assessment* (pp. 35–36). Edmonton, AB: Faculty of Nursing, University of Alberta.

STUDENT: _____ DATE: _____
INSTRUCTOR: _____ DATE: _____

Skill 32–11 Assessing Neck Veins and Arteries and Range of Motion

	S	U	NP	Comments

INSPECTION

Neck fully exposed. Sitting position or supine at 30-degree angle.

Neck, carotid arteries, jugular veins

1. Use tangential lighting on neck. ____ ____ ____ _____
2. Inspect neck. ____ ____ ____ _____
3. Inspect carotid arteries and jugular veins. ____ ____ ____ _____

PALPATION

Carotid arteries

1. Palpate each carotid artery separately (at the level of the cricoid cartilage) using thumb or index and middle fingers. ____ ____ ____ _____
2. Assess amplitude, contour, and presence of thrills (humming vibrations). ____ ____ ____ _____
3. Avoid carotid sinus. ____ ____ ____ _____
4. Avoid pressing too hard. ____ ____ ____ _____

AUSCULTATION

Carotid arteries

1. Instruct client to hold breath while holding own breath. ____ ____ ____ _____
2. Use bell of stethoscope to auscultate over each carotid artery. ____ ____ ____ _____

INSPECTION

Jugular veins

Neck and upper thorax exposed. Client in supine position with head on pillow and elevated 45 degrees.
1. Use tangential lighting on neck. ____ ____ ____ _____
2. Locate external jugular first and then the internal jugular veins. ____ ____ ____ _____
3. Repeat on other side. ____ ____ ____ _____
4. Locate sternal angle (angle of Louis). ____ ____ ____ _____
5. Use (R) internal jugular vein to measure jugular venous pressure. ____ ____ ____ _____
6. Line up bottom edge of ruler with the top of the highest point of pulsations of the (R) internal jugular vein, holding it horizontal. ____ ____ ____ _____
7. Stand a second ruler on end on the sternal angle (angle of Louis), perpendicular to the first ruler. ____ ____ ____ _____
8. Measure the vertical distance between the sternal angle and the second ruler and the highest level of internal jugular vein pulsation (first ruler). ____ ____ ____ _____
9. Repeat on other side. ____ ____ ____ _____

Range of motion of neck

Client in sitting or standing position.
1. Inspect range of motion of cervical vertebrae by instructing client to ____ ____ ____ _____
   A. Touch chin to chest (flexion) ____ ____ ____ _____
   B. Look up at ceiling (extension) ____ ____ ____ _____
   C. Touch ear to shoulder bilaterally (lateral flexion) while examiner restricts shoulder movement ____ ____ ____ _____
   D. Turn head to each side, looking over shoulder (rotation) ____ ____ ____ _____

From Skillen, D. L., & Day, R. A. (Eds.). (2004). *A syllabus for adult health assessment* (pp. 36–37). Edmonton, AB: Faculty of Nursing, University of Alberta.

Skill 32–12 Assessing Lymph Nodes of the Neck, Trachea, and Thyroid Gland

	S	U	NP	Comments
INSPECTION				
Lymph nodes				
1. Inspect area of each set of lymph nodes.	___	___	___	_____
PALPATION				
Lymph nodes				
1. Palpate lymph nodes (bilaterally) using finger pads in circular (rotary) motion to move the skin over the underlying structure. May palpate simultaneously	___	___	___	_____
• Preauricular	___	___	___	_____
• Postauricular	___	___	___	_____
• Occipital	___	___	___	_____
• Tonsillar	___	___	___	_____
• Submaxillary	___	___	___	_____
• Submental (braces top of head with one hand)	___	___	___	_____
• Superficial cervical	___	___	___	_____
• Deep cervical	___	___	___	_____
• Posterior cervical	___	___	___	_____
• Supraclavicular	___	___	___	_____
PALPATION				
Trachea				
Client sitting or supine.				
1. Locate trachea above suprasternal notch with index finger and compare spacing from sternomastoid on each side.	___	___	___	_____
INSPECTION				
Cricoid cartilage and below thyroid				
1. Instruct client to extend head slightly.	___	___	___	_____
2. Direct tangential lighting from tip of chin toward thyroid region.	___	___	___	_____
3. Inspect region below cricoid cartilage at rest.	___	___	___	_____
4. Ask client to hold water in mouth.	___	___	___	_____
5. Instruct client to extend head slightly again.	___	___	___	_____
Thyroid gland movement; cranial nerve (CN) IX, X				
6. Inspect for isthmus and thyroid gland movement during swallowing.	___	___	___	_____
PALPATION				
Thyroid				
1. From the front, palpate down midline to identify each structure.	___	___	___	_____
2. From behind, place index fingers just below cricoid cartilage on neck.	___	___	___	_____
3. Instruct client to flex head slightly toward the side being examined.	___	___	___	_____
4. Instruct client to swallow water while palpating for glandular tissues (isthmus and lobes) first on one side and then the other.	___	___	___	_____
AUSCULTATION				
Thyroid gland				
1. Place bell of stethoscope lightly over thyroid lobe.	___	___	___	_____
2. Ask client to hold breath while holding own breath.	___	___	___	_____
3. Listen for bruit.	___	___	___	_____
4. Let client breathe and then ask to hold breath again.	___	___	___	_____
5. Repeat auscultation on other side.	___	___	___	_____

Continued

	S	U	NP	Comments

Test motor function of CN XI (spinal accessory)

Client in sitting position.
1. Observe client shrug shoulders.
2. Instruct client to shrug shoulders while applying resistance with hands on client's shoulders.
3. Instruct client to look straight ahead.
4. Place hand on side of face, then instruct client to turn head to the same side against resistance. Observe opposite sternomastoid contraction and force against hand.
5. Repeat on other side.

From Skillen, D. L., & Day, R. A. (Eds.). (2004). *A syllabus for adult health assessment* (pp. 36–37). Edmonton, AB: Faculty of Nursing, University of Alberta.

STUDENT: _____   DATE: _____
INSTRUCTOR: _____   DATE: _____

Skill 32–13 Assessing the Spine

	S	U	NP	Comments

Client should be standing, loosely draped, feet together. Pants should rest just below sacroiliac joints.

INSPECTION

Curvatures

1. Inspect from side (profile). ___ ___ ___ _____
2. Inspect from back, midline. ___ ___ ___ _____

Vertical alignment

1. Inspect symmetry of shoulders, scapulae, iliac crests, sacroiliac joints, and gluteal folds. ___ ___ ___ _____

Horizontal alignment

1. Inspect symmetry of shoulders, scapulae, iliac crests, sacroiliac joints, and gluteal folds. ___ ___ ___ _____

PALPATION

2. Palpate structures to confirm symmetry. ___ ___ ___ _____

INSPECTION

Range of motion

1. Instruct client to touch toes (flexion). ___ ___ ___ _____
2. Place hand on posterior superior iliac spine, fingers pointing toward midline. ___ ___ ___ _____
3. Instruct client to bend backward as far as possible (extension). ___ ___ ___ _____
4. Place hands on client's hips. ___ ___ ___ _____
5. Instruct client to bend sideways as far as possible (lateral bending). ___ ___ ___ _____
6. Repeat on other side. ___ ___ ___ _____
7. Place hand on client's hip and other hand on opposite shoulder. ___ ___ ___ _____
8. Rotate trunk by pulling shoulder, then hip (rotation). ___ ___ ___ _____
9. Repeat on other side. ___ ___ ___ _____

PALPATION

Spinous processes

Client standing.
1. Palpate spinous processes from C1 to L5. ___ ___ ___ _____
2. Use finger pads or thumbs in rotary motion. ___ ___ ___ _____
3. Inquire about tenderness. ___ ___ ___ _____
4. Assess alignment by running two fingers down spine C1 to L5. ___ ___ ___ _____

Paravertebral muscles

1. Palpate paravertebral muscles bilaterally from level of C1 to L5. ___ ___ ___ _____
2. Use finger pads or thumbs. ___ ___ ___ _____
3. Inquire about tenderness. ___ ___ ___ _____

From Skillen, D. L., & Day, R. A. (Eds.). (2004). *A syllabus for adult health assessment* (p. 38). Edmonton, AB: Faculty of Nursing, University of Alberta.

STUDENT: _____   DATE: _____

INSTRUCTOR: _____   DATE: _____

Skill 32–14 Examination of the Posterior Thorax and Lungs

	S	U	NP	Comments

INSPECTION

Thorax; anteroposterior/lateral; posterior lung fields

Client sitting disrobed to waist.
1. Inspect from side (profile).
2. Inspect posterior thorax from midline.

PALPATION

Chest expansion

1. Place thumbs at level of and parallel to tenth ribs.
2. Wrap hands loosely around lateral rib cage.
3. Slide hands medially to raise skin folds between thumb and spine.
4. Instruct client to inhale deeply and exhale.
5. Compare sides.

Tactile fremitus

1. Instruct client to round shoulders with arms folded across chest, hands on shoulders.
2. Palpate and compare symmetrical areas:
   • Upper (apices and interscapular)
   • Lower
   • Lateral (in midaxillary line)
3. Ask client to repeat "99" **OR** words "blue moon" in a deep voice.
4. Use ball of hand (palm at base of fingers) **OR** ulnar aspect of hand.
5. Use one **OR** two hands to assess fremitus in symmetrical areas (upper, lower, and lateral).

PERCUSSION

Posterior chest

1. Instruct client to continue rounding shoulders.
2. Percuss and compare symmetrical areas at 5-cm intervals over
   • Upper (apices and interscapular)
   • Lower
   • Lateral (in midaxillary line)
3. Press distal phalanx and joint of middle (pleximeter) finger firmly over intercostal space (avoiding contact with other fingers).
4. Aim at distal phalanx or interphalangeal joint.
5. Strike pleximeter a sharp perpendicular blow with tip of middle (plexor) finger (may support plexor finger with thumb).
6. Use wrist action only.

AUSCULTATION

Posterior lung fields

1. Instruct client to continue rounding shoulders.
2. Auscultate with diaphragm of stethoscope.
3. Instruct client to breathe through open mouth, more deeply than usual, and inform if dizzy.
4. Listen to at least ONE full breath in each area.
5. Listen to and compare symmetrical areas:
   • Upper (apices and interscapular)
   • Lower
   • Lateral (in midaxillary line)

From Skillen, D. L., & Day, R. A. (Eds.). (2004). *A syllabus for adult health assessment* (pp. 39–40). Edmonton, AB: Faculty of Nursing, University of Alberta.

STUDENT: _____   DATE: _____

INSTRUCTOR: _____   DATE: _____

Skill 32–15 Assessing the Heart

	S	U	NP	Comments
INSPECTION				
Client in supine position with head elevated 30 degrees, anterior thorax and epigastric area exposed, examiner at client's right side.				
Precordium				
1. Inspect precordium tangentially using penlight.	___	___	___	_____
PALPATION				
1. Landmark using sternal angle.	___	___	___	_____
2. Palpate, proceeding from the apex to the base **OR** the base to the apex.	___	___	___	_____
Apical area				
1. Use finger pads to palpate fifth interspace medial to (L) midclavicular line.	___	___	___	_____
2. Ask client to exhale and hold if unable to locate apical area in 1 above.				
3. Analyze impulses in apical area using fingertips, then one finger.	___	___	___	_____
Right ventricular area				
1. Place tips of curved fingers in (L) third, fourth, and fifth interspaces close to sternum.	___	___	___	_____
2. Ask client to exhale and hold breath.	___	___	___	_____
Epigastric area (subxiphoid)				
1. Press index finger of flattened hand under (L) costal margin and up toward left shoulder.	___	___	___	_____
2. Ask client to inhale and hold.	___	___	___	_____
Left second interspace (pulmonic area)				
1. Place index finger pad in second (L) interspace.	___	___	___	_____
2. Ask client to exhale and hold breath, palpate firmly.	___	___	___	_____
Right second interspace (aortic area)				
1. Place index finger pad in second (R) interspace.	___	___	___	_____
2. Ask client to exhale and hold breath; palpate firmly.	___	___	___	_____
AUSCULTATION				
1. Use diaphragm and bell to listen to all six areas.	___	___	___	_____
2. Apply bell lightly to the chest wall.	___	___	___	_____
3. Auscultate proceeding from apex to base **OR** base to apex.	___	___	___	_____
4. Listen for 5 seconds in each area with diaphragm and bell.	___	___	___	_____
Right second interspace; left second, third, fourth, fifth interspace; apex; apical rate				
5. Auscultate				
• Right second interspace close to sternum	___	___	___	_____
• Left second interspace close to sternum	___	___	___	_____
• Left third interspace close to sternum	___	___	___	_____
• Left fourth interspace close to sternum	___	___	___	_____
• Left fifth interspace close to sternum	___	___	___	_____
• Apex	___	___	___	_____
6. Listen for 1 minute at apex for rate, using diaphragm.	___	___	___	_____

STUDENT: _____ DATE: _____
INSTRUCTOR: _____ DATE: _____

Skill 32–16 Assessing Breasts and Axillae

	S	U	NP	Comments

INSPECTION

Breast, areola, nipple

Client in sitting position, disrobed to waist.
1. Inspect breast, areola, and nipple bilaterally from anterior and lateral view ___ ___ ___ _____
   - With arms at side ___ ___ ___ _____
   - With arms raised over head ___ ___ ___ _____
   - With hands pressed against hips **OR** with hands pressed together, not obstructing view of breasts ___ ___ ___ _____
2. Inspect with client leaning forward and then with breasts lifted. ___ ___ ___ _____

PALPATION

Large breasts

1. With the client leaning forward, palpate breast tissue between the examiner's hands. ___ ___ ___ _____

INSPECTION

Axillae

1. Inspect skin of axillae with arms raised over head. ___ ___ ___ _____
2. *Only* if signs of infection, put on gloves for palpation. ___ ___ ___ _____

PALPATION

Axillary lymph nodes

1. Assist client to dry axillae. ___ ___ ___ _____
2. Support client's (L) hand and wrist with examiner's (L) hand to examine (L) axilla and reverse for (R) axilla. ___ ___ ___ _____
3. Instruct client to relax arm. ___ ___ ___ _____

Central lymph nodes

4. Cup fingers together. ___ ___ ___ _____
5. Reach as high as possible into apex of (L) axilla. ___ ___ ___ _____
6. Press fingers against chest wall. ___ ___ ___ _____
7. Bring finger pads down over ribs and feel for central nodes. ___ ___ ___ _____

Pectoral lymph nodes

8. Slide fingers under anterior axillary fold, palpating chest wall with finger pads for pectoral nodes. ___ ___ ___ _____
9. Grasp anterior axillary folds (pectoral) and palpate with finger pads, using thumbs as anchor. ___ ___ ___ _____
10. Slide fingers under posterior axillary fold, palpating chest wall with finger pads for subscapular nodes. ___ ___ ___ _____

Subscapular lymph nodes

11. Turn hands and feel inside posterior axillary folds with finger pads (subscapular). ___ ___ ___ _____

Lateral lymph nodes

12. Feel along upper humerus with finger pads (lateral). ___ ___ ___ _____
13. Repeat on (R) side. ___ ___ ___ _____

PALPATION

Infraclavicular lymph nodes

1. Palpate bilaterally for infraclavicular nodes below clavicle in first interspace with finger pads. ___ ___ ___ _____

Supraclavicular lymph nodes

1. Palpate bilaterally for supraclavicular nodes above clavicle with finger pads. ___ ___ ___ _____

Continued

	S	U	NP	Comments

INSPECTION

Breast, areola, nipple

Client supine, with pillow removed from under head. Use small pillow under client's shoulder on side examined *only if breasts are large.*

	S	U	NP	Comments
1. Inspect breasts bilaterally.	___	___	___	_____

PALPATION

Breast, areola, nipple, and tail of Spence

Ask client to move arm away from chest on side being examined.

	S	U	NP	Comments
1. Palpate each breast.	___	___	___	_____
2. Use flat of second, third, and fourth fingers in a rotary motion to compress breast tissue.	___	___	___	_____
3. Flex from the wrist, not the fingers.	___	___	___	_____
4. Apply moderate pressure, keeping constant contact with skin.	___	___	___	_____
5. Move back and forth across breast in straight lines, making constant small circles.	___	___	___	_____
6. Slide hand down one finger width for each pass.	___	___	___	_____
7. Cover full area from below clavicle to 3 cm below breast, from midaxillary line to midsternal line:	___	___	___	_____
• Glandular tissue	___	___	___	_____
• Areolar area	___	___	___	_____
• Nipple	___	___	___	_____
• Tail of Spence	___	___	___	_____

From Skillen, D. L., & Day, R. A. (Eds.). (2004). *A syllabus for adult health assessment* (pp. 43–44). Edmonton, AB: Faculty of Nursing, University of Alberta.

STUDENT: _____ DATE: _____

INSTRUCTOR: _____ DATE: _____

Skill 32–17 Inspecting and Auscultating the Abdomen

	S	U	NP	Comments

INSPECTION

Abdomen

Abdomen fully exposed, bladder empty, draped; client with arms at sides
OR folded across chest.

	S	U	NP	Comments
1. Inspect tangentially from "R" side and from foot of table.	___	___	___	_____
2. Inspect across abdomen.	___	___	___	_____
3. Ask client to inhale deeply and hold breath.	___	___	___	_____
4. Inspect for symmetry.	___	___	___	_____

AUSCULTATION

Bowel sounds

	S	U	NP	Comments
1. Inquire about abdominal tenderness and ask to indicate area.	___	___	___	_____
2. Auscultate prior to percussion and palpation.	___	___	___	_____
3. Place diaphragm gently.	___	___	___	_____
4. Listen in all four quadrants.	___	___	___	_____

AUSCULTATION

	S	U	NP	Comments
1. Press diaphragm *gently* against abdomen.	___	___	___	_____

Aorta

	S	U	NP	Comments
2. Listen slightly "L" of midline in epigastric region (aorta).	___	___	___	_____

Renal arteries

	S	U	NP	Comments
3. Listen to "L" and "R" of midline just superior to umbilicus (renal).	___	___	___	_____

Iliac arteries

	S	U	NP	Comments
4. Listen just above inguinal ligament midway between anterior superior iliac spine and symphysis pubis (iliac).	___	___	___	_____

From Skillen, D. L., & Day, R. A. (Eds.). (2004). *A syllabus for adult health assessment* (p. 45). Edmonton, AB: Faculty of Nursing, University of Alberta.

STUDENT: _____ DATE: _____

INSTRUCTOR: _____ DATE: _____

Skill 32–18 Percussing the Abdomen

	S	U	NP	Comments
PERCUSSION				
Abdomen				
1. Place distal phalanx and joint of middle (pleximeter) finger on abdominal wall (avoiding contact with other fingers).	___	___	___	_____
2. Aim at distal phalanx or interphalangeal joint.	___	___	___	_____
3. Strike pleximeter a sharp, light blow with tip of middle (plexor) finger.	___	___	___	_____
4. Percuss lightly over entire abdomen.	___	___	___	_____
5. Inquire about areas of tenderness.	___	___	___	_____
6. Observe client's facial reactions during percussion.	___	___	___	_____
Liver				
1. Percuss in right midclavicular line from lung resonance to liver dullness (upper border); mark level.	___	___	___	_____
2. Start at level below umbilicus in right midclavicular line and percuss upward to liver dullness (lower border); mark level.	___	___	___	_____
3. Measure vertical span of liver dullness in centimetres.	___	___	___	_____
4. Request client to inhale deeply.	___	___	___	_____
5. Percuss upward toward lower border.	___	___	___	_____
Splenic percussion sign				
1. Percuss lowest interspace in left anterior axillary line.	___	___	___	_____
2. Instruct client to take a deep breath and repeat percussion in lowest interspace of left anterior axillary line.	___	___	___	_____
3. Note any change in percussion.	___	___	___	_____
Bladder				
Percuss downward in midline from umbilicus to the pelvic brim.				
Kidney				
Client sitting or standing. Inform client of procedure.				
1. Inquire about kidney tenderness.				
2. If tender, press in each costovertebral angle in turn with fingertips.	___	___	___	_____
3. Inquire about tenderness.	___	___	___	_____
4. If not tender, place palm (fingers not touching client) of nondominant hand over each costovertebral angle in turn.	___	___	___	_____
5. Strike dorsum of hand with ulnar surface of fist.	___	___	___	_____
6. Inquire about tenderness.	___	___	___	_____

From Skillen, D. L., & Day, R. A. (Eds.). (2004). *A syllabus for adult health assessment* (pp. 38–39, 45–46). Edmonton, AB: Faculty of Nursing, University of Alberta.

STUDENT: _____ DATE: _____

INSTRUCTOR: _____ DATE: _____

Skill 32–19 Palpating the Abdomen

	S	U	NP	Comments

PALPATION

1. Use flat of four fingers held together, in a light dipping motion.

Light abdominal palpation

2. Palpate over entire abdomen, more than once in each of four quadrants.
3. Inquire about tenderness.

Deep abdominal palpation

1. Palpate deeply after light palpation.
2. Palpate over entire abdomen, more than once in each quadrant. Use flat of four fingers of one hand **OR** use two hands, one placed on top of the other and pressure exerted with top hand.
3. Inquire about tenderness.
4. Observe client's facial reactions during palpation.

PALPATION

Liver

1. Place (L) hand behind client parallel to and supporting eleventh and twelfth ribs and soft tissue below.
2. Press (L) hand forward while client relaxes.
3. Place (R) hand on client's abdomen
   • Below lower border of liver dullness percussed upon deep inspiration
   • Lateral to rectus muscle with hand held parallel or obliquely to midline of body **OR** parallel to costal margin
4. Palpate deeply with flat of four fingers.
5. Instruct client to take a deep breath and try to feel liver edge as it comes down to meet fingertips **OR** lateral edge of index finger.
6. If liver not palpable,
   • Inch hand closer to (R) costal margin and repeat procedure
   • Exert more pressure inward upon expiration and repeat procedure

Inguinal nodes; horizontal

1. Palpate inferior to inguinal ligament from symphysis pubis to anterior superior iliac spine.

Inguinal nodes; vertical

2. Palpate medial to femoral canal from superior ramus to an area 5 cm distally.

From Skillen, D. L. & Day, R. A. (Eds.). (2004). *A syllabus for adult health assessment* (p. 46). Edmonton, AB: Faculty of Nursing, University of Alberta.

STUDENT: _____   DATE: _____
INSTRUCTOR: _____   DATE: _____

Skill 32–20 Assessing the External Female Genitalia

	S	U	NP	Comments

Client in lithotomy position, with feet in stirrups, draped with pubis and genitalia exposed, nurse gloved, and light coming over nurse's shoulder.

INSPECTION

Pubic hair

1. Inspect hair, hair distribution, and skin of pubis. ___ ___ ___ _____

Labia majora

1. Inspect labia majora. ___ ___ ___ _____
2. Use thumb and index finger of nondominant hand inside labia minora to gently but firmly retract tissues forward. ___ ___ ___ _____
3. Inspect labia minora. ___ ___ ___ _____

PALPATION

Labia minora

1. With other hand, palpate labia minora between thumb and index finger on one side. ___ ___ ___ _____
2. Repeat on other side. ___ ___ ___ _____

INSPECTION

Clitoris

1. Inspect clitoris. ___ ___ ___ _____

Urethral meatus

1. Locate urethral meatus above vaginal canal. ___ ___ ___ _____
2. Inspect meatus. ___ ___ ___ _____

Vaginal orifice (introitus)

1. With the labia minora still retracted, inspect the introitus. ___ ___ ___ _____
2. With the labia minora still retracted, and using the dominant hand, first dip the index finger into a basin of warm water for lubrication. ___ ___ ___ _____
3. With the palm facing upward, insert index finger into the vagina as far as the proximal interphalangeal joint (second finger joint). ___ ___ ___ _____

PALPATION

Skene's glands

4. Exert upward pressure by moving fingers outward (milking action) on either side of urethra and directly over the urethra. ___ ___ ___ _____
5. Inquire about tenderness. ___ ___ ___ _____
6. Culture any discharge. ___ ___ ___ _____
7. Remove retracting hand. ___ ___ ___ _____
8. Insert index finger into posterior vaginal opening toward the (L) side and palpate the posterior labia majora between the index finger and the thumb. ___ ___ ___ _____
9. Repeat on other side. ___ ___ ___ _____
10. Culture any discharge. ___ ___ ___ _____
11. Change gloves. ___ ___ ___ _____

Bartholin's glands, perineum, vaginal orifice

1. Insert first two fingers into vagina and instruct client to squeeze examiner's fingers. ___ ___ ___ _____
2. Instruct client to strain downward as if voiding. Determine if any structures touch examining fingers. ___ ___ ___ _____
3. Remove fingers from vagina and use first two fingers of both hands to separate the vaginal orifice. ___ ___ ___ _____
4. Instruct client to bear down. ___ ___ ___ _____
5. Inspect vaginal orifice. ___ ___ ___ _____

Continued

	S	U	NP	Comments

INSPECTION

Anus

See Skill 32–24, "Assessing the Anus, Rectum, Prostate, and Cervix"   ___   ___   ___   _____

From Day, R. A. (2004). Female external and internal genital examination. In D. L. Skillen & R. A. Day (Eds.), *A syllabus for adult health assessment* (pp. 92–95). Edmonton, AB: Faculty of Nursing, University of Alberta.

STUDENT: _____ DATE: _____

INSTRUCTOR: _____ DATE: _____

Skill 32–21 Assessing Male Genitalia and Inguinal Regions

	S	U	NP	Comments

INSPECTION

Client standing or supine, pubis and genitalia exposed, nurse gloved.

Pubic hair

1. Inspect hair and skin of pubis.

Penis

1. Inspect shaft of penis.

Skin prepuce, glans, corona, urethral meatus

2. Ask client to retract prepuce (foreskin) if present.
3. Inspect glans and corona.
4. Inspect location of meatus.
5. Compress glans gently.
6. Inspect meatus.
7. Replace prepuce if retracted.

PALPATION

Shaft

1. Palpate shaft between thumb and first two fingers.
2. Inquire about tenderness.

INSPECTION

Scrotum

1. Inspect anterior and lateral surfaces.
2. Lift scrotum gently to inspect posterior surface.

PALPATION

1. Use thumb and first two fingers of examining hand.
2. Palpate one side in sequence:
   A. Testis
   B. Epididymis
   C. Spermatic cord (and vas deferens)
3. Repeat on other side.

INSPECTION

Client standing.

Inguinal region; pubic tubercle to anterior superior iliac spine (inguinal canal)

1. Inspect (L) (R) inguinal regions.
2. Instruct client to strain or bear down.
3. Inspect regions using tangential lighting.
4. Compare regions.

Femoral canal

1. Inspect (L) (R) femoral regions.
2. Use tangential lighting.

PALPATION

3. Instruct client to cough or strain down (R) (L).
4. Use tangential lighting.
5. Compare regions.

Inguinal ring, inguinal canal

Client remains standing.
1. Stand on (R) side of client.
2. Place index finger of (R) hand against scrotal skin on (R) side.
3. Place finger low on scrotum.

Continued

	S	U	NP	Comments
4. Move finger toward inguinal ring by invaginating scrotal skin over finger.	___	___	___	_____
5. Assess possibility of passage through inguinal ring.	___	___	___	_____
6. Insert index finger superiorly and obliquely along vas deferens into inguinal canal, following spermatic cord.	___	___	___	_____
7. When index finger cannot move further, instruct client to cough and strain down.	___	___	___	_____
8. Assess for bulging pressure against finger.	___	___	___	_____
9. Observe relationship to pubic tubercle.	___	___	___	_____
10. Repeat on (L) side with (L) index finger.	___	___	___	_____

Femoral canal

	S	U	NP	Comments
1. Place finger pads on anterior thigh in region of femoral canal.	___	___	___	_____
2. Instruct client to cough and strain down.	___	___	___	_____
3. Assess for bulge or impulse against fingers.	___	___	___	_____
4. Observe relationship to pubic tubercle.	___	___	___	_____
5. Repeat on opposite thigh.	___	___	___	_____

Inguinal lymph nodes

See Skill 32–20   ___ ___ ___ _____

From Skillen, D. L. (2004). Male genitalia examination. In D. L. Skillen & R. A. Day (Eds.), *A syllabus for adult health assessment* (pp. 89–90). Edmonton, AB: Faculty of Nursing, University of Alberta.

STUDENT: _____ DATE: _____
INSTRUCTOR: _____ DATE: _____

Skill 32–22 Assessing the Anus and Rectum

	S	U	NP	Comments

INSPECTION

Client bending forward or in Sims' position.

PALPATION

Anus

Anal area exposed. Nurse gloved.

	S	U	NP	Comments
1. Spread buttocks apart.	___	___	___	_____
2. Inspect perianal and sacrococcygeal regions.	___	___	___	_____
3. Lubricate index finger of dominant hand by dropping lubricant onto gloved finger.	___	___	___	_____
4. Place finger pad across anus.	___	___	___	_____
5. Instruct client to bear down.	___	___	___	_____
6. Assess tone of anal sphincter.	___	___	___	_____

Rectum

	S	U	NP	Comments
1. Flex fingertip and insert gently into anal canal.	___	___	___	_____
2. Insert finger in direction of umbilicus.	___	___	___	_____

Adapted from Skillen, D. L. (2004). Anus, rectum, and prostate examination. In D. L. Skillen & R. A. Day (Eds.), *A syllabus for adult health assessment* (p. 96). Edmonton, AB: Faculty of Nursing, University of Alberta.

Skill 32–23 Inspecting the Upper Extremities

	S	U	NP	Comments

SKIN, NAILS, HAIR, SYMMETRY

	S	U	NP	Comments
1. Fully expose the hands and arms of the seated or supine client.	___	___	___	_____
2. Inspect skin, nails, and symmetry of both arms and hands.	___	___	___	_____

RANGE OF MOTION (ROM)

	S	U	NP	Comments
The examiner inspects the ROM. Each arm is tested, either separately or simultaneously, and compared. Only if the client is unable to perform active ROM does the examiner attempt passive ROM.	___	___	___	_____

THUMBS

	S	U	NP	Comments
1. Instruct client to supinate hands and	___	___	___	_____
2. Touch base of fifth finger with thumb (flexion).	___	___	___	_____
3. Move thumb back and forth away from fingers (extension).	___	___	___	_____
4. Move thumb anteriorly away from palm (abduction).	___	___	___	_____
5. Move thumb back down (adduction).	___	___	___	_____
6. Touch tip of thumb to each fingertip (opposition).	___	___	___	_____

FINGERS

	S	U	NP	Comments
1. Instruct client to make a fist (flexion), thumb across knuckles.	___	___	___	_____
2. Straighten fingers (extension).	___	___	___	_____
3. Spread extended fingers (abduction).	___	___	___	_____
4. Close extended fingers together (adduction).	___	___	___	_____

WRISTS

	S	U	NP	Comments
1. Instruct client to flex wrist and	___	___	___	_____
2. Extend wrist.	___	___	___	_____
3. Stabilize client's forearm and hand in supination and instruct client to	___	___	___	_____
• Move hand medially (ulnar deviation) and	___	___	___	_____
• Move hand laterally (radial deviation).	___	___	___	_____

ELBOWS

	S	U	NP	Comments
1. Instruct client to bend elbows (flexion) and	___	___	___	_____
2. Straighten elbows (extension).	___	___	___	_____
3. Instruct client to hold flexed elbows close to sides and turn palms upward (supination) and	___	___	___	_____
4. Turn palms downward (pronation).	___	___	___	_____

SHOULDERS

	S	U	NP	Comments
1. Instruct client to extend arms forward (flexion) and	___	___	___	_____
2. Extend straightened arms as far back as possible (extension).	___	___	___	_____
3. Instruct client to bring straightened arms across anterior midline (adduction).	___	___	___	_____
4. Instruct client to lift arms laterally in an arc starting from sides and ending with both arms extended above head, palms facing (abduction).	___	___	___	_____
5. Instruct client to place hands behind own neck (external rotation) and	___	___	___	_____
6. Place hands behind small of back (internal rotation).	___	___	___	_____

From Skillen, D. L., & Day, R. A. (Eds.). (2004). *A syllabus for adult health assessment* (pp. 47–48). Edmonton, AB: Faculty of Nursing, University of Alberta.

STUDENT: _____ DATE: _____

INSTRUCTOR: _____ DATE: _____

Skill 32–24 Palpating Temperature and Joints of the Upper Extremities

	S	U	NP	Comments
PALPATION				
Temperature				
1. Use dorsum of hands or fingers to compare temperature of each hand with forearm and upper arm above it.	___	___	___	_____
2. Compare sides.	___	___	___	_____
Joints				
Examiner instructs the client to indicate if there is any tenderness during joint palpation. Both limbs are palpated separately and compared.				
Fingers: interphalangeal (IP) joints				
1. Palpate with thumb and index finger of one hand all of the distal and proximal IP joints of fingers and thumb of both hands at the medial and lateral aspects of each joint.	___	___	___	_____
Fingers: metacarpophalangeal (MCP) joints				
1. Palpate with thumbs of both hands the MCP joints of both hands just distal to and on each side of the knuckle.	___	___	___	_____
Wrists				
1. Palpate medial and lateral surfaces of each wrist (distal radius and ulna).	___	___	___	_____
2. Palpate each wrist with thumbs dorsally and fingers ventrally.	___	___	___	_____
Elbows				
1. Support the left slightly flexed arm with the left hand and forearm.	___	___	___	_____
2. Palpate	___	___	___	_____
A. The olecranon process	___	___	___	_____
B. The groove on either side of the olecranon process	___	___	___	_____
C. The lateral and medial epicondyles	___	___	___	_____
3. Inquire about tenderness.	___	___	___	_____
4. Repeat on the right side.	___	___	___	_____
Shoulders				
1. Cup a hand over each of the client's exposed shoulders and	___	___	___	_____
2. Feel for crepitus during adduction, abduction, external and internal rotation.	___	___	___	_____
3. Palpate the sternoclavicular joint.	___	___	___	_____
4. Palpate the acromioclavicular joint.	___	___	___	_____
5. Palpate the biceps groove for long head of biceps tendon.	___	___	___	_____
6. Inquire about tenderness during 3, 4, 5 above.	___	___	___	_____

From Skillen, D. L., & Day, R. A. (Eds.). (2004). *A syllabus for adult health assessment.* Edmonton, AB: Faculty of Nursing, University of Alberta.

STUDENT: _____   DATE: _____

INSTRUCTOR: _____   DATE: _____

Skill 32–25 Assessing Muscle Tone and Strength of the Upper Extremities

	S	U	NP	Comments

PALPATION

Muscle tone

1. Support the relaxed arm at the hand and elbow.
2. Move each arm (fingers, wrist, elbow, shoulder) through a modified passive range of motion.
3. Attend to the resistance offered.
4. Test muscle tone prior to testing muscle strength.

Muscle strength: fingers

1. Place two crossed fingers in each hand of client.
2. Instruct client to squeeze firmly (grip).
3. Compare sides; may test simultaneously.
4. Try, against resistance, to force client's outspread fingers of each hand together (abduction).
5. Instruct client to touch thumb to little fingertip.
6. Resist pull of examiner's thumb against client's thumb (opposition).
7. Compare sides; may test simultaneously.

Muscle strength: wrists

1. Instruct client to hold flexed elbows close to sides with forearm in pronation.
2. Instruct client to make a fist and flex wrists.
3. Try to pull client's fist up against resistance (flexion).
4. Instruct client to make a fist and extend wrist.
5. Try to pull client's fist down against resistance (extension).
6. Compare sides; may test simultaneously.

Muscle strength: elbows

1. Instruct client to flex arm at the elbow.
2. Try, against resistance, to extend client's flexed elbows (biceps).
3. Instruct client to flex arm at the elbow.
4. Try, against resistance, to further flex client's elbows (triceps).
5. Compare sides; may test simultaneously.

Muscle strength: shoulders

1. Instruct client to raise both extended arms above the head.
2. Try, against resistance, to force client's arms to sides.
3. Compare sides; may test simultaneously.

From Skillen, D. L., & Day, R. A. (Eds.). *A syllabus for adult health assessment* (pp. 49–50). Edmonton, AB: Faculty of Nursing, University of Alberta.

STUDENT: _____ DATE: _____

INSTRUCTOR: _____ DATE: _____

Skill 32–26 Palpating Pulses and Epitrochlear Nodes in the Upper Extremities

	S	U	NP	Comments
PALPATION				
Brachial pulse				
1. Palpate brachial artery with finger pads or thumbs at the antecubital crease (fossa) **OR** above elbow in groove between biceps and triceps muscles.	___	___	___	_____
2. Compare sides.	___	___	___	_____
Radial pulse				
1. Palpate radial artery with finger pads on the lateral flexor surface of wrist.	___	___	___	_____
2. Compare sides.	___	___	___	_____
Epitrochlear nodes				
1. Support client's right forearm with examiner's right hand as client flexes elbow about 90 degrees.	___	___	___	_____
2. Palpate for epitrochlear node in groove between biceps and triceps muscles with finger pads of the left hand medially and approximately 3 cm above the medial epicondyle.	___	___	___	_____
3. Reverse hand position to examine client's left arm.	___	___	___	_____

From Skillen, D. L., & Day, R. A. (Eds.). *A syllabus for adult health assessment* (p. 50). Edmonton, AB: Faculty of Nursing, University of Alberta.

STUDENT: _____ DATE: _____

INSTRUCTOR: _____ DATE: _____

Skill 32–27 Inspecting Coordination in the Upper Extremities

	S	U	NP	Comments

COORDINATION

Test each hand separately.

RAPID ALTERNATING TESTING

	S	U	NP	Comments
1. Instruct client to pat thigh as rapidly as possible, alternating between palm and dorsum of hand.	___	___	___	_____
2. Compare sides.	___	___	___	_____
3. Instruct client to touch distal joint of thumb with index fingertip repeatedly as rapidly as possible.	___	___	___	_____
4. Compare sides.	___	___	___	_____

POINT-TO-POINT TESTING

	S	U	NP	Comments
1. Instruct client to extend arm.	___	___	___	_____
2. Instruct client to alternately touch client's nose, then examiner's finger with fully extended arm.	___	___	___	_____
3. Alter finger position.	___	___	___	_____
4. Hold finger in one place.	___	___	___	_____
5. Instruct client to raise extended arm over head and lower it to touch finger.	___	___	___	_____
6. After several tries, instruct client to close eyes and repeat.	___	___	___	_____
7. Repeat 5 and 6 with other arm.	___	___	___	_____

From Skillen, D. L., & Day, R. A. (Eds.). (2004). *A syllabus for adult health assessment* (p. 50). Edmonton, AB: Faculty of Nursing, University of Alberta.

STUDENT: _____   DATE: _____

INSTRUCTOR: _____   DATE: _____

Skill 32–28 Assessing Sensation in the Upper Extremities

	S	U	NP	Comments

INSPECTION AND PALPATION

Both arms are tested. The examiner demonstrates how sharp, dull, and light touch feel before beginning tests.

Sensation: superficial pain

1. Instruct client to close eyes and report with each touch whether it is "sharp" or "dull."
2. Touch client's arms lightly and alternately in corresponding areas with sharp end of splintered tongue blade (occasionally using blunt end), covering C4 to C8 and T1 dermatomes in upper arms, forearms, and hands.
3. Compare sides.

Sensation: light touch

1. Instruct client to close eyes and report each time touch of the cotton wisp is perceived.
2. Touch client's arms lightly, avoiding pressure, alternately in corresponding areas with cotton wisp, testing C4 to C8 and T1 dermatomes in upper arms, forearms, and hands.
3. Vary the intervals between touches.
4. Compare sides.

Sensation: vibration

1. Instruct client to close eyes and describe the sensation felt.
2. Place vibrating 128 Hz tuning fork firmly over distal interphalangeal joint of one finger and proceed proximally to proximal interphalangeal and metacarpophalangeal joints, etc., until vibrations are felt and reported.
3. Stop vibration and ask what is felt.
4. Compare sides.

Sensation: position sense

1. Demonstrate "up" and "down" position of a finger.
2. Instruct client to close eyes and identify position of finger.
3. Grasp distal phalanx by medial and lateral aspects and move it "up" or "down." Ensure that adjacent digits are not involved.
4. Compare sides.

INSPECTION AND PALPATION

Tactile discrimination

Both sides are tested.

Stereognosis

1. Instruct client to close eyes and identify object placed in palm.
2. Place a small familiar object in each palm in turn. The object can only be manipulated by the hand being tested.
3. Compare sides.

Graphesthesia

1. Instruct client to close eyes and identify what number is drawn on the skin.
2. With palm facing client, draw number with a blunt object on palm of hand.
3. Compare sides.

Extinction

1. Instruct client to close eyes and identify where touched.
2. Touch client in corresponding area of both arms simultaneously.
3. Ask client where touched.

From Skillen, D. L., & Day, R. A. (Eds.). (2004). *A syllabus for adult health assessment* (pp. 50–52). Edmonton, AB: Faculty of Nursing, University of Alberta.

STUDENT: _____   DATE: _____

INSTRUCTOR: _____   DATE: _____

Skill 32–29 Assessing Deep Tendon Reflexes of the Upper Extremities

	S	U	NP	Comments

INSPECTION AND PERCUSSION

Deep tendon reflexes

Both sides are tested and compared. *Only if* responses are symmetrically diminished or absent does examiner use reinforcement (augmentation). The examiner strikes the slightly stretched tendon briskly with reflex hammer held loosely and swung freely in an arc.

Biceps reflex

1. Position client with arm supported and relaxed, elbow flexed, and palm downward on thigh (seated client) or abdomen (supine client).   ___ ___ ___ _____
2. Use hammer to tap own thumb placed over biceps tendon at antecubital fossa (crease).   ___ ___ ___ _____
3. Compare flexion of forearm on each side.   ___ ___ ___ _____

Triceps reflex

1. Position client with arm supported and relaxed, elbow flexed **OR** abducted and flexed in a right angle, in "hang-to-dry" position.   ___ ___ ___ _____
2. Use hammer to tap the triceps tendon 2 to 5 cm above elbow.   ___ ___ ___ _____
3. Compare extension of forearm on each side.   ___ ___ ___ _____

Brachioradialis reflex

1. Position client with arm resting on lap (sitting) or abdomen (supine) and palm down.   ___ ___ ___ _____
2. Use hammer to tap the brachioradialis tendon 2 to 5 cm above wrist.   ___ ___ ___ _____
3. Compare flexion and supination of hand on each side.   ___ ___ ___ _____

From Skillen, D. L., & Day, R. A. (Eds.). (2004). *A syllabus for adult health assessment* (pp. 50–52). Edmonton, AB: Faculty of Nursing, University of Alberta.

STUDENT: _____ DATE: _____

INSTRUCTOR: _____ DATE: _____

Skill 32–30 Inspecting the Lower Extremities, Including Range of Motion

	S	U	NP	Comments
SKIN, NAILS, HAIR, SYMMETRY				
1. Fully expose legs and feet of supine client.	____	____	____	_____
2. Inspect skin, nails, muscle mass, and symmetry of both legs and feet.	____	____	____	_____
3. Inspect knee for expected depressions on either side of patella.	____	____	____	_____

RANGE OF MOTION (ROM)

Test each leg either separately or simultaneously and compare. Only if client is unable to perform active ROM does the examiner attempt passive ROM.

	S	U	NP	Comments
TOES				
1. Instruct client to bend toes downward (flexion).	____	____	____	_____
2. Instruct client to straighten toes and point upward (extension).	____	____	____	_____
ANKLES				
1. Instruct client to bring foot upward toward shin (dorsiflexion).	____	____	____	_____
2. Instruct client to bend foot downward away from shin (plantar flexion).	____	____	____	_____
3. Stabilize ankle and hold heel and instruct client to tilt foot inward with sole toward midline (inversion).	____	____	____	_____
4. Stabilize ankle and hold heel and instruct client to tilt foot outward with sole facing laterally (eversion).	____	____	____	_____
5. Repeat on other foot.	____	____	____	_____
HIPS AND KNEES				
1. Place hand under lumbar spine.	____	____	____	_____
2. Instruct client to bring each knee in turn up toward chest and press firmly onto the abdomen (flexion at hip and knee).	____	____	____	_____
3. Note when back touches hand.	____	____	____	_____
4. Observe that opposite thigh remains flat on table.	____	____	____	_____
5. Instruct client to straighten leg (extension).	____	____	____	_____
HIPS				
1. Stabilize pelvis by pressing on one anterior superior iliac crest with left hand.	____	____	____	_____
2. Grasp opposite ankle with right hand and move leg over other leg (adduction).	____	____	____	_____
3. Repeat on other side.	____	____	____	_____
4. Stabilize pelvis by pressing on one anterior superior iliac crest with left hand.	____	____	____	_____
5. Grasp opposite leg at ankle and abduct leg until iliac spine moves (abduction).	____	____	____	_____
6. Repeat on other side.	____	____	____	_____
7. Flex leg at hip and knee to 90 degrees.	____	____	____	_____
8. Support thigh with left hand and ankle with right hand.	____	____	____	_____
9. Turn lower leg medially (external rotation), then laterally (internal rotation).	____	____	____	_____
10. Repeat on other side.	____	____	____	_____

From Skillen, D. L., & Day, R. A. (Eds.). (2004). *A syllabus for adult health assessment* (pp. 52–53). Edmonton, AB: Faculty of Nursing, University of Alberta.

STUDENT: _____ DATE: _____

INSTRUCTOR: _____ DATE: _____

Skill 32–31 Palpating Joints and Skin Surface for Temperature and Edema

	S	U	NP	Comments

TEMPERATURE

1. Use dorsum of hands or fingers to compare temperature of each foot with lower leg and thigh above it.
2. Compare sides.

EDEMA

1. Press firmly and gently with thumb for 5 seconds over dorsum of each foot and/or medial malleolus.
2. Assess for extent of depression in the skin.
3. Press firmly and gently with thumb for 5 seconds over each shin.
4. Assess for extent of depression in the skin.

FEET

Interphalangeal (IP) joints

1. Palpate with thumb and index finger of one hand all of the distal and proximal IP joints of the toes.

Metatarsophalangeal (MTP) joints

2. Compress each forefoot just proximal to MTP joints with thumb and fingers placed on medial and lateral surfaces.

Heel

3. Palpate each heel.

Ankles: ankle joint and Achilles tendon

1. Place thumbs dorsally and fingers ventrally.
2. Palpate anterior aspect of each ankle joint.
3. Palpate along each Achilles tendon with thumb and fingers.

KNEES

1. Instruct client to bend knees (flexion).
2. Cup hands over each knee in turn as client returns leg to resting position (extension).

Suprapatellar pouch

3. Note any crepitations.
4. Palpate each side of quadriceps in progressive steps, from 10 cm above superior border of patella to patellar pouch.

Patella

5. Continue palpation along sides of patella.

Tibiofemoral joint

6. Instruct client to slightly flex knee.
7. Palpate tibiofemoral joints (inferior, medial, and lateral to patella).

From Skillen, D. L., & Day, R. A. (Eds.). (2004). *A syllabus for adult health assessment* (pp. 53–54). Edmonton, AB: Faculty of Nursing, University of Alberta.

STUDENT: _____ DATE: _____

INSTRUCTOR: _____ DATE: _____

Skill 32–32 Assessing Muscle Tone and Muscle Strength of the Lower Extremities

	S	U	NP	Comments
MUSCLE TONE: LEGS				
1. Support the leg at the foot and lower thigh.	___	___	___	_____
2. Move each leg (ankle, knee, hip) through a modified range of motion.	___	___	___	_____
3. Assess resistance offered.	___	___	___	_____
4. Test muscle tone prior to testing muscle strength.	___	___	___	_____
MUSCLE STRENGTH: FEET				
1. May test separately or simultaneously.	___	___	___	_____
2. Place hands on client's soles of feet.	___	___	___	_____
3. Ask client to plantar-flex foot against the resistance offered.	___	___	___	_____
4. Compare sides.	___	___	___	_____
5. Place hands on dorsum of client's feet.	___	___	___	_____
6. Ask client to dorsiflex feet against resistance offered.	___	___	___	_____
7. Compare sides.	___	___	___	_____
MUSCLE STRENGTH: LEGS				
1. Instruct client to flex knee.	___	___	___	_____
2. Place left hand at knee and grasp client's ankle with right hand.	___	___	___	_____
3. Instruct client to keep foot in contact with table as you attempt to straighten client's leg (flexion at knee).	___	___	___	_____
4. Compare sides.	___	___	___	_____
5. Instruct client to flex knee.	___	___	___	_____
6. Support client's flexed knee with left hand and push against lower shin with right hand as client attempts to straighten leg (extension at knee).	___	___	___	_____
7. Compare sides.	___	___	___	_____
MUSCLE STRENGTH: HIP				
1. Place both hands on client's thigh.	___	___	___	_____
2. Try to force thigh downward as client raises leg against hand (flexion).	___	___	___	_____
3. Place hand under client's thigh.	___	___	___	_____
4. Instruct client to force thigh downward on examiner's hand (extension).	___	___	___	_____
5. Compare sides.	___	___	___	_____
6. Place both hands firmly on surface between client's knees.	___	___	___	_____
7. Instruct client to bring legs together (adduction).	___	___	___	_____
8. Place hands firmly on surface at lateral aspect of client's knees.	___	___	___	_____
9. Instruct client to spread legs (abduction).	___	___	___	_____
10. Compare sides.	___	___	___	_____

From Skillen, D. L., & Day, R. A. (Eds.). (2004). *A syllabus for adult health assessment* (pp. 54–55). Edmonton, AB: Faculty of Nursing, University of Alberta.

STUDENT: _____   DATE: _____

INSTRUCTOR: _____   DATE: _____

Skill 32–33 Assessing Pulses in the Lower Extremities

	S	U	NP	Comments

POPLITEAL PULSES

1. Instruct client to flex leg slightly and relax muscles.
2. Palpate popliteal artery with fingertips of both hands midline in popliteal fossa, pressing deeply.
3. Compare sides.
4. If unable to palpate, ask client to lie prone on examining surface with legs flexed at knee and palpate.

POSTERIOR TIBIAL PULSES

1. Palpate posterior tibial artery behind and below medial malleolus with finger pads.
2. Compare sides. May palpate simultaneously.

DORSALIS PEDIS PULSES

1. Palpate dorsalis pedis artery with finger pads on dorsum of foot just lateral to extensor tendon of great toe.
2. Compare sides. May palpate simultaneously.

From Skillen, D. L., & Day, R. A. (Eds.). (2004). *A syllabus for adult health assessment* (p. 55). Edmonton, AB: Faculty of Nursing, University of Alberta.

STUDENT: _____ DATE: _____

INSTRUCTOR: _____ DATE: _____

Skill 32–34 Assessing Coordination of the Lower Extremities

	S	U	NP	Comments

COORDINATION

Test each leg separately.

RAPID ALTERNATING MOVEMENTS

1. Instruct client to pat foot against examiner's hand as rapidly as possible (rhythmic patting).   ___ ___ ___ _____

POINT-TO-POINT TEST

2. Instruct client to place heel on opposite knee and run heel down shin and off great toe.   ___ ___ ___ _____

POSITION SENSE

3. Repeat each side with eyes closed.   ___ ___ ___ _____
4. Compare sides.   ___ ___ ___ _____

From Skillen, D. L., & Day, R. A. (Eds.). (2004). *A syllabus for adult health assessment* (p. 55). Edmonton, AB: Faculty of Nursing, University of Alberta.

STUDENT: _____   DATE: _____

INSTRUCTOR: _____   DATE: _____

Skill 32–35 Assessing Deep Tendon and Superficial Reflexes of the Lower Extremities

	S	U	NP	Comments

DEEP TENDON REFLEXES

Both sides are tested. *Only if* responses are symmetrically diminished or absent does examiner use reinforcement (augmentation). Strike tendon briskly with hammer held loosely and swung freely in an arc.

Patellar reflex

1. Position client so that leg is relaxed and knee is flexed.
2. Use hammer to tap patellar tendon just below patella.
3. Compare extension on each side.

Ankle reflex

1. Position client so that knee is flexed and foot is supported in dorsiflexed position by examiner.
2. Use hammer to tap Achilles tendon just above the heel.
3. Compare plantar flexion on each side.

SUPERFICIAL REFLEX

Plantar reflex

1. Stroke the lateral aspect of sole with blunt pointed object beginning at heel, laterally along sole, and curving medially across ball of the foot.
2. Compare toe movement on each side.

From Skillen, D. L., & Day, R. A. (Eds.). (2004). *A syllabus for adult health assessment* (p. 56). Edmonton, AB: Faculty of Nursing, University of Alberta.

STUDENT: _____ DATE: _____

INSTRUCTOR: _____ DATE: _____

Skill 32–36 Inspecting the Legs and Assessing Coordination With the Client in the Standing Position

	S	U	NP	Comments
LEGS AND FEET				
Symmetry, veins, arches, and popliteal fossae				
1. Inspect both legs, noting symmetry, veins, arches, and popliteal fossae.	___	___	___	_____
2. Palpate popliteal fossae.	___	___	___	_____
Cerebellar tests, position sense				
1. Instruct client to stand without support, arms at sides and feet together, first with eyes open, then closed for 20 seconds (Romberg test).	___	___	___	_____
2. Protect client from falling.	___	___	___	_____
3. Instruct client to walk in straight line by placing heel of foot directly before toes of other foot (tandem walking).	___	___	___	_____
Muscle strength				
4. Instruct client to hop in place on one foot, then the other.	___	___	___	_____
Shallow knee bend				
5. Instruct client to stand on one foot and do a shallow knee bend, first on one leg, then the other.	___	___	___	_____
6. Support elbow if risk of falling.	___	___	___	_____
Heel walk				
7. Instruct client to walk on heels.	___	___	___	_____
Toe walk				
8. Instruct client to walk on toes.	___	___	___	_____
Gait, balance, and posture				
1. Instruct client to walk away and then back toward examiner.	___	___	___	_____
2. Inspect during walking for posture, gait (stance and swing), balance, arm swing, leg movement, and position of head on turning.	___	___	___	_____

From Skillen, D. L., & Day, R. A. (Eds.). (2004). *A syllabus for adult health assessment* (p. 57). Edmonton, AB: Faculty of Nursing, University of Alberta.

STUDENT: _____ DATE: _____
INSTRUCTOR: _____ DATE: _____

Skill 33–1 Hand Hygiene

	S	U	NP	Comments
1. Inspect surfaces of hands for breaks or cuts in skin or cuticles. Report and cover lesions before providing client care.				
2. Inspect hands for heavy soiling.				
3. Inspect nails for length and presence of artificial acrylics or chipped nail polish.				
4. Assess client's risk for or extent of infection.				
5. Place wristwatch in pocket and roll long uniform sleeves above elbows. Remove rings during washing.				
6. If hands are visibly dirty or contaminated with protein-containing material, use plain or antimicrobial soap and water.				
A. Stand in front of sink, keeping hands and uniform away from sink surface.				
B. Turn on water. Turn faucet on or push knee pedals laterally or press foot pedals to regulate water flow and temperature.				
C. Avoid splashing water onto uniform.				
D. Regulate flow of water so that temperature is warm.				
E. Wet hands and wrists thoroughly under running water. Keep hands and forearms lower than elbows during washing.				
F. Apply a small amount of soap, lathering thoroughly.				
G. Wash hands using plenty of lather and friction for at least 15 seconds. Interlace fingers and rub palms and back of hands with circular motion at least 5 times each. Keep fingertips down. Rub knuckles of one hand into the palm of the other; repeat with other hand.				
H. Rub thumb on one hand with the palm of the other hand; repeat with other hand.				
I. Work the fingertips on one hand into the palm of the other. Massage soap into nail spaces. Repeat with other hand.				
J. Clean fingernails of both hands with additional soap or clean orangewood stick.				
K. Rinse hands and wrists thoroughly, keeping hands down and elbows up.				
L. Optional: Repeat steps A through J and extend period of washing if hands are heavily soiled.				
M. Dry hands thoroughly from fingers to wrists and forearms with paper towel, single-use cloth, or warm air dryer.				
N. Discard paper towel, if used, in proper receptacle.				
O. Turn off water with foot or knee pedals. To turn off hand faucet, use clean, dry paper towel. Avoid touching handles with hands.				
P. If hands are dry or chapped, a small amount of lotion or barrier cream can be applied.				
Q. Inspect surfaces of hands for obvious signs of soil or other contaminants.				
R. Inspect hands for dermatitis or cracked skin.				
7. If hands are not visibly soiled, use an alcohol-based waterless antiseptic for routine decontamination in all clinical situations.				
A. Apply an ample amount of product to the palm of one hand.				
B. Rub hands together, covering all surfaces.				
C. Rub hands together until alcohol is dry. Allow hands to dry before applying gloves.				
D. If hands are dry or chapped, a small amount of lotion or barrier cream can be applied.				

STUDENT: _____ DATE: _____

INSTRUCTOR: _____ DATE: _____

Skill 33–2 Preparation of a Sterile Field

	S	U	NP	Comments
1. Prepare sterile field just before planned procedure.	___	___	___	_____
2. Select clean work surface above waist level.	___	___	___	_____
3. Assemble equipment.	___	___	___	_____
4. Check dates on supplies.	___	___	___	_____
5. Perform hand hygiene.	___	___	___	_____
6. Place pack with sterile drape on work surface and open pack.	___	___	___	_____
7. With fingertips of one hand, pick up folded top edge.	___	___	___	
8. Lift drape from its outer cover and let it unfold by itself without touching anything. Discard outer cover with other hand.	___	___	___	_____
9. With other hand, grasp adjacent corner of drape and hold it straight up and away from your body.	___	___	___	_____
10. Holding drape, first position and lay bottom half over intended work surface.	___	___	___	_____
11. Allow top half of drape to be placed over work surface last.	___	___	___	
12. Grasp 2.5 cm border around edge to position as needed.	___	___	___	_____

ADDING STERILE ITEMS

	S	U	NP	Comments
13. Open sterile item.	___	___	___	_____
14. Peel wrapper.	___	___	___	_____
15. Being sure wrapper does not fall down on sterile field, place item onto field at angle. Do not hold arm over field.	___	___	___	_____
16. Dispose of wrapper.	___	___	___	_____
17. Perform procedure using sterile technique.	___	___	___	_____

STUDENT: _____   DATE: _____

INSTRUCTOR: _____   DATE: _____

Skill 33–3 Surgical Hand Hygiene: Preparing for Gowning

	S	U	NP	Comments
1. Consult agency policy for length of time for handwashing.	___	___	___	_____
2. Keep fingernails short, clean, and healthy. Remove artificial nails.	___	___	___	_____
3. Inspect hands for presence of abrasions, cuts, or open lesions.	___	___	___	_____
4. Apply surgical shoe covers, cap or hood, face mask, and protective eyewear.	___	___	___	_____
5. Surgical handwashing:				
A. Turn on water using knee or foot controls and adjust water to comfortable temperature.	___	___	___	_____
B. Wet hands and arms under running lukewarm water and lather with detergent to 5 cm above elbows. Keep hands above elbows.	___	___	___	_____
C. Rinse hands and arms thoroughly under running water, keeping hands above elbows.	___	___	___	_____
D. Under running water, clean under nails of both hands with nail pick. Discard nail pick after use.	___	___	___	_____
E. Wet clean sponge and apply antimicrobial detergent. Scrub the nails of one hand with 15 strokes. Holding sponge perpendicular, scrub the palm, each side of the thumb and all fingers, and the posterior side of the hand with 10 strokes each. Scrub each section of the arm 10 times. Check manufacturer's recommendations for the duration of the scrub, usually 2 to 6 minutes. Rinse sponge and repeat for other arm.	___	___	___	_____
F. Discard sponge and rinse hands and arms thoroughly. Turn off water with foot or knee controls and back into room entrance with hands elevated in front of and away from the body.	___	___	___	_____
G. Bend slightly forward at the waist to pick up a sterile towel. Dry one hand thoroughly, moving from fingers to elbow. Dry in a rotating motion from cleanest to least clean area.	___	___	___	_____
H. Repeat drying method for other hand, using a different area of the towel or a new sterile towel.	___	___	___	_____
I. Discard towel.	___	___	___	_____
J. Proceed with sterile gowning.	___	___	___	_____
6. Alternate method of surgical hand hygiene using alcohol-based antiseptic:	___	___	___	_____
A. Wash hands with soap and water for 15 seconds.	___	___	___	_____
B. Clean nails of both hands under running water with nail pick. Discard nail pick after use and dry hands with a paper towel.	___	___	___	_____
C. Apply enough alcohol-based waterless antiseptic to one palm to cover both hands thoroughly. Spread antiseptic over all hand and nail surfaces. Allow to air-dry.	___	___	___	_____
D. Repeat the process and allow hands to air-dry before applying sterile gloves.	___	___	___	_____

STUDENT: _____ DATE: _____

INSTRUCTOR: _____ DATE: _____

Skill 33–4 Applying a Sterile Gown and Performing Closed Gloving

	S	U	NP	Comments
1. Apply cap, face mask, eyewear, and foot covers.	___	___	___	_____
2. Perform surgical hand hygiene.	___	___	___	_____
3. Have circulating nurse open pack containing sterile gown.	___	___	___	_____
4. Have circulating nurse prepare glove package.	___	___	___	_____
5. Reach down to sterile gown package; lift gown directly upward and step back from table.	___	___	___	_____
6. Holding folded gown, locate neckband. Grasp inside front of gown just below neckband.	___	___	___	_____
7. Allow gown to unfold, keeping inside of gown toward body. Do not touch outside of gown.	___	___	___	_____
8. Insert each hand through armholes simultaneously. Ask circulating nurse to bring gown over shoulders, leaving sleeves covering hands.	___	___	___	_____
9. Have circulating nurse tie back of gown at neck and waist.	___	___	___	_____
10. Closed gloving procedure:	___	___	___	_____
A. With hands covered by sleeves, open glove package.	___	___	___	_____
B. With dominant hand inside gown cuff, pick up glove for nondominant hand.	___	___	___	_____
C. Extend nondominant forearm with palm up and place palm of glove against palm of nondominant hand. Glove fingers will point toward elbow.	___	___	___	_____
D. Grasp back of glove cuff with covered dominant hand and turn glove cuff over end of nondominant hand and gown cuff.	___	___	___	_____
E. Grasp top of glove and underlying gown sleeve with covered dominant hand. Carefully extend fingers into glove, being sure glove's cuff covers gown's cuff.	___	___	___	_____
F. Repeat steps A through E to glove dominant hand.	___	___	___	_____
G. Adjust fingers until fully extended into both gloves.	___	___	___	_____
11. For wraparound sterile gowns, release front fastener with gloved hand.	___	___	___	_____
12. Handing tie to stationary team member, turn 360 degrees to left and secure tie to gown.	___	___	___	_____

STUDENT: _____ DATE: _____

INSTRUCTOR: _____ DATE: _____

Skill 33–5 Open Gloving

	S	U	NP	Comments
1. Perform thorough hand hygiene.	___	___	___	_____
2. Peel apart sides of outer package of glove wrapper.	___	___	___	_____
3. Lay inner package on clean, flat surface just above waist level. Open package, keeping gloves on inside surface of wrapper.	___	___	___	_____
4. If gloves are not prepowdered, apply powder lightly to hands over sink or wastebasket.	___	___	___	_____
5. Identify right and left gloves.	___	___	___	_____
6. Start by applying glove to dominant hand. With thumb and first two fingers of nondominant hand, grasp edge of cuff of glove for dominant hand, touching only inside surface.	___	___	___	_____
7. Carefully pull glove over dominant hand, ensuring cuff does not roll up wrist.	___	___	___	_____
8. With gloved dominant hand, slip fingers underneath second glove's cuff.	___	___	___	_____
9. Carefully pull second glove over nondominant hand and do not allow gloved hand to touch any part of exposed nondominant hand.	___	___	___	_____
10. When both gloves are on, interlock fingers of both hands to secure gloves in position, being careful to touch only sterile sides.	___	___	___	_____

GLOVE DISPOSAL

	S	U	NP	Comments
11. Without touching wrist, grasp outside of one cuff with other gloved hand.	___	___	___	_____
12. Pull glove off, turning it inside out. Discard in receptacle.	___	___	___	_____
13. Tuck fingers of bare hand inside remaining glove cuff. Peel glove off, inside out. Discard in receptacle.	___	___	___	_____

STUDENT: _____ DATE: _____

INSTRUCTOR: _____ DATE: _____

Skill 34–1 Administering Oral Medications

	S	U	NP	Comments
1. Check accuracy and completeness of each medication administration record (MAR) or computer printout against the prescriber's original medication order. Check the client's name and medication name, dosage, route and time for administration. Copy or rewrite any portion of the MAR that is difficult to read.	___	___	___	_____
2. Assess client for any contraindications to receiving oral medication. Is the client experiencing nausea or vomiting? Has the client received a diagnosis of bowel inflammation or reduced peristalsis? Has client undergone recent gastrointestinal (GI) surgery? Does client have gastric suction? Is the client restricted to nothing by mouth (NPO)? Check the client's reflexes for swallowing, coughing, and gagging.	___	___	___	_____
3. Assess the client's medical history, history of allergies, medication history, and diet history. List the client's food and drug allergies on each page of the MAR and prominently display the allergies on the client's medical record. This information may also be added to an identification bracelet.	___	___	___	_____
4. Gather information from the client's physical examination and laboratory data that may influence medication administration (e.g., vital signs, blood glucose levels, electrolyte levels, laboratory findings related to blood clotting times and to renal and liver function).	___	___	___	_____
5. Assess client's knowledge regarding health and medication usage.	___	___	___	_____
6. Assess client's preferences for fluids. Maintain fluid restriction when applicable.	___	___	___	_____
7. Prepare medications:				
A. Perform hand hygiene.				
B. If medication cart is used, move it outside client's room.	___	___	___	_____
C. Unlock medicine drawer or cart or log on to the automated medication dispensing system.	___	___	___	_____
D. Prepare medication for one client at a time. If you are using paper copies of the MAR, keep all pages for one client together. If you are using the client's medication administration on the computer, view only one computer screen at a time.	___	___	___	_____
E. Select correct medication from a stock supply or a unit-dose drawer. Compare the label on the medication with the MAR or the computer screen. Check expiration date on all medication labels.	___	___	___	_____
F. Calculate the medication dose as necessary. Double-check all calculations, and verify your calculations with another nurse.	___	___	___	_____
G. If you are preparing a controlled substance, check the client's MAR or computer record to determine the last time the medication was administered. Check the record for the previous medication count and compare the current count with the supply available.	___	___	___	_____
H. To prepare tablets or capsules from a floor stock bottle, pour required number into the bottle cap and transfer medication to a medication cup. Do not touch the medication with your fingers. Return extra tablets or capsules to the bottle. Break prescored medications. If necessary, use a gloved hand or clean pillating device. Identify prescored tablets by looking for a line that divides the tablet in half.	___	___	___	_____
I. To prepare unit-dose tablets or capsules, place the packaged tablet or capsule directly into a medicine cup. Do not remove the wrapper.	___	___	___	_____
J. Place all tablets or capsules to be given to client in one medicine cup, with the client's identification label attached, except for those medications that require preadministration assessments (e.g., pulse rate or blood pressure); keep medications in their wrappers. After medication administration, remove the client's identification label and discard the label in the appropriate confidential waste disposal receptacle.	___	___	___	_____

Continued

	S	U	NP	Comments

K. If the client has difficulty swallowing, and liquid medications are not an option, use a pill-crushing device, such as a mortar and pestle to grind the pills. Before using a mortar and pestle, clean them. If a pill-crushing device is not available, place the tablet inside a medication cup, place another cup on top of it, and press on the top cup with a blunt instrument until the pill is crushed. Mix the ground tablet in small amount of soft food (custard or applesauce).

L. To prepare liquids:
  (1) Gently shake the container. If the medication is in a unit-dose container with the correct amount to administer, no further preparation is needed. If medication is in a multidose bottle, remove the bottle cap from container and place the cap so that the inside of cap is not exposed.
  (2) Hold a multidose bottle with the label against the palm of your hand while pouring.
  (3) Hold medication cup at eye level and fill to the desired level on the scale. The scale should be even with fluid level at its surface or the base of the meniscus, not at its edges. Draw up volumes of less than 10 mL in a syringe without a needle.
  (4) Discard any excess liquid into a sink. Wipe lip and neck of the multidose bottle with a paper towel.

M. Compare the MAR, computer printout, or computer screen with the prepared medication and container.

N. Return stock containers or unused unit-dose medications to the storage shelf or drawer and read the labels again.

O. Do not leave medications unattended.

8. Administering medications:

A. Bring medications to the client at the correct time.

B. Identify the client by using at least two client identifiers. Compare the client's name and one other identifier (e.g., the hospital identification number) on the MAR, computer printout, or computer screen against information on the client's identification bracelet. Ask the client to state his or her name, if possible, for a third identifier.

C. Compare the labels of the medications with the MAR at the client's bedside.

D. Explain to client the purpose of each medication and its action. Encourage client to ask any questions about the drugs.

E. Assist the client to a sitting position (or side-lying position if sitting is contraindicated).

F. Administer medications:
  (1) *For tablets:* The client may wish to hold solid medications in the hand or in a cup before placing in the mouth.
  (2) Offer water or juice to help the client swallow medications. Give cold carbonated water if it is available and not contraindicated.
  (3) *For sublingual-administered medications:* Have the client place the medication under the tongue and allow it to dissolve completely. Caution the client against swallowing tablet.
  (4) *For buccal medications:* Have the client place the medication in the mouth against the mucous membranes of the cheek until it dissolves. Avoid administering liquids until the buccal medication has dissolved.
  (5) *For powdered medications:* Mix with liquids at bedside and give to the client to drink.
  (6) Caution the client against chewing or swallowing lozenges.
  (7) Give effervescent powders and tablets immediately after they have dissolved.

G. If the client is unable to hold medications in the hand or in a cup, place the medication cup to the client's lips and gently introduce each drug into the mouth, one at a time. Do not rush.

H. If a tablet or capsule falls to the floor, discard it and repeat the preparation.

I. Stay at the bedside until the client has completely swallowed each medication. If you are uncertain whether the medication was swallowed, ask the client to open the mouth.

Continued

	S	U	NP	Comments
J. For highly acidic medications (e.g., aspirin), offer the client a nonfat snack (e.g., crackers) if it is not contraindicated by the client's condition.	____	____	____	_____
K. Assist the client in returning to a comfortable position.	____	____	____	_____
L. Dispose of soiled supplies and perform hand hygiene.	____	____	____	_____
M. Replenish the stock, such as cups and straws. If a medication cart was used, return the cart to the medication room. Clean the work area.	____	____	____	_____
9. Evaluate the client's response to medication at times that correlate with the medication's onset, peak, and duration.	____	____	____	_____
10. Ask the client or the client's family member to identify the medication name and explain the purpose, action, dosage schedule, and potential side effects of drug.	____	____	____	_____
11. Notify prescriber if the client exhibits a toxic effect or allergic reaction or if side effects occur. If any of these occur, withhold further doses of medication.	____	____	____	_____
12. Record administration (or withholding) of oral medications.	____	____	____	_____

STUDENT: _____ DATE: _____

INSTRUCTOR: _____ DATE: _____

Skill 34–2 Administering Ophthalmic Medications

	S	U	NP	Comments
1. Check the accuracy and completeness of each MAR or computer printout against the prescriber's medication order. Check the client's name, the medication name and dosage (e.g., number of drops, if a liquid) the eye to be treated (e.g., right, left, or both eyes), and the route and time of administration. Copy or rewrite any portion of the MAR that is difficult to read.	___	___	___	_____
2. Assess the condition of the client's external eye structures. (This may also be assessed just before drug instillation.)	___	___	___	_____
3. Determine whether the client has any known allergies to eye medications. Also ask whether the client has an allergy to latex.	___	___	___	_____
4. Determine whether the client has any symptoms of visual alterations.	___	___	___	_____
5. Assess the client's level of consciousness and ability to follow directions.	___	___	___	_____
6. Assess the client's knowledge regarding medication therapy and the desire to self-administer medication.	___	___	___	_____
7. Assess the client's ability to manipulate and hold an eye dropper.	___	___	___	_____
8. Prepare medication. Ensure that you check the label of the medication against the MAR at least two times while preparing medication.	___	___	___	_____
9. Bring the medication to the client at correct time and perform hand hygiene.	___	___	___	_____
10. Identify the client by using at least two client identifiers. Compare the client's name and one other identifier (e.g., the hospital identification number) on the MAR, computer printout, or computer screen against information on the client's identification bracelet. Ask the client to state his or her name, if possible, for a third identifier.	___	___	___	_____
11. Compare the labels of the medications with the MAR or computer printout at the client's bedside.	___	___	___	_____
12. Arrange the medication supplies at bedside and put on clean gloves. If eye drops are stored in the refrigerator, allow them to reach room temperature before instilling them.	___	___	___	_____
13. Gently roll the container.	___	___	___	_____
14. Explain the procedure to the client, including positioning and sensations to expect, such as burning or stinging.	___	___	___	_____
15. Ask the client to lie supine or to sit back in a chair with the head slightly hyperextended.	___	___	___	_____
16. If crusts or drainage are present along the eyelid margins or the inner canthus, gently wash them away. Soak any crusts that are dried and difficult to remove by applying a damp washcloth or cotton ball over the eye for a few minutes. Always wipe from the inner to the outer canthus.	___	___	___	_____
17. Hold a cotton ball or clean tissue in your nondominant hand on the client's cheekbone just below the lower eyelid.	___	___	___	_____
18. With the tissue or cotton ball resting below the lower lid, gently press downward with thumb or forefinger against the bony orbit.	___	___	___	_____
19. Ask the client to look at ceiling, and explain steps to the client.	___	___	___	_____
A. Instill the eye drops:				
(1) With your dominant hand resting on the client's forehead, hold the filled medication eyedropper or ophthalmic solution approximately 1–2 cm above the conjunctival sac.	___	___	___	_____
(2) Instill the prescribed number of medication drops into the conjunctival sac.	___	___	___	_____
(3) If the client blinks or closes the eye, or if the drops land on the outer lid margins, repeat the procedure.	___	___	___	_____
(4) After instilling drops, ask the client to close the eye gently.	___	___	___	_____
(5) When administering medications that cause systemic effects, apply gentle pressure with your finger and a clean tissue on the client's nasolacrimal duct for 30–60 seconds.	___	___	___	_____

Continued

	S	U	NP	Comments

B. Instill eye ointment:
   (1) Ask the client to look at the ceiling. ____ ____ ____ _____
   (2) Holding the ointment applicator above the lower lid margin, apply thin stream of ointment evenly along the inner edge of the lower eyelid on conjunctiva from inner canthus to outer canthus. ____ ____ ____ _____
   (3) Have the client close the eye and use a cotton ball to rub lid gently in a circular motion, if rubbing is not contraindicated. ____ ____ ____ _____

C. Intraocular disc
   (1) Application:
      (a) Open the package containing the disc. Gently press your fingertip against the disc so it adheres to your finger. Position the convex side of the disc on your fingertip. ____ ____ ____ _____
      (b) With other hand, gently pull the client's lower eyelid away from the eye. Ask the client to look up. ____ ____ ____ _____
      (c) Place the disc in the conjunctival sac, so that it floats on the sclera between the iris and the lower eyelid. ____ ____ ____ _____
      (d) Pull the client's lower eyelid out and over the disc. ____ ____ ____ _____
   (2) Removal:
      (a) Perform hand hygiene and put on gloves. ____ ____ ____ _____
      (b) Explain procedure to client. ____ ____ ____ _____
      (c) Gently pull on the client's lower eyelid to expose the intraocular disc. ____ ____ ____ _____
      (d) Using your forefinger and thumb of the opposite hand, pinch the disc and lift it out of the client's eye. ____ ____ ____ _____

20. If excess medication is on eyelid, gently wipe it from inner canthus to outer canthus. ____ ____ ____ _____

21. If client wears an eye patch, apply a clean patch by placing it over the affected eye so entire eye is covered. Tape securely without applying pressure to eye. ____ ____ ____ _____

22. If client receives eye medication to both eyes at the same time, use a different tissue or cotton ball for each eye. ____ ____ ____ _____

23. Remove gloves, dispose of soiled supplies in proper receptacle, and perform hand hygiene. ____ ____ ____ _____

24. Note the client's response to instillation; ask whether the client felt any discomfort. ____ ____ ____ _____

25. Observe client's response to medication by assessing any visual changes and noting any side effects. ____ ____ ____ _____

26. Ask the client to discuss the medication's purpose, action, side effects, and the technique of administration. ____ ____ ____ _____

27. Have client demonstrate self-administration of next dose. ____ ____ ____ _____

STUDENT: _____ DATE: _____

INSTRUCTOR: _____ DATE: _____

Skill 34–3 Using Metered-Dose or Dry Powder Inhalers

	S	U	NP	Comments
1. Check the accuracy and completeness of each MAR or computer printout against the prescriber's original medication order. Check the client's name and medication name, route, dosage, and time of administration. Copy or rewrite any portion of the MAR that is difficult to read.	___	___	___	_____
2. Assess client's respiratory pattern, and auscultate the client's breath sounds.	___	___	___	_____
3. If the client has been previously instructed in self-administration, assess the client's technique in using the inhaler.	___	___	___	_____
4. Assess the client's ability to hold, manipulate, and depress canister and inhaler. Assess the client's strength of inhalation.	___	___	___	_____
5. Assess the client's readiness to learn: for example, whether the client asks questions about the medication, disease, or complications; requests education in use of inhaler; is mentally alert; participates in self-care.	___	___	___	_____
6. Assess client's ability to learn: The client should not be fatigued, in pain, or in respiratory distress; assess the client's level of understanding of technical terms.	___	___	___	_____
7. Assess the client's knowledge and understanding of the disease and the purpose and action of the prescribed medications.	___	___	___	_____
8. Determine the medication schedule and the number of inhalations prescribed for each dose.	___	___	___	_____
9. Prepare the medication. Ensure that you compare the medication label with the MAR two times during medication preparation.	___	___	___	_____
10. Identify the client by using at least two client identifiers. Compare the client's name and one other identifier (e.g., the hospital identification number) on the MAR, computer printout, or computer screen against information on the client's identification bracelet. Ask the client to state his or her name, if possible, for a third identifier.	___	___	___	_____
11. Compare the label of medications with the MAR one more time at the client's bedside.	___	___	___	_____
12. Instruct the client in a comfortable environment by sitting in a chair in the hospital room or by sitting at a kitchen table in the client's home.	___	___	___	_____
13. Provide adequate time for the teaching session.	___	___	___	_____
14. Perform hand hygiene and arrange the equipment needed.	___	___	___	_____
15. Allow the client an opportunity to manipulate the inhaler, the canister, and the spacer device. Explain and demonstrate how the canister fits into the inhaler.	___	___	___	_____
16. Explain what a metered dose is, and warn the client about overuse of the inhaler, including medication side effects.	___	___	___	_____
17. Explain the steps for administering squeeze-and-breathe inhaled dose of medication of metered-dose inhaler (MDI) (demonstrate steps when possible).	___	___	___	_____
A. Insert the MDI canister into the holder.	___	___	___	_____
B. Remove the mouthpiece cover from the inhaler.	___	___	___	_____
C. Shake the inhaler vigorously five or six times.	___	___	___	_____
D. Have the client take a deep breath and exhale.	___	___	___	_____
E. Instruct the client to position the inhaler in one of two ways:				
(1) Close the mouth around the MDI, with the opening toward the back of the throat.	___	___	___	_____
(2) Position the device 2–4 cm in front of the mouth.	___	___	___	_____
F. With the inhaler properly positioned, have the client hold it with thumb at the mouthpiece and middle finger at the top. This arrangement is called a three-point or lateral hand position.	___	___	___	_____
G. Instruct client to tilt the head back slightly, inhale slowly and deeply through mouth for 3–5 seconds while depressing the canister fully.	___	___	___	_____

Continued

	S	U	NP	Comments

H. Instruct the client to hold the breath for approximately 10 seconds.

I. Have the client remove the MDI from the mouth and to exhale through pursed lips.

18. Explain steps to administer MDI by using a spacer, such as an AeroChamber (demonstrate when possible):

    A. Remove the mouthpiece cover from the MDI and the mouthpiece of spacer. Inspect the spacer for foreign objects. If the spacer has a valve, ensure the valve is intact.

    B. Insert the MDI into the end of the spacer.

    C. Shake the inhaler vigorously five or six times.

    D. Have the client exhale completely before closing the mouth around the mouthpiece of the spacer. Avoid covering small exhalation slots with the lips.

    E. Have the client depress the medication canister, spraying one puff into the spacer.

    F. Instruct the client to inhale deeply and slowly through the mouth for 3–5 seconds.

    G. Instruct the client to hold the breath for 10 seconds.

    H. Instruct the client to remove the MDI and spacer before exhaling.

19. Explain the steps to administer dry powder inhaler (DPI) or breath-activated MDI (demonstrate when possible):

    A. Remove the cover from the mouthpiece. Do not shake the inhaler.

    B. Prepare medication as directed by the manufacturer (e.g., hold inhaler upright and turn the wheel to the right and then to the left until a click is heard; load the medication pellet).

    C. Instruct the client to exhale away from inhaler before inhalation.

    D. Position mouthpiece between the client's lips.

    E. Instruct the client to inhale deeply and forcefully through the mouth.

    F. Instruct the client to hold breath for 5–10 seconds.

20. Instruct client to wait at least 20–30 seconds between inhalations.

21. Instruct the client against repeating inhalations before the next scheduled dose.

22. Explain that the client may feel a gagging sensation in the throat, caused by droplets of medication on the pharynx or tongue.

23. Instruct client in cleaning the inhaler:

    A. Once a day, the inhaler and its cap should be rinsed in warm running water. The inhaler must be completely dry before use.

    B. Twice a week, the L-shaped plastic mouthpiece should be washed with mild dishwashing soap and warm water. Rinse and dry well before placing the canister back inside the mouthpiece.

24. Ask whether the client has any questions.

25. Have the client explain and demonstrate the steps in the use of an inhaler.

26. Ask the client to explain the medication schedule, side effects, and when to call health care professionals

27. Ask the client to calculate how many days the inhaler will last.

28. After the medication has been taken, assess the client's respiratory status, including the ease of respirations; auscultate the lungs, and use pulse oximetry to assess the client's oxygenation status.

STUDENT: _____ DATE: _____

INSTRUCTOR: _____ DATE: _____

Skill 34–4 Preparing Injections

	S	U	NP	Comments

1. Check the accuracy and completeness of each MAR or computer printout against the prescriber's original medication order. Check the client's name and the medication name, route, dosage, and time of administration. Copy or rewrite any portion of the MAR that is difficult to read. ___ ___ ___ _____
2. Review pertinent information related to medication, including its action, purpose, side effects, and nursing implications. ___ ___ ___ _____
3. Assess the client's body build, muscle size, and weight. ___ ___ ___ _____
4. Perform hand hygiene and assemble the medication supplies. ___ ___ ___ _____
5. Check the date of expiration on the medication vial or ampule. . ___ ___ ___ _____
6. Prepare medication: Ensure that you compare the label of the medication with the MAR at least two times while preparing the medication. ___ ___ ___ _____
   A. Ampule preparation:
      (1) Tap top of ampule lightly and quickly with your finger until the fluid moves from the neck of ampule. ___ ___ ___ _____
      (2) Place a small gauze pad or an unopened alcohol swab around the neck of the ampule. ___ ___ ___ _____
      (3) Snap the neck of the ampule quickly and firmly away from the hands. ___ ___ ___ _____
      (4) Draw up medication quickly, using a filter needle long enough to reach the bottom of the ampule. ___ ___ ___ _____
      (5) Hold the ampule upside down, or set it on a flat surface. Insert the filter needle into centre of the ampule opening. Do not allow the needle tip or shaft to touch the rim of the ampule. ___ ___ ___ _____
      (6) Aspirate the medication into the syringe by gently pulling back on the plunger. ___ ___ ___ _____
      (7) Keep the needle tip under the surface of the liquid. Tip the ampule to bring all fluid within reach of the needle. ___ ___ ___ _____
      (8) If air bubbles are aspirated, do not expel the air into the ampule. ___ ___ ___ _____
      (9) To expel excess air bubbles, remove the needle from the ampule. Hold the syringe with the needle pointing up. Tap the side of the syringe to cause the bubbles to rise toward the needle. Draw back slightly on the plunger, then push the plunger upward to eject the air. Do not eject any fluid. ___ ___ ___ _____
      (10) If the syringe contains excess fluid, dispose of it in a sink. Hold the syringe vertically with the needle tip up and slanted slightly toward the sink. Slowly eject the excess fluid into the sink. Recheck the fluid level in the syringe by holding it vertically. ___ ___ ___ _____
      (11) Cover the needle with its safety sheath or cap. Replace the filter needle with a needle or a needleless access device for injection. ___ ___ ___ _____
   B. Vial containing a solution:
      (1) Remove the cap covering the top of the unused vial to expose the sterile rubber seal. If a multidose vial has been previously used, the cap has already been removed. Firmly and briskly wipe the surface of the rubber seal with an alcohol swab and allow it to dry. ___ ___ ___ _____
      (2) Pick up the syringe and remove the needle cap or the cap covering the needleless vial access device. Pull back on the plunger to draw an amount of air into the syringe equivalent to the volume of medication to be aspirated from the vial. ___ ___ ___ _____
      (3) With the vial on a flat surface, insert the tip of the needle. Ensure the bevelled tip enters first, through the centre of the rubber seal. Apply pressure to the tip of the needle during insertion. ___ ___ ___ _____

Continued

	S	U	NP	Comments

(4) Inject air into the vial's airspace, holding on to the plunger. Hold the plunger with firm pressure; the plunger may be forced backward by air pressure within the vial.   ____ ____ ____ _____

(5) Invert the vial while keeping a firm hold on the syringe and plunger. Hold the vial between the thumb and middle fingers of your nondominant hand. Grasp the end of the syringe barrel and plunger with the thumb and forefinger of your dominant hand to counteract pressure in the vial.   ____ ____ ____ _____

(6) Keep the tip of the needle below the fluid level.   ____ ____ ____ _____

(7) Allow air pressure from the vial to fill the syringe gradually with medication. If necessary, pull back slightly on the plunger to obtain the correct amount of solution.   ____ ____ ____ _____

(8) When the desired volume is obtained, position the needle into the vial's airspace. Tap the side of the syringe barrel carefully to dislodge any air bubbles. Eject any air remaining at the top of the syringe into the vial.   ____ ____ ____ _____

(9) Remove the needle from the vial by pulling back on the barrel of the syringe.   ____ ____ ____ _____

(10) Hold the syringe at eye level, at a 90-degree angle, to ensure the correct volume has been obtained and no air bubbles are present. Remove any remaining air by tapping the barrel to dislodge the air bubbles. Draw back slightly on the plunger; then push the plunger upward to eject the air. Do not eject the fluid. Recheck the volume of medication.   ____ ____ ____ _____

(11) If medication is to be injected into a client's tissue, change needle to one of the appropriate gauge and length according to the route of medication and the client's size and weight.   ____ ____ ____ _____

(12) For a multidose vial, make a label that includes the date of mixing, the concentration of the medication per millilitre, and your initials.   ____ ____ ____ _____

C. Vial containing a powder (reconstituting medications):

(1) Remove the cap covering the vial of powdered medication and the cap covering the vial of proper diluent. Firmly wipe both seals with an alcohol swab and allow to dry.   ____ ____ ____ _____

(2) Draw up diluent into the syringe by following Steps 6B(2) through 6B(10).   ____ ____ ____ _____

(3) Insert the tip of the needle through the centre of the rubber seal on the vial of powdered medication. Inject the diluent into the vial. Remove the needle.   ____ ____ ____ _____

(4) Mix the medication thoroughly. Roll the vial in your palms. Do not shake the vial.   ____ ____ ____ _____

(5) Reconstituted medication in the vial is ready to be drawn into a new syringe. Read the label carefully to determine the dose after reconstitution.   ____ ____ ____ _____

(6) Prepare medication in syringe, following Steps 6B(2) through 6B(12).   ____ ____ ____ _____

7. Dispose of all soiled supplies. Place broken ampule vials, used vials, and used needles in a puncture-proof and leak-proof container. Clean medication work area and perform hand hygiene.   ____ ____ ____ _____

STUDENT: _____   DATE: _____

INSTRUCTOR: _____   DATE: _____

Skill 34–5 Administering Injections

	S	U	NP	Comments
1. Check accuracy and completeness of each MAR or computer printout against the prescriber's original medication order. Check the client's name and the medication name, route, dosage, and time of administration. Copy or rewrite any portion of the MAR that is difficult to read.	___	___	___	_____
2. Assess the client's medical history, medication history, and history of allergies. Determine whether the client is allergic to any substances and the usual allergic reaction experienced.	___	___	___	_____
3. Check the date of expiration for the medication.	___	___	___	_____
4. Observe client's verbal and nonverbal responses to receiving an injection.	___	___	___	_____
5. Assess the client for contraindications:				
A. For subcutaneous injections: Assess the client for factors such as circulatory shock and reduced local tissue perfusion. Assess the adequacy of the client's adipose tissue.	___	___	___	_____
B. For intramuscular injections: Assess the client for muscle atrophy, reduced blood flow, and circulatory shock.	___	___	___	_____
6. Perform hand hygiene. Aseptically prepare the correct medication dose from an ampule or vial. Ensure all air is expelled from the syringe. Check the label of medication against the MAR two times while preparing the medication. Create a removable label that shows the client's name, the name of the drug, and the dosage. Apply the label to the removable needle cap.	___	___	___	_____
7. Bring the medication to the client at the right time, and perform hand hygiene.	___	___	___	_____
8. Close the room curtain or door.	___	___	___	_____
9. Identify the client by using at least two client identifiers. Compare the client's name and one other identifier (e.g., the hospital identification number) on the MAR, computer printout, or computer screen against information on the client's identification bracelet. Ask the client to state his or her name, if possible, for a third identifier.	___	___	___	_____
10. Compare the label of the medication with the MAR one more time at the client's bedside.	___	___	___	_____
11. Describe the steps of the procedure, and inform the client that the injection will cause a slight burning or stinging sensation.	___	___	___	_____
12. Perform hand hygiene; put on disposable gloves.	___	___	___	_____
13. Keep a sheet or gown draped over the client's body parts that do not need to be exposed.	___	___	___	_____
14. Select appropriate injection site. Inspect the skin surface over the injection site for bruises, inflammation, and edema.	___	___	___	_____
A. *Subcutaneous injection:* Palpate the injection site for masses or tenderness. Avoid these areas. For clients who require daily insulin, rotate the injection site daily. Ensure the needle is the correct size by grasping a skinfold at the injection site with your thumb and forefinger. Measure the fold from top to bottom. The needle should be half the length of the skinfold.	___	___	___	_____
B. *Intramuscular injection:* Note the integrity and size of muscle and palpate for tenderness or hardness. Avoid these areas. If injections are given frequently, rotate the injection sites. Use the ventrogluteal site if possible.	___	___	___	_____
C. *Intradermal injection:* Note any lesions or discoloration of client's forearm. Select an injection site three to four fingerwidths below the antecubital space and a handwidth above the wrist. If the forearm cannot be used, inspect the client's upper back. If necessary, sites for subcutaneous injections may be used.	___	___	___	_____
15. Assist client to a comfortable position:				
A. *Subcutaneous injection:* Have the client relax the arm, leg, or abdomen, depending on the site chosen for injection.	___	___	___	_____

Continued

	S	U	NP	Comments

B. *Intramuscular injection:* Position the client depending on the site chosen (e.g., have the client sit, lie flat, lie on one side, or lie prone).   ___ ___ ___ _____

C. *Intradermal injection:* Have the client extend the elbow and support the elbow and forearm on a flat surface.   ___ ___ ___ _____

D. Speak with the client about a subject of interest.   ___ ___ ___ _____

16. Relocate the injection site by using anatomical landmarks.   ___ ___ ___ _____

17. Clean the injection site with an antiseptic swab. Touch the swab to the centre of the site and rotate it outward in a circular direction for about 5 cm.   ___ ___ ___ _____

18. Hold the swab or gauze between the third and fourth fingers of your nondominant hand.   ___ ___ ___ _____

19. Remove the needle cap or sheath from the needle by pulling it straight off.   ___ ___ ___ _____

20. Hold the syringe between the thumb and forefinger of your dominant hand:

A. *Subcutaneous injection:* Hold the syringe as if you were holding a dart, palm down; or hold the syringe across tops of your fingertips.   ___ ___ ___ _____

B. *Intramuscular injection:* Hold the syringe as if you were holding a dart, palm down.   ___ ___ ___ _____

C. *Intradermal injection:* Hold the bevel of the needle pointing up.   ___ ___ ___ _____

21. Administer injection.

A. Subcutaneous injection:

(1) For an average-size client, spread the skin tightly across the injection site or pinch the skin with your nondominant hand.   ___ ___ ___ _____

(2) Inject the needle quickly and firmly at a 45- to 90-degree angle. Then release the skin, if pinched.   ___ ___ ___ _____

(3) For an obese client, pinch the skin at the injection site and inject the needle at a 90-degree angle below the tissue fold.   ___ ___ ___ _____

(4) Inject medication slowly.   ___ ___ ___ _____

B. Intramuscular injection:

(1) Position your nondominant hand at the proper anatomical landmarks and pull the skin down approximately 2.5–3.5 cm or laterally with the ulnar side of your hand to administer the injection in a Z-track. Hold this position until the medication is injected. Use your dominant hand to insert the needle quickly at a 90-degree angle into the muscle.   ___ ___ ___ _____

(2) If the client's muscle mass is small, grasp a body of muscle between your thumb and fingers.   ___ ___ ___ _____

(3) After needle pierces the skin, grasp the lower end of the syringe barrel with your nondominant hand to stabilize the syringe. Continue to hold the skin tightly with your nondominant hand. Move your dominant hand to the end of the plunger. Do not move the syringe.   ___ ___ ___ _____

(4) Pull back on the plunger. If no blood appears, inject the medicine slowly, at a rate of 1 mL per 10 seconds.   ___ ___ ___ _____

(5) Wait 10 seconds, and then smoothly and steadily withdraw the needle and release the skin. Apply gentle pressure with dry gauze if desired.   ___ ___ ___ _____

C. Intradermal injection:

(1) With your nondominant hand, stretch the skin over the injection site with your forefinger or thumb.   ___ ___ ___ _____

(2) With the needle almost against the client's skin, insert it slowly at a 5- to 15-degree angle until resistance is felt. Advance the needle through the epidermis to approximately 3 mm below skin surface. The needle tip can be seen through the skin.   ___ ___ ___ _____

(3) Inject the medication slowly. Normally, resistance is felt. If resistance is not felt, the needle is in too deep; remove and begin again. Your nondominant hand can stabilize the needle during the injection.   ___ ___ ___ _____

(4) While injecting medication, notice that a small bleb approximately 6 mm in diameter (resembling a mosquito bite) appears on the skin's surface. Instruct the client that this bleb is a normal finding.   ___ ___ ___ _____

Continued

	S	U	NP	Comments
22. Withdraw the needle while applying an alcohol swab or gauze gently over the injection site.	____	____	____	_____
23. Apply gentle pressure. Do not massage the injection site. Put on a bandage if needed.	____	____	____	_____
24. Assist the client to a comfortable position.	____	____	____	_____
25. Discard the uncapped needle or the needle enclosed in safety shield and attached syringe into a puncture- and leak-proof receptacle. Do *not* recap the needle.	____	____	____	
26. Remove disposable gloves and perform hand hygiene.	____	____	____	_____
27. Stay with the client 3–5 minutes to observe for any allergic reactions.	____	____	____	_____
28. Periodically return to the client's room to ask whether the client feels any acute pain, burning, numbness, or tingling at the injection site.	____	____	____	_____
29. Inspect the injection site, noting any bruising or induration.	____	____	____	_____
30. Observe the client's response to medication at times that correlate with the medication's onset, peak, and duration.	____	____	____	_____
31. Ask the client to explain the purpose and effects of the medication.	____	____	____	_____
32. For intradermal injections, use a skin pencil and draw a circle around the perimeter of the injection site. Read the site within an appropriate amount of time, which is determined by the type of medication or skin test administered.	____	____	____	_____

STUDENT: _____ DATE: _____

INSTRUCTOR: _____ DATE: _____

Skill 34–6 Adding Medications to Intravenous Fluid Containers

	S	U	NP	Comments
1. Check the accuracy and completeness of each MAR or computer printout against the prescriber's original medication order. Check the client's name and the medication name, route, dosage, and time of administration. Copy or rewrite any portion of the MAR that is difficult to read.	___	___	___	_____
2. Assess the client's medical history.				
3. Collect information necessary to administer the drug safely, including the medication's action, purpose, side effects, normal dose, time of peak onset, and nursing implications.	___	___	___	_____
4. When more than one medication is to be added to the intravenous (IV) solution, assess for compatibility of the medications.	___	___	___	_____
5. Assess client's systemic fluid balance, as reflected by skin hydration and turgor, body weight, pulse, blood pressure, and ratio of fluid intake to urinary output.	___	___	___	_____
6. Assess client's history of medication allergies.	___	___	___	_____
7. Perform hand hygiene.	___	___	___	_____
8. Assess the IV insertion site for signs of infiltration or phlebitis.	___	___	___	_____
9. Assess the client's understanding of the purpose of the medication therapy.	___	___	___	_____
10. Prepare prescribed medication; use aseptic techniques. Ensure that you compare the label of the medication with the MAR two times while preparing the medication.	___	___	___	_____
11. Perform hand hygiene.	___	___	___	_____
12. Compare the labels of the medication and the IV fluid bag with the MAR or computer printout.	___	___	___	_____
13. Add the medication to a new container (usually in the medication room or at medication cart):	___	___	___	_____
A. *Solution in a bag:* Locate the medication injection port on the plastic IV solution bag. The port has a small rubber stopper at the end. Do not select the port for the IV tubing insertion or the air vent.	___	___	___	_____
B. *Solution in a bottle:* Locate the injection site on the IV solution bottle, which is often covered by a metal or plastic cap.	___	___	___	_____
C. Wipe the port or injection site with alcohol or an antiseptic swab.	___	___	___	_____
D. Remove the needle cap or sheath from the syringe and insert the needle of the syringe or the needleless device through the centre of the injection port or site. Inject the medication.	___	___	___	_____
E. Withdraw the syringe from the bag or bottle.	___	___	___	_____
F. Mix the medication and the IV solution by holding the bag or bottle and turning it gently end to end.	___	___	___	_____
G. Complete the medication label by printing the client's name and dose of medication, date and time of administration, and your initials. Apply the label to the bottle or bag; do not cover essential information on the bottle or bag. Spike the bag or bottle with the IV tubing.	___	___	___	_____
14. Take the assembled items to client's bedside at the right time and perform hand hygiene.	___	___	___	_____
15. Identify the client by using at least two client identifiers. Compare the client's name and one other identifier (e.g., the hospital identification number) on the MAR, computer printout, or computer screen against information on the client's identification bracelet. Ask the client to state his or her name, if possible, for a third identifier.	___	___	___	_____
16. Prepare the client by explaining that the medication is to be given through the existing IV line or a new line that will be started. Explain that no discomfort should be felt during the medication infusion. Encourage client to report symptoms of discomfort.	___	___	___	_____
17. Connect infusion tubing or spike container to the existing tubing. Regulate infusion at ordered rate.	___	___	___	_____

Continued

	S	U	NP	Comments

18. Add the medication to the existing container:
   A. Prepare a vented IV bottle or plastic bag:
      (1) Check the volume of the solution remaining in the bottle or bag. ___ ___ ___ _____
      (2) Close off IV infusion clamp. ___ ___ ___ _____
      (3) Wipe the medication port with an alcohol or antiseptic swab. ___ ___ ___ _____
      (4) Remove the needle cap or sheath from the syringe; insert the syringe needle or needleless device through the injection port and inject the medication. ___ ___ ___ _____
      (5) Withdraw the syringe from the bag or bottle. ___ ___ ___ _____
      (6) Lower the bag or bottle from the IV pole and gently mix the medication and IV solution by holding the bag or bottle and turning it gently from end to end. Rehang the bag or bottle.
   B. Complete the medication label and apply it to the unprinted side of the IV solution bag or bottle. Do not cover the imprinted label of the solution. ___ ___ ___ _____
   C. Regulate the infusion to the desired rate. Use an IV pump if indicated. ___ ___ ___ _____
19. Properly dispose of equipment and supplies. Do not recap the needle or syringe. Discard sheathed needles as a unit with the needle covered. ___ ___ ___ _____
20. Perform hand hygiene.
21. Observe the client for signs or symptoms of medication reaction. ___ ___ ___ _____
22. Observe the client for signs and symptoms of fluid volume excess. ___ ___ ___ _____
23. Periodically return to the client's room to assess the IV insertion site and the rate of infusion. ___ ___ ___ _____
24. Observe the client for signs or symptoms of IV infiltration. ___ ___ ___ _____
25. Ensure that a label is applied to the IV tubing; the label must state the date and time that the IV tubing was opened and must be attached to the IV infusion system. Consult agency policy regarding frequency of changing IV tubing.
26. Assess the IV tubing frequently for integrity and occlusions. ___ ___ ___ _____
27. Ask the client to explain the purpose and effects of the medication therapy. ___ ___ ___ _____

STUDENT: _____ DATE: _____

INSTRUCTOR: _____ DATE: _____

Skill 34–7 Administering Medications by Intravenous Bolus

	S	U	NP	Comments
1. Check the accuracy and completeness of each MAR or computer printout against the prescriber's original medication order. Check the client's name and the medication name, route, dosage, and time of administration. Copy or rewrite any portion of the MAR that is difficult to read.	___	___	___	_____
2. Collect the information necessary to administer the medication safely, including action, purpose, side effects, normal dose, time of peak onset, the pace at which to give the medication, and nursing implications, such as the need to dilute the medication or to administer it through a filter.	___	___	___	_____
3. If pushing medication into an IV line, determine the compatibility of the medication both with the IV fluids ordered and any additives in the IV solution.	___	___	___	_____
4. Perform hand hygiene. Assess the IV or saline (heparin) lock insertion site for signs of infiltration or phlebitis.	___	___	___	_____
5. Check the client's medical history and allergies.	___	___	___	_____
6. Check the date of expiration for the medication vial or ampule.	___	___	___	_____
7. Assess the client's understanding of the purpose of medication therapy.	___	___	___	_____
8. Prepare the ordered medication from the vial or ampule by using aseptic technique. Check the label of the medication carefully with the MAR two times. Apply a removable label indicating the client's name and the medication name and dosage to the removable needle cap.	___	___	___	_____
9. Bring the medication to the client at the correct time.	___	___	___	_____
10. Identify the client by using at least two client identifiers. Compare the client's name and one other identifier (e.g., the hospital identification number) on the MAR, computer printout, or computer screen against information on the client's identification bracelet. Ask the client to state his or her name, if possible for a third identifier.	___	___	___	_____
11. Compare the label of the medications with the MAR at the client's bedside.	___	___	___	_____
12. Explain the procedure to the client. Encourage the client to report symptoms of discomfort at the IV site.	___	___	___	_____
13. Perform hand hygiene. Put on gloves.	___	___	___	_____
14. Administer the medication by IV push (through the existing IV line):				
A. Select the injection port of the IV tubing closest to the client. Whenever possible, the injection port should accept a needleless syringe. Use the IV filter if required by a medication reference manual or agency policy.	___	___	___	_____
B. Wipe the injection port with an antiseptic swab. Allow to dry.	___	___	___	_____
C. Connect the syringe to the IV line. Insert the needleless tip or a small-gauge needle of a syringe containing the prepared drug through the centre of the injection port.	___	___	___	_____
D. Occlude the IV line by pinching the tubing just above the injection port. Pull back gently on the syringe's plunger to aspirate the blood return.	___	___	___	_____
E. Release the tubing and inject the medication within the amount of time recommended by institutional policy, the pharmacist, or a medication reference manual. Use your watch to time the administration. The IV line may be pinched while medication is being pushed and released when medication is not being pushed. Allow IV fluids to infuse when the medication is not being pushed.	___	___	___	_____
F. After injecting the medication, release the tubing, withdraw the syringe, and recheck the fluid infusion rate.	___	___	___	_____

Continued

434

15. Administer medication by IV push (IV lock or needleless system):
    A. Prepare flush solutions according to agency policy. Ensure that a syringe with the correct barrel width is used. Consult agency policy regarding syringes used for delivering IV bolus medications.
        (1) *Saline flush method (preferred):*
            (a) Prepare two appropriate sized syringes with 2–3 mL of normal saline (0.9%).   ____ ____ ____ _____
        (2) *Heparin flush method (traditional method):*
            (a) Prepare one appropriate size syringe with the ordered amount of heparin flush solution.   ____ ____ ____ _____
            (b) Prepare two syringes with 2–3 mL of normal saline (0.9%).   ____ ____ ____ _____
    B. Administer medication:
        (1) Wipe the lock's injection port with an antiseptic swab.   ____ ____ ____ _____
        (2) Insert a syringe containing normal saline into the injection port of the IV lock.   ____ ____ ____ _____
        (3) Pull back gently on the syringe plunger and look for blood return.   ____ ____ ____ _____
        (4) Flush the IV lock with normal saline by pushing slowly on plunger.   ____ ____ ____ _____
        (5) Remove the saline-filled syringe.   ____ ____ ____ _____
        (6) Clean the lock's injection port with an antiseptic swab.   ____ ____ ____ _____
        (7) Insert the syringe containing the prepared medication into the injection port of the IV lock.   ____ ____ ____ _____
        (8) Inject the medication within the amount of time recommended by institutional policy, the pharmacist, or a medication reference manual. Use a watch to time the administration.   ____ ____ ____ _____
        (9) After administering the bolus, withdraw the syringe.   ____ ____ ____ _____
        (10) Clean the lock's injection port with an antiseptic swab.   ____ ____ ____ _____
        (11) Attach the syringe with normal saline and inject the normal saline flush at the same rate that the medication was delivered.   ____ ____ ____ _____
        (12) *Heparin flush option:* Insert the needle of the syringe containing the heparin through the diaphragm.   ____ ____ ____ _____
16. Dispose of uncapped needles and syringes in a puncture-proof and leak-proof container.   ____ ____ ____ _____
17. Remove and dispose of gloves. Perform hand hygiene.   ____ ____ ____ _____
18. Observe the client closely for adverse reactions while the medication is administered and for several minutes thereafter.   ____ ____ ____ _____
19. Observe the IV site during injection for sudden swelling.   ____ ____ ____ _____
20. Observe the client's status after the medication is administered, to evaluate effectiveness of medication.   ____ ____ ____ _____
21. Consult agency policy with regard to the frequency of saline flushes.   ____ ____ ____ _____
22. Ask the client to explain the medication's purposes and side effects.   ____ ____ ____ _____

STUDENT: _____ DATE: _____

INSTRUCTOR: _____ DATE: _____

Skill 34–8 Administering Intravenous Medications by Piggyback, Intermittent Intravenous Infusion Sets, and Mini-Infusion Pumps

	S	U	NP	Comments
1. Check the accuracy and completeness of each MAR or computer printout against the prescriber's original medication order. Check the client's name and the medication name, route, dosage, and time of administration. Copy or rewrite any portion of the MAR that is difficult to read.	___	___	___	_____
2. Determine the client's medical history.				
3. Collect the information necessary to administer the medication safely, including the action, purpose, side effects, normal dose, time of peak onset, and nursing implications, such as the need to dilute the medication or administer it through a filter.	___	___	___	_____
4. Assess the compatibility of the drug with the existing IV solution.	___	___	___	_____
5. Assess patency of the client's existing IV infusion line by the noting infusion rate of the main IV line.	___	___	___	_____
6. Perform hand hygiene. Assess IV insertion site for signs of infiltration or phlebitis: redness, pallor, swelling, tenderness on palpation.	___	___	___	_____
7. Assess the client's history of medication allergies.	___	___	___	_____
8. Assess the client's understanding of the purpose of medication therapy.	___	___	___	_____
9. Prepare the medication. Ensure that you compare the label of the medication with the MAR two times while preparing the medication.	___	___	___	_____
10. Assemble supplies at the client's bedside. Prepare the client by explaining that the medication will be given through the IV equipment.	___	___	___	_____
11. Perform hand hygiene.				
12. Identify the client by using at least two client identifiers. Compare the client's name and one other identifier (e.g., the hospital identification number) on the MAR, computer printout, or computer screen against information on the client's identification bracelet. Ask the client to state his or her name, if possible, for a third identifier.	___	___	___	_____
13. Compare medication label with MAR at the client's bedside.	___	___	___	_____
14. Explain to the client the purpose of the medication and its side effects. Encourage the client to report symptoms of discomfort at the injection site.	___	___	___	_____
15. Administer the infusion:				
A. Piggyback or tandem infusion:				
(1) Connect the infusion tubing to the medication bag. Allow the solution to fill the tubing by opening the regulator flow clamp. Once the tubing is full, close the clamp and cap the end of the tubing.	___	___	___	_____
(2) Hang the piggyback medication bag above the level of the primary fluid bag. (A hook may be used to lower the main bag.) Hang the tandem infusion bag at the same level as the primary fluid bag.	___	___	___	_____
(3) Connect the tubing of the piggyback or tandem infusion to the appropriate connector on the primary infusion line:				
(a) *Stopcock:* Wipe the stopcock port with an alcohol swab and connect the tubing. Turn the stopcock to the open position.	___	___	___	_____
(b) *Needleless system:* Wipe the needleless port, and insert the tip of the piggyback or tandem infusion tubing.	___	___	___	_____
(c) *Tubing port:* Connect the sterile needle to the end of the piggyback or tandem infusion tubing, remove the cap, clean the injection port on the main IV line, and insert the needle or needleless access device through the centre of the port. Secure by taping the connection.	___	___	___	_____

Continued

		S	U	NP	Comments

(4) Regulate the flow rate of the medication solution by adjusting the regulator clamp. (Infusion times vary. Refer to a medication reference manual or institutional policy for the safe flow rate.)   ___ ___ ___ _____

(5) After medication has infused, check the flow regulator on the primary infusion. The primary infusion should automatically begin to flow after the piggyback or tandem solution is empty.   ___ ___ ___ _____

(6) Regulate the main infusion line to the desired rate, if necessary.   ___ ___ ___ _____

(7) Leave the IV piggyback bag and tubing in place for future medication administration or discard in appropriate containers.   ___ ___ ___ _____

B. Volume-control administration set (e.g., Volutrol):

(1) Assemble the supplies in the medication room.   ___ ___ ___ _____

(2) Prepare medication from a vial or ampule.   ___ ___ ___ _____

(3) Fill the Volutrol with the desired amount of fluid (50–100 mL) by the opening clamp between the Volutrol and the main IV bag.   ___ ___ ___ _____

(4) Close the clamp and ensure the clamp on the air vent of the Volutrol chamber is open.   ___ ___ ___ _____

(5) Clean the injection port on the top of the Volutrol with an antiseptic swab.   ___ ___ ___ _____

(6) Remove the needle cap or sheath and insert the syringe needle through the port, then inject medication. Gently rotate the Volutrol between your hands.   ___ ___ ___ _____

(7) Regulate the IV infusion rate to allow the medication to infuse in time recommended by institutional policy, a pharmacist, or a medication reference manual.   ___ ___ ___ _____

(8) Label the Volutrol with the name of the medication, the dosage, the total volume (including the diluent), and the time of administration.   ___ ___ ___ _____

(9) Dispose of the uncapped needle or the needle enclosed in the safety shield and syringe in a proper container. Perform hand hygiene.   ___ ___ ___ _____

C. Mini-infusion administration:

(1) Connect prefilled syringe to the mini-infusion tubing.   ___ ___ ___ _____

(2) Carefully apply pressure to the syringe plunger, allowing the tubing to fill with medication.   ___ ___ ___ _____

(3) Place the syringe into mini-infusor pump (follow product directions). Ensure the syringe is secure.   ___ ___ ___ _____

(4) Connect the mini-infusion tubing to the main IV line:

(a) *Stopcock:* Wipe the stopcock port with an alcohol swab and connect the tubing. Turn the stopcock to the open position.   ___ ___ ___ _____

(b) *Needleless system:* Wipe the needleless port and insert the tip of the mini-infusor tubing.   ___ ___ ___ _____

(c) *Tubing port:* Connect the sterile needle to the mini-infusion tubing, remove the cap, clean the injection port on the main IV line, and insert the needle through the centre of port. Consider placing tape where the IV tubing enters the port to secure the connection.   ___ ___ ___ _____

(5) Explain the purpose of the medication and the side effects to the client, and explain that the medication is to be given through the existing IV line. Ask the client to report any symptoms of discomfort at the injection site.   ___ ___ ___ _____

(6) Hang the infusion pump with the syringe on the IV pole alongside the main IV bag. Set the pump to deliver medication within the time recommended by institutional policy, the pharmacist, or a medication reference manual. Press the button on the pump to begin infusion. Optional: Set the alarm.   ___ ___ ___ _____

(7) After medication has infused, check the flow regulator on the primary infusion. The infusion should automatically begin to flow once the pump stops. Regulate the main infusion line to the desired rate as needed. (Note: If the stopcock is used, turn off the mini-infusion line.)   ___ ___ ___ _____

16. Observe the client for signs of adverse reactions.   ___ ___ ___ _____

17. During infusion, periodically check the infusion rate and the condition of the IV site.   ___ ___ ___ _____

18. Ask the client to explain the purpose and side effects of the medication.   ___ ___ ___ _____

STUDENT: _____ DATE: _____

INSTRUCTOR: _____ DATE: _____

Skill 37–1 Applying Physical Restraints

	S	U	NP	Comments
1. Assess whether the client needs a restraint. Does the client continually try to interrupt needed therapy? Is the client at risk for injuring self or others?	___	___	___	_____
2. Assess the client's behaviour, such as confusion, disorientation, agitation, restlessness, combativeness, or inability to follow directions.	___	___	___	_____
3. Review your agency's policies regarding restraints. Consider the purpose, type, location, and duration of restraint. Determine whether signed consent for the use of restraint is needed.	___	___	___	_____
4. Review restraint manufacturer's instructions before entering the client's room. Determine the most appropriate size of restraint.	___	___	___	_____
5. Perform hand hygiene, and gather equipment.	___	___	___	_____
6. Introduce yourself to the client and family. Assess their feelings about restraint use. Explain that restraint is temporary and designed to protect the client from injury.	___	___	___	_____
7. Inspect the area of the client's body where the restraint is to be placed. Assess the condition of skin underlying where the restraint is to be applied.	___	___	___	_____
8. Approach client in a calm, confident manner. Check the client's identification by using two identifiers. Explain what you plan to do.	___	___	___	_____
9. Adjust the bed to proper height and lower the side rail on the side of client contact.	___	___	___	_____
10. Provide privacy. Make sure the client is comfortable and in proper body alignment. Drape the client as needed.	___	___	___	_____
11. Pad the skin and bony prominences (if necessary) before applying restraints.	___	___	___	_____
12. Apply the appropriate-size restraint, making sure it does not cover an IV line or other device (e.g., dialysis shunt) and that it does not cover the client's identification or allergy bracelet.				
A. *Belt restraint:* This device secures the client to a bed or stretcher. Apply it over the client's clothes or gown. Remove wrinkles from the front and back of the restraint while placing it around the client's waist. Bring ties through slots in the belt. Avoid placing the belt across the chest or too tightly across the abdomen.	___	___	___	_____
B. *Extremity (ankle or wrist) restraint:* This restraint is designed to immobilize one or all extremities. Commercially available limb restraints are composed of sheepskin or foam padding. Wrap the limb restraint around the wrist or ankle with the soft part toward the skin and is secured snugly in place with Velcro straps.	___	___	___	_____
C. *Mitten restraint:* This thumbless mitten device is used to restrain the client's hands. Place a hand in the mitten, being sure the mitten end is brought all the way over the wrist.	___	___	___	_____
D. *Elbow restraint:* This piece of fabric with slots has tongue blades placed so that elbow joint remains rigid.	___	___	___	_____
E. *Mummy restraint:* The mummy restraint consists of a blanket or sheet. It is opened on the bed or crib with one corner folded toward the centre. Place the child on the blanket with shoulders at the fold and feet toward the opposite corner. With child's right arm straight down against the body, pull the right side of the blanket firmly across the right shoulder and chest, and secure it beneath the left side of the body. Place the left arm straight against the body, and bring the left side of the blanket across the shoulder and chest and beneath the child's body on right side. Fold lower corner, bring it over the child's body, and tuck or fasten it securely with safety pins.	___	___	___	_____
13. Attach restraints to the bed frame, which moves when the head of the bed is raised or lowered. Do not attach them to side rails.	___	___	___	_____
14. Secure restraints with a quick-release tie. Do not tie in a knot.	___	___	___	_____

Continued

		S	U	NP	Comments
15.	Make sure two fingers will fit under secured restraint.	___	___	___	_____
16.	The proper placement of the restraint, skin integrity, pulses, temperature, colour, and sensation of the restrained body part should be assessed at least every hour or per your agency's policy.	___	___	___	_____
17.	Restraints should be removed at regular intervals (see agency policy). If the client is violent and noncompliant, remove one restraint at a time or have staff assist while removing restraints. The client should not be left unattended at this time.	___	___	___	_____
18.	Secure a call light or intercom system within the client's reach.	___	___	___	_____
19.	Leave the client's bed or chair with wheels locked. The bed should be in its lowest position.	___	___	___	_____
20.	Perform hand hygiene.	___	___	___	_____
21.	Reassess the client's status and needs:				
	A. Inspect the client for any injuries, including all hazards of immobility, while restraints are in use.	___	___	___	_____
	B. Observe IV catheters, urinary catheters, and drainage tubes to ensure that they are positioned correctly and that therapy remains uninterrupted.	___	___	___	_____
	C. Regularly reassess the client's need for continued use of the restraint (for medical or surgical reason) with the intent of discontinuing the restraint at the earliest possible time.	___	___	___	_____
	D. Provide sensory stimulation and reorient client as needed.	___	___	___	_____

STUDENT: _____   DATE: _____

INSTRUCTOR: _____   DATE: _____

Skill 37–2 Seizure Precautions

	S	U	NP	Comments
1. Assess seizure history, noting the frequency of seizures, presence of aura, and sequence of events, if known. Assess for medical and surgical conditions that may lead to seizures or exacerbate existing seizure condition. Assess medication history.	___	___	___	_____
2. Inspect the client's environment for potential safety hazards if risk for seizure exists, such as a bedside stand or table, an intravenous (IV) pole, or other medical equipment.	___	___	___	_____
3. Perform hand hygiene and prepare bed with padded side rails and headboard. Set the bed in the low position, and place the client in side-lying position when possible.	___	___	___	_____
4. For clients with a history of seizures, ensure that items such as an airway, suction apparatus, disposable gloves, and pillows are visible in the hospital setting for immediate use.	___	___	___	_____
5. When a seizure begins, position the client safely. If the client is standing or sitting, guide the client to the floor And protect his or her head by cradling it in your lap or placing a pillow under the head. Clear the surrounding area of furniture. If the client is in bed, raise the side rails, add padding, and put the bed in low position.	___	___	___	_____
6. Provide privacy.				
7. If possible, turn the client on the side, with the head flexed slightly forward.	___	___	___	_____
8. Do not restrain the client. Loosen the client's clothing.	___	___	___	_____
9. Do not put anything into the client's mouth, such as fingers, tongue depressor, or medicine.	___	___	___	_____
10. Stay with the client. Observe the sequence and timing of seizure activity.	___	___	___	_____
11. After the seizure is over, explain what happened and answer the client's questions. Foster an atmosphere of acceptance and respect.	___	___	___	_____
12. After the seizure, assist the client to a position of comfort in bed with padded side rails up and the bed in low position. Place a call light within reach, and provide a quiet, nonstimulating environment. Perform hand hygiene before leaving the room.	___	___	___	_____

STATUS EPILEPTICUS

For a client experiencing status epilepticus, the following actions are required:

	S	U	NP	Comments
13. Put on disposable gloves and insert an oral airway when the jaw is relaxed between seizure activities. Hold the airway with curved side up, insert downward until airway reaches the back of the throat, and then rotate and follow the natural curve of the tongue.	___	___	___	_____
14. Access oxygen and suction equipment. Prepare for IV insertion.	___	___	___	_____
15. Use pillows or pads to protect the client from injuring self.	___	___	___	_____

STUDENT: _____ DATE: _____

INSTRUCTOR: _____ DATE: _____

Skill 38–1 Bathing a Client

	S	U	NP	Comments
1. Review orders for specific safety measures concerning the client's movement, positioning, or isolation precautions.	___	___	___	_____
2. Explain the procedure to the client and ask the client for suggestions on how to prepare supplies. Encourage and promote independence by asking the client how much of the bath he or she wishes to complete.	___	___	___	_____
3. Assess the client's ability to perform self-care and allow the client to perform as much of the bath as he or she can.	___	___	___	_____
4. Assess the client's tolerance for activity, comfort level, cognitive ability, and musculoskeletal function.	___	___	___	_____
5. Assess the client's bathing preferences: frequency, type of hygiene products, and other factors.	___	___	___	_____
6. Ask whether client has noticed any skin problems or unusual marks on the skin. Observe the skin throughout the procedure, paying particular attention to areas that were previously soiled, reddened, or showed early signs of breakdown.	___	___	___	_____
7. Begin complete or partial bed bath, tub bath, whirlpool bath, or shower.				
A. *Complete or partial bed bath:*				
(1) Close room doors and draw room divider curtain.	___	___	___	_____
(2) Prepare equipment and supplies.	___	___	___	_____
(3) For nonambulatory clients, offer a bedpan or urinal. Provide a towel and washcloth for perineal care afterward.	___	___	___	_____
(4) Perform hand hygiene. If the client's skin is soiled with drainage or body secretions, put on disposable gloves. Ensure the client is not allergic to latex.	___	___	___	_____
(5) Place hospital bed at appropriate level, and lower side rail closest to you. Assist the client in assuming a comfortable position that maintains body alignment, preferably supine. Bring the client, or have the client move, toward the side of the bed closest to you.	___	___	___	_____
(6) Loosen the top covers. Place the bath blanket over the top sheet. Remove the top sheet from under the blanket. If possible, have the client hold the bath blanket while you withdraw the sheet. Optional: Use the top sheet when a bath blanket is not available.	___	___	___	_____
(7) If the top sheet is to be reused, fold it for replacement later. If not, place it in linen bag, taking care not to allow linen to contact uniform.	___	___	___	_____
(8) Assist the client with oral hygiene. See Skill 38–3.	___	___	___	_____
(9) Remove the client's gown or pyjamas. If the client has an IV infusing and the gown has snaps, simply unsnap and remove the gown without disconnecting the IV tubing. If the gown does not have snaps, remove gown from the arm without the IV first; then lower the IV container or remove from the pump and slide the gown covering the affected arm over the tubing and container. Rehang the IV container and check flow rate or reset pump rate. Do not disconnect the tubing. If an extremity is injured or has reduced mobility, begin removal from the unaffected side.	___	___	___	_____
(10) Raise the side rail. Fill a wash basin two-thirds full with warm water. Have the client place fingers in the water to test temperature.	___	___	___	_____
(11) Remove the pillow, if allowed, and raise the head of the bed 30–45 degrees. Place the bath towel under the client's head. Place a second bath towel over the client's chest.	___	___	___	_____
(12) Immerse the washcloth in warm water and wring it thoroughly. If desired, fold the washcloth around the fingers of your hand to form a mitt.	___	___	___	_____

Continued

442

	S	U	NP	Comments

(13) Inquire whether the client is wearing contact lenses. Wash the client's eyes with plain warm water. Use a different section of the mitt for each eye. Move the mitt from inner to outer canthus. Soak any crusts on eyelid for 2–3 minutes with the damp cloth before attempting removal. Dry eye thoroughly but gently.

(14) Ask whether the client prefers to use soap on his or her face. Wash, rinse, and thoroughly dry all areas of the face, neck, and ears. Men may wish to shave at this point or after the bath.

(15) Expose the client's arm that is farthest from you, and place the bath towel lengthwise under that arm.

(16) Bathe the client's arm with soap and water, using long, firm strokes from distal to proximal areas. Raise and support the arm as needed while washing the axilla.

(17) Rinse and dry the arm and axilla thoroughly. If the client uses deodorant or talcum powder, apply it.

(18) Fold the bath towel in half and lay it on the bed beside the client. Place a basin on the towel. Immerse the client's hand in water. Allow the hand to soak for 3–5 minutes before washing hand and fingernails. Remove the basin and dry the hand well.

(19) Cover the arm with a bath blanket or towel. Repeat steps 15 through 18 for other arm.

(20) Cover the client's chest with a bath towel, and fold the bath blanket down to the umbilicus. With one hand, lift the edge of the towel away from the client's chest. With washcloth or mitted hand, bathe the client's chest, using long, firm strokes. Take special care to wash skinfolds under a female client's breasts. Keep the client's chest covered between wash and rinse periods. Dry well.

(21) Place bath towel lengthwise over the client's chest and abdomen. (Two towels may be needed.) Fold blanket down to just above the client's pubic region.

(22) With one hand, lift the bath towel. With the mitted hand, bathe the client's abdomen, giving special attention to bathing the umbilicus and abdominal folds. Keep the client's abdomen covered between washing and rinsing. Dry well.

(23) Cover the client's chest and abdomen with the top of the bath blanket. Expose the client's far leg by folding the blanket toward the midline. Be sure the other leg and perineum are covered.

(24) Place the bath towel lengthwise under the far leg and, using firm strokes, wash, rinse, and dry thoroughly. Support the leg with one hand if the client is unable to support it.

(25) Cleanse the foot, making sure to bathe between toes. Clean and clip nails as per physician orders. Dry well. If the skin is dry, apply lotion. Do not massage any reddened area on the client's skin.

(26) Repeat steps 23–25 for the client's other leg and foot.

(27) Assist the client in assuming a prone or side-lying position (as applicable). Place towel lengthwise along the client's side. Put on disposable gloves if you have not done so already.

(28) Wash, rinse, and dry the client's back from neck to buttocks, using long, firm strokes. Pay special attention to folds of the buttocks and the anus for redness or skin breakdown. Give a back rub. Change bath water if necessary, and put on disposable gloves.

(a) *Female perineal care:*

(a1) Assist client in assuming a dorsal recumbent position, if not contraindicated. Cover the chest and upper extremities with a towel and the lower extremities with a bath blanket. Expose only the genitalia. (If the client can wash, covering entire body with a bath blanket may be preferable.) Clean the perineal area. Pay special attention to skin folds. If fecal material is present, enclose in a fold of underpad and remove with disposable wipes.

Continued

	S	U	NP	Comments

(a2) Wash labia majora. Wipe from the perineum to the rectum. Repeat on the opposite side, using a different section of the washcloth.

(a3) Separate the labia with your nondominant hand, exposing the urethral meatus and vaginal orifice. Wash downward from the pubic area toward the rectum in one smooth stroke. Use a separate section of cloth for each stroke. Cleanse thoroughly around the labia minora, clitoris, and vaginal orifice.

(a4) Assist the client to a comfortable position.

(a5) Remove disposable gloves and perform hand hygiene.

(b) *Male perineal care:*

(b1) Lower the side rails, and assist the client to a supine position. Note restriction in mobility.

(b2) Gently raise the penis, and place a bath towel underneath. Gently grasp the shaft of the penis. If the client is uncircumcised, retract the foreskin. If the client has an erection, defer perineal care until later.

(b3) Wash the tip of the penis at the urethral meatus first, using a circular motion. Cleanse from the meatus outward. Rinse and dry gently.

(b4) Return the foreskin to its natural position.

(b5) Wash the shaft of the penis with gentle but firm downward strokes. Pay special attention to the underlying surface of the penis. Rinse and dry thoroughly.

(b6) Gently cleanse the scrotum, making sure to wash underlying skinfolds. Rinse and dry thoroughly.

(b7) Inspect the surface of the external genitalia after cleansing.

(b8) If the client has bowel or urinary incontinence, apply a thin layer of skin barrier cream to the buttock, anus, and perineal area.

(b9) Assist the client to a comfortable position and cover with the bath blanket.

(29) Assist the client in dressing. Comb the client's hair. Women may want to apply makeup, and men may wish to shave at this point. Assist the client to a chair or wheelchair.

(30) Make the client's bed.

(31) Remove soiled linen and place it in a linen bag. Clean and replace the bathing equipment. Replace the call light and the client's personal possessions. Leave the room as clean and comfortable as possible.

(32) Remove disposable gloves and perform hand hygiene.

B. *Tub or whirlpool bath or shower (verify with agency policy whether a physician's order is needed):*

(1) Check the tub or shower for cleanliness. Use cleaning techniques outlined in agency policy. Place a rubber mat on the tub or shower bottom. Place a disposable bath mat or towel on the floor in front of the tub or shower.

(2) Collect all hygienic aids, toiletry items, and linens requested by the client. Place within easy reach of the tub or shower.

(3) Assist the client to the bathroom if necessary. Have the client wear a robe and slippers to the bathroom.

(4) Demonstrate how to use the call signal for assistance.

(5) Place an "occupied" sign on the bathroom door.

(6) Provide a shower seat or tub chair if needed. Fill the bathtub halfway with warm water. If the client's sensation is normal, ask the client to test the water, and adjust the temperature if needed. Explain which faucet controls hot water. If the client is taking a shower, turn it on and adjust the water temperature before the client enters the shower stall.

(7) Instruct the client to use safety bars when getting in and out of the tub or shower. Caution the client against the use of bath oil in tub water.

Continued

		S	U	NP	Comments

(8) Instruct the client not to remain in tub >20 minutes. Check on the client every 5 minutes. For clients at risk for falls or for debilitated clients, remain in the room with them during the bath. Observe client's range of motion during the bath.   ____ ____ ____ _____

(9) Return to the bathroom when the client signals, and knock before entering.   ____ ____ ____ _____

(10) For the client who is unsteady, drain the tub of water before the client attempts to get out of it. Place a bath towel over the client's shoulders. Assist the client in getting out of the tub as needed, and assist with drying. If the client is weak or unstable, have another person assist.   ____ ____ ____ _____

(11) Observe the client's skin, paying particular attention to areas that were previously soiled, reddened, or showed early signs of breakdown.   ____ ____ ____ _____

(12) Assist the client as needed in donning a clean gown or pyjamas, slippers, and robe. (In a home setting, the client may don regular clothing.)   ____ ____ ____ _____

(13) Assist the client to his or her room and a comfortable position in a bed or chair.   ____ ____ ____ _____

(14) Clean the tub or shower according to agency policy. Whirlpool baths may require special cleaning. Remove soiled linen and place it in a linen bag. Discard disposable equipment in the proper receptacle. Place an "unoccupied" sign on the bathroom door. Return supplies to the storage area.   ____ ____ ____ _____

(15) Perform hand hygiene.   ____ ____ ____ _____

STUDENT: _____ DATE: _____

INSTRUCTOR: _____ DATE: _____

Skill 38–2 Performing Nail and Foot Care

	S	U	NP	Comments
1. Identify clients at risk for foot or nail problems:				
A. Older adult				
B. Diabetes mellitus				
C. Heart failure or renal disease				
D. Cerebrovascular accident (stroke)				
2. Assess the client's knowledge of foot and nail care practices.				
3. Ask female clients whether they use nail polish and polish remover frequently.				
4. Assess the client's ability to care for nails or feet: Consider visual alterations, fatigue, and musculoskeletal weakness.				
5. Assess the types of home remedies (e.g., aloe vera, herbal preparations) that the client uses for existing foot problems:				
A. Over-the-counter liquid preparations to remove corns				
B. Cutting of corns or calluses with razor blade or scissors				
C. Use of oval corn pads				
D. Application of adhesive tape				
6. Assess the type of footwear worn by the client: Are socks worn? Are shoes tight or ill fitting? Are garters or knee-high nylons worn? Is footwear clean?				
7. Observe client's walking gait. Have the client walk down a hall or in a straight line (if able).				
8. Assist an ambulatory client to sit in a bedside chair. Help a bedbound client to a supine position with the head of the bed elevated. Place a disposable bath mat on the floor under the client's feet, or place a towel on the mattress.				
9. Obtain a physician's order for cutting client's nails if your agency policy requires it.				
10. Explain the procedure to the client, including the fact that proper soaking requires several minutes.				
11. Perform hand hygiene. Arrange equipment on an overbed table.				
12. Fill wash basin with warm water. Test water temperature.				
13. Place the basin on the bath mat or towel.				
14. Fill an emesis basin with warm water, and place the basin on paper towels on the overbed table.				
15. Pull the curtain around the bed or close the room door (if desired).				
16. Inspect all surfaces of the fingers, toes, feet, and nails. Pay particular attention to areas of dryness, inflammation, or cracking. Also inspect areas between toes, heels, and soles of the feet.				
17. Assess the colour and temperature of toes, feet, and fingers. Assess capillary refill. Palpate radial and ulnar pulses of each hand and dorsalis pedis pulses of feet.				
18. Instruct the client to place his or her fingers in the emesis basin and to place arms in a comfortable position. Assist the client in placing feet in the wash basin.				
19. Allow the client's feet and fingernails to soak for 10–20 minutes (unless the client has diabetes). Rewarm the water after 10 minutes.				
20. Clean gently under the fingernails with an orange stick or the wooden end of a cotton-tipped swab while the client's fingers are immersed. Remove fingers from emesis basin, and dry fingers thoroughly.				
21. Using nail clippers, clip fingernails straight across and even with tops of the fingers. Using a file, shape the nails straight across. If the client has circulatory problems, do not cut the nail; only file the nail.				
22. Push the client's cuticles back gently with the orange stick. Thoroughly dry the client's hands.				
23. Move the overbed table away from the client.				
24. Put on disposable gloves, and scrub callused areas of the feet with a washcloth, unless contraindicated.				
25. Clean gently under the toenails with the orange stick. Remove the client's feet from the basin and dry thoroughly, especially between the toes.				

Continued

446

	S	U	NP	Comments
26. Clean and trim toenails, using the procedures described in Steps 21 and 22. Do not file the corners of toenails.	___	___	___	_____
27. Apply lotion to feet (not between the toes) and hands, and assist the client back to bed and into a comfortable position.	___	___	___	_____
28. Remove disposable gloves and place in a receptacle. Clean and return equipment and supplies to the proper place. Dispose of soiled linen in a hamper. Perform hand hygiene.	___	___	___	_____
29. Inspect the client's nails and surrounding skin surfaces after soaking and nail trimming.	___	___	___	_____
30. Ask the client to explain or demonstrate nail care.	___	___	___	_____
31. Observe client's walk or gait after toenail care.	___	___	___	_____

STUDENT: _____ DATE: _____

INSTRUCTOR: _____ DATE: _____

Skill 38–3 Providing Oral Hygiene

	S	U	NP	Comments
1. Determine the client's oral hygiene practices:				
A. Frequency of toothbrushing and flossing	___	___	___	_____
B. Type of toothpaste or dentifrice used	___	___	___	_____
C. Last dental visit	___	___	___	_____
D. Frequency of dental visits	___	___	___	_____
E. Type of mouthwash or moistening preparation such as over-the-counter saliva substitutes or sugar-free gum with xylitol	___	___	___	_____
2. Assess the risk for oral hygiene problems.				
3. Assess the client's risk for aspiration: impaired swallowing, reduced gag reflex.	___	___	___	_____
4. Assess the client's ability to grasp and manipulate a toothbrush. (For older adults, try a 30-second toothbrushing assessment.)	___	___	___	_____
5. Prepare equipment at the bedside.	___	___	___	_____
6. Perform hand hygiene and put on disposable gloves.	___	___	___	_____
7. Inspect integrity of the lips, teeth, buccal mucosa, gums, palate, and tongue.	___	___	___	_____
8. Identify the presence of common oral problems:			___	_____
A. Dental caries—chalky white discoloration of a tooth or the presence of brown or black discoloration	___	___	___	_____
B. Gingivitis—inflammation of gums				_____
C. Periodontitis—receding gum lines, inflammation, gaps between teeth	___	___	___	_____
D. Halitosis—bad breath	___	___	___	_____
E. Cheilosis—cracking of the lips	___	___	___	_____
F. Stomatitis—inflammation of the mouth	___	___	___	_____
G. Dry, cracked, coated tongue	___	___	___	_____
9. Explain the procedure to the client and discuss preferences regarding the use of hygienic aids.	___	___	___	_____
10. Raise the bed to a comfortable working position. Raise the head of the bed (if allowed) and lower the side rail. Move the client, or help the client move closer. A side-lying position can be used.	___	___	___	_____
11. Place paper towels on overbed table, and arrange other necessary equipment within easy reach.	___	___	___	_____
12. Place a towel over the client's chest.	___	___	___	_____
13. Apply toothpaste to the toothbrush while holding the brush over the emesis basin. Pour a small amount of water over toothpaste.	___	___	___	_____
14. Client may assist by brushing. Hold (or have client hold if able to) the toothbrush bristles at a 45-degree angle to the gum line. Be sure tips of bristles rest against and penetrate under gum line. Brush inner and outer surfaces of upper and lower teeth by brushing from gum to crown of each tooth. Clean the biting surfaces of teeth by holding the top of the bristles parallel with teeth and brushing gently back and forth. Brush sides of the teeth by moving bristles back and forth.	___	___	___	_____
15. Have the client hold the brush at a 45-degree angle and lightly brush over the surface and sides of the tongue. Avoid initiating gag reflex.	___	___	___	_____
16. Allow the client to rinse the mouth thoroughly by taking several sips of water, swishing water across all tooth surfaces, and spitting into the emesis basin.	___	___	___	_____
17. Allow the client to gargle and rinse the mouth with mouthwash as desired.	___	___	___	_____
18. Assist in wiping the client's mouth.	___	___	___	_____
19. Allow the client to floss, or assist client with flossing.	___	___	___	_____
20. Allow the client to rinse the mouth thoroughly with cool water and spit into the emesis basin. Assist in wiping the client's mouth.	___	___	___	_____
21. Ask the client whether any area of the oral cavity feels uncomfortable or irritated. Inspect the oral cavity.	___	___	___	_____
22. Assist the client to a comfortable position, remove the emesis basin and bedside table, raise the side rail (if used), and lower the bed to the original position.	___	___	___	_____
23. Wipe off overbed table. Discard soiled linens and paper towels in appropriate containers. Remove and dispose of soiled gloves. Return equipment to the proper place.	___	___	___	_____
24. Remove gloves and perform hand hygiene.	___	___	___	_____
25. Ask the client to describe proper hygiene techniques.	___	___	___	_____

STUDENT: _____ DATE: _____

INSTRUCTOR: _____ DATE: _____

Skill 38–4 Performing Mouth Care for an Unconscious or Debilitated Client

	S	U	NP	Comments
1. Assess the client's risk for oral hygiene problems.	___	___	___	_____
2. Explain the procedure to the client.	___	___	___	_____
3. Test for the presence of a gag reflex by placing a tongue blade on the back half of the client's tongue.	___	___	___	_____
4. Raise the bed to the appropriate working height; lower the head of bed and then lower the side rail.	___	___	___	_____
5. Pull the curtain around the bed, or close the room door.	___	___	___	_____
6. Perform hand hygiene and put on disposable gloves.	___	___	___	_____
7. Place paper towels on an overbed table and arrange equipment. If needed, turn on a suction machine and connect tubing to the suction catheter.	___	___	___	_____
8. Position the client on the side (Sims' position), close to the side of the bed. Turn the client's head toward the dependent side. Raise the side rail.	___	___	___	_____
9. Place a towel under the client's head and place an emesis basin under the chin.	___	___	___	_____
10. Carefully separate upper and lower teeth with padded tongue blade by inserting the blade, quickly but gently, between the back molars. Do not use your fingers. Insert blade when client is relaxed, if possible. Do not use force.	___	___	___	_____
11. Inspect the condition of the oral cavity.	___	___	___	_____
12. Clean the mouth, using a toothbrush or sponge Toothette swabs moistened with a chlorhexidine solution (if client can tolerate it); otherwise, moisten with water. Clean chewing and inner and outer tooth surfaces. Swab the roof of the mouth, gums, insides of cheeks, and tongue, but avoid stimulating the gag reflex (if present). Moisten a clean swab or a Toothette swab with water to rinse. (A bulb syringe may also be used to rinse.) Repeat rinse several times.	___	___	___	_____
13. Suction secretions as they accumulate, if necessary.	___	___	___	_____
14. Apply a thin layer of water-soluble jelly to the lips.	___	___	___	_____
15. Inform the client that the procedure is completed.	___	___	___	_____
16. Put on clean gloves, and inspect the oral cavity.	___	___	___	_____
17. Ask the debilitated client whether his or her mouth feels clean.	___	___	___	_____
18. Reposition client comfortably, raise the side rail as appropriate or as ordered, and return the bed to the original position.	___	___	___	_____
19. Clean equipment and return it to the proper place. Place soiled linen in the proper receptacle.	___	___	___	_____
20. Remove and discard gloves. Perform hand hygiene.	___	___	___	_____
21. Assess the client's respirations on an ongoing basis.	___	___	___	_____

STUDENT: _____   DATE: _____

INSTRUCTOR: _____   DATE: _____

Skill 38–5 Making an Occupied Bed

	S	U	NP	Comments
1. Assess the potential for client incontinence or for excess drainage on bed linen.	___	___	___	_____
2. Check the chart for orders or specific precautions concerning movement and positioning.	___	___	___	_____
3. Explain the procedure to the client, noting that he or she will be asked to turn on the side and to roll over linen.	___	___	___	_____
4. Perform hand hygiene and put on gloves. (Gloves are worn only if linen is soiled or if contact with body secretions is possible.)	___	___	___	_____
5. Assemble equipment and arrange it on a bedside chair or table. Remove unnecessary equipment such as a dietary tray or items used for hygiene.	___	___	___	_____
6. Draw the room curtain around the bed, or close the room door.	___	___	___	_____
7. Adjust the bed height to a comfortable working position. Lower any raised side rail on one side of the bed. Remove the call light.	___	___	___	_____
8. Loosen top linen at the foot of the bed.	___	___	___	_____
9. Remove bedspread and blanket separately. If they are soiled, place them in a soiled linen bag. Do not allow soiled linen to contact uniform. Do not fan or shake linen.	___	___	___	_____
10. If the blanket and bedspread are to be reused, fold them by bringing the top and bottom edges together. Fold the farthest side over onto the nearer bottom edge. Bring top and bottom edges together again. Place folded linen over the back of a chair.	___	___	___	_____
11. Cover the client with a bath blanket in the following manner: Unfold the bath blanket over the top sheet. Ask the client to hold the top edge of the bath blanket. If the client is unable to help, tuck the top of the bath blanket under the client's shoulder. Grasp the top sheet under the bath blanket at the client's shoulders and bring the sheet down to the foot of the bed. Remove the sheet and discard it in a linen bag.	___	___	___	_____
12. With assistance from another person, slide the mattress toward the head of the bed.	___	___	___	_____
13. Position the client on the far side of the bed, turned onto his or her side and facing away from you. Be sure the side rail in front of the client is up. Adjust the pillow under the client's head.	___	___	___	_____
14. Loosen bottom bed linens, moving from head to foot of the bed. With seam side down (facing the mattress), fan-fold first drawsheet and then bottom sheet toward the client. Tuck edges of linen just under buttocks, back, and shoulders. Do not fan-fold the mattress pad if it is to be reused.	___	___	___	_____
15. Wipe off any moisture on the exposed mattress with a towel and appropriate disinfectant.	___	___	___	_____
16. Put clean linen on the exposed half of the bed:				
A. Place a clean mattress pad on the bed by folding it lengthwise with centre crease in the middle of the bed. Fan-fold the top layer over the mattress. (If pad part is reused, simply smooth out any wrinkles.)	___	___	___	_____
B. Unfold bottom sheet lengthwise so that centre crease is situated lengthwise along the centre of the bed. Fan-fold the sheet's top layer toward the centre of the bed alongside the client. Smooth the bottom layer of the sheet over the closest side of the mattress. Pull the fitted sheet smoothly over mattress ends. Allow the edge of the flat unfitted sheet to hang about 25 cm over the mattress edge. The lower hem of the bottom flat sheet should lie seam down and even with the bottom edge of the mattress.	___	___	___	_____
17. Mitre the bottom flat sheet at the head of the bed:				
A. Face the head of the bed diagonally. Place your hand away from the head of the bed under the top corner of the mattress, near the mattress edge, and lift.	___	___	___	_____
B. With your other hand, tuck the top edge of the bottom sheet smoothly under the mattress so that side edges of the sheet above and below the mattress would meet if brought together.	___	___	___	_____

Continued

452

	S	U	NP	Comments

C. Face the side of the bed and pick up the top edge of the sheet approximately 45 cm from top of mattress.

D. Lift the sheet, and lay it on top of the mattress to form a neat triangular fold, with the lower base of the triangle even with the mattress side edge.

E. Tuck the lower edge of sheet, which is hanging free below the mattress, under the mattress. Tuck with your palms down, without pulling triangular fold.

F. Hold the portion of the sheet covering the side of mattress in place with one hand. With the other hand, pick up the top of triangular linen fold and bring it down over the side of the mattress. Tuck this portion under the mattress.

18. Tuck the remaining portion of the sheet under the mattress, moving toward the foot of the bed. Keep the linen smooth.

19. (Optional) Open drawsheet so that it unfolds in half. Lay centre fold along the middle of the bed lengthwise, and position the sheet so that it will be under the client's buttocks and torso. Fan-fold the top layer toward the client, with the edge along the client's back. Smooth the bottom layer out over the mattress, and tuck the excess edge under the mattress (keep your palms down).

20. Place waterproof pad over drawsheet, with centre fold against the client's side. Fan-fold the top layer toward the client.

21. Have the client roll slowly toward you, over the layers of linen. Raise the side rail on the working side of the bed, and go to the other side of the bed.

22. Lower the side rail. Assist the client in positioning on the other side, over the folds of linen. Loosen the edges of soiled linen from under the mattress.

23. Remove soiled linen by folding it into a bundle or square, with soiled side turned in. Discard in a linen bag. If necessary, wipe the mattress with antiseptic solution, and dry the mattress surface before putting on new linen.

24. Pull clean, fan-folded linen smoothly over the edge of the mattress from head to foot of the bed.

25. Assist the client in rolling back into the supine position. Reposition pillow.

26. Pull the fitted sheet smoothly over the mattress ends. Mitre the top corner of the bottom sheet. When tucking the corner, be sure the sheet is smooth and free of wrinkles.

27. Facing the side of the bed, grasp the remaining edge of the bottom flat sheet. Lean back; keeping your back straight, pull while tucking excess linen under the mattress. Proceed from head to foot of the bed. (Avoid lifting the mattress during tucking to ensure fit.)

28. Smooth the fan-folded drawsheet or waterproof pad out over the bottom sheet. Grasp the edge of the sheet with your palms down, lean back, and tuck the sheet under the mattress. Tuck from middle to top and then to bottom.

29. Place the top sheet over the client with centre fold lengthwise down the middle of the bed. Open the sheet from head to foot, and unfold it over the client.

30. Ask the client to hold the clean top sheet, or tuck the sheet around the client's shoulders. Remove the bath blanket and discard in the linen bag.

31. Place a blanket on the bed, unfolding it so that the crease runs lengthwise along the middle of the bed. Unfold the blanket to cover the client. The top edge should be parallel with the edge of the top sheet and 15–20 cm from the top sheet's edge.

32. Place the bedspread over the bed according to Step 31. Be sure that the top edge of the bedspread extends about 2.5 cm above the blanket's edge. Tuck the top edge of the bedspread over and under the top edge of the blanket.

33. Make a cuff by turning the edge of the top sheet down over the edge of the blanket.

34. Standing on one side at the foot of the bed, lift the mattress corner slightly with one hand and tuck top linens under the mattress. Tuck the top sheet and blanket under together. Be sure that linens are loose enough to allow movement of the client's feet. Making a horizontal toe pleat is an option.

Continued

	S	U	NP	Comments

35. Make a modified mitred corner with the top sheet, blanket, and bedspread:
    A. Pick up the side edge of the top sheet, blanket, and bedspread approximately 45 cm from the foot of the mattress. Lift the linen to form a triangular fold, and lay it on the bed. ____ ____ ____ _____
    B. Pick up the lower edge of the sheet, which is hanging free below the mattress, and tuck it under the mattress. Do not pull the triangular fold. ____ ____ ____ _____
    C. Pick up the triangular fold, and bring it down over the mattress while holding the linen in place along the side of the mattress. Do not tuck the tip of the triangle. ____ ____ ____ _____
36. Raise the side rail. Make the other side of the bed; spread sheet, blanket, and bedspread out evenly. Fold the top edge of the sheet over the blanket and make a cuff with the top sheet (see Step 33). Make a modified mitred corner at foot of bed (see Step 35). ____ ____ ____ _____
37. Change pillowcase and fit pillow corners evenly in corners of pillowcase.
    A. Have the client raise his or her head. While supporting the client's neck with one hand, remove the pillow. Allow the client to lower the head. ____ ____ ____ _____
    B. Remove soiled pillowcase by grasping the pillow at the open end with one hand and pulling the case back over the pillow with the other hand. Discard the case in the linen bag. ____ ____ ____ _____
    C. Grasp the clean pillowcase at the centre of the closed end. Gather the case, turning it inside out of the hand holding it. With the same hand, pick up the middle of one end of the pillow. Pull the pillowcase down over the pillow with the other hand. ____ ____ ____ _____
    D. Be sure pillow corners fit evenly into the corners of the pillowcase. Place the pillow under the client's head. ____ ____ ____ _____
38. Place the call bell within the client's reach, and return the bed to a comfortable position. ____ ____ ____ _____
39. Open the room curtains, and rearrange furniture. Place personal items within the client's easy reach on the overbed table or bedside stand. Return the bed to a comfortable height. ____ ____ ____ _____
40. Discard dirty linen in a hamper or chute, remove your gloves, and perform hand hygiene. ____ ____ ____ _____
41. Ask whether the client feels comfortable. ____ ____ ____ _____
42. While you are performing this skill, inspect the client's skin for areas of irritation. ____ ____ ____ _____
43. Observe the client for signs of fatigue, dyspnea, pain, or discomfort throughout the skill. ____ ____ ____ _____

STUDENT: _____ DATE: _____

INSTRUCTOR: _____ DATE: _____

Skill 39–1 Suctioning

	S	U	NP	Comments
1. Assess for signs and symptoms of upper and lower airway obstruction necessitating nasotracheal or orotracheal suctioning; abnormal respiratory rate; adventitious sounds; nasal secretions, gurgling, drooling; restlessness; gastric secretions or vomitus in the mouth; and coughing without clearing secretions from the airway.	___	___	___	_____
2. Assess for signs and symptoms associated with hypoxia and hypercapnia: decreased SpO_2, increased pulse and blood pressure, increased respiratory rate, apprehension, anxiety, decreased ability to concentrate, lethargy, decreased level of consciousness (especially acute), increased fatigue, dizziness, behavioural changes (especially irritability), dysrhythmias, pallor, and cyanosis.	___	___	___	_____
3. Determine factors that normally influence upper or lower airway functioning: fluid status; lack of humidity; pulmonary disease, chronic obstructive pulmonary disorder, and pulmonary infection; anatomy; changes in level of consciousness; and decreased cough or gag reflex.	___	___	___	_____
4. Identify contraindications to nasotracheal suctioning: occluded nasal passages; nasal bleeding, epiglottitis, or croup; acute head, facial, or neck injury or surgery, coagulopathy, or bleeding disorder; irritable airway or laryngospasm or bronchospasm; gastric surgery with high anastomosis; or myocardial infarction.	___	___	___	_____
5. Examine sputum microbiology data.	___	___	___	_____
6. Assess the client's understanding of the procedure.	___	___	___	_____
7. Obtain a physician's order if indicated by agency policy.	___	___	___	_____
8. Explain to the client how the procedure will help clear the airway and relieve breathing problems and that temporary coughing, sneezing, gagging, or shortness of breath is normal. Encourage the client to cough out secretions. Have the client practise coughing, if able. Splint surgical incisions, if necessary.	___	___	___	_____
9. Explain the importance of coughing, and encourage coughing during the procedure.	___	___	___	_____
10. Help the client to assume a position comfortable for you and the client (usually semi-Fowler's or sitting upright with head hyperextended, unless contraindicated).	___	___	___	_____
11. Place a pulse oximeter on the client's finger. Take a reading, and leave the pulse oximeter in place.	___	___	___	_____
12. Place a towel across the client's chest.	___	___	___	_____
13. Perform hand hygiene. Put on a face shield if splashing is likely.	___	___	___	_____
14. Connect one end of the connecting tubing to the suction machine, and place the other end in a convenient location near the client. Turn on the suction device, and set the vacuum regulator to appropriate negative pressure (120–150 mm Hg). Appropriate pressure may vary; check agency policy.				
15. If indicated, increase supplemental oxygen therapy to 100% or as ordered by the physician. Encourage the client to breathe deeply.				
16. Preparation for all types of suctioning:				
A. Open the suction kit or catheter, using aseptic technique. If a sterile drape is available, place it across the client's chest or on the overbed table. Do not allow the suction catheter to touch any nonsterile surfaces.	___	___	___	_____
B. Unwrap or open a sterile basin and place it on the bedside table. Fill it with about 100 mL of sterile normal saline solution or water. Connect one end of connecting tubing to suction machine. Place other end in convenient location near client. Check that equipment is functioning properly by suctioning a small amount of water from basin.	___	___	___	_____
C. Turn on suction device. Set regulator to appropriate negative pressure: 100–150 mm Hg for adults.	___	___	___	_____
17. Suction airway.				
A. Oropharyngeal suctioning:				
(1) Put on clean disposable glove to your dominant hand. Put on mask or face shield.	___	___	___	_____

Continued

	S	U	NP	Comments

(2) Attach the suction catheter to connecting tubing. Check that equipment is functioning properly by suctioning a small amount of water or normal saline from the basin. ___ ___ ___ _____

(3) Remove oxygen mask, if present. Keep the oxygen mask near the client's face. A nasal cannula may remain in place (if present). ___ ___ ___ _____

(4) Insert the catheter into the client's mouth. With suction applied, move the catheter around the mouth, including pharynx and gum line, until secretions are cleared. ___ ___ ___ _____

(5) Encourage the client to cough, and repeat suctioning if needed. Replace oxygen mask, if used. ___ ___ ___ _____

(6) Suction water from the basin through the catheter until the catheter is cleared of secretions. ___ ___ ___ _____

(7) Place the catheter in a clean, dry area for reuse, with suction turned off, or within the client's reach, with suction on, if the client is capable of suctioning self. ___ ___ ___ _____

B. Nasopharyngeal and nasotracheal suctioning:

(1) Increase supplemental oxygen therapy to 100% as indicated or as ordered. Encourage client to breathe deeply. Open the lubricant. Squeeze a small amount onto the open sterile catheter package. ___ ___ ___ _____

(2) Put a sterile glove on each hand, or put a nonsterile glove on your nondominant hand and a sterile glove on your dominant hand. ___ ___ ___ _____

(3) Pick up the suction catheter with your dominant hand without touching nonsterile surfaces. Pick up connecting tubing with your nondominant hand. Secure the catheter to the tubing. ___ ___ ___ _____

(4) Check that the equipment is functioning properly by suctioning a small amount of normal saline solution from the basin. ___ ___ ___ _____

(5) Lightly coat the distal 6–8 cm of the catheter with water-soluble lubricant. ___ ___ ___ _____

(6) Remove the oxygen delivery device, if applicable, with your nondominant hand. Without applying suction and using your dominant thumb and forefinger, gently insert the catheter into the client's naris during inhalation. ___ ___ ___ _____

(7) *Nasopharyngeal:* Follow the natural course of the naris; slightly slant the catheter downward and advance to the back of the pharynx. In adults, insert the catheter about 16 cm; in older children, 8–12 cm; in infants and young children, 4–8 cm. The rule of thumb is to insert the catheter a distance from the tip of the nose (or mouth) to the base of the earlobe. ___ ___ ___ _____

   (a) Apply intermittent suction for up to 10–15 seconds by placing and releasing your nondominant thumb over the catheter vent. Slowly withdraw the catheter while rotating it back and forth between your thumb and forefinger. ___ ___ ___ _____

(8) *Nasotracheal:* Follow the natural course of the naris and advance the catheter slightly slanted and downward to just above the entrance into the trachea. Allow the client to take a breath. Quickly insert catheter approximately 16–20 cm (in adult) into the trachea. The client will begin to cough. *Note:* In older children, advance 14–20 cm; in young children and infants, 8–14 cm. ___ ___ ___ _____

   (a) *Positioning option for nasotracheal suctioning:* In some instances, turning the client's head to the right helps you suction the left mainstem bronchus; turning the head to the left helps you suction the right mainstem bronchus. If resistance is felt after insertion of the catheter for the maximum recommended distance, the catheter has probably hit the carina. Pull the catheter back 1–2 cm before applying suction. ___ ___ ___ _____

   (b) Apply intermittent suction for up to 10–15 seconds by placing and releasing your nondominant thumb over the vent of the catheter and slowly withdrawing the catheter while rotating it back and forth between your dominant thumb and forefinger. Encourage the client to cough. Replace the oxygen device, if applicable. ___ ___ ___ _____

Continued

	S	U	NP	Comments

(9) Rinse the catheter and connecting tubing with normal saline or water until cleared.

(10) Assess for need to repeat the suctioning procedure. Allow adequate time (1–2 minutes) between suction passes for ventilation and oxygenation. Ask the client to breathe deeply and cough.

C. Artificial airway suctioning:

(1) Put on face shield.

(2) Put one sterile glove on each hand, or put a nonsterile glove on your nondominant hand and a sterile glove on your dominant hand.

(3) Pick up the suction catheter with your dominant hand without touching nonsterile surfaces. Pick up the connecting tubing with your nondominant hand. Secure the catheter to the tubing.

(4) Check that equipment is functioning properly by suctioning a small amount of saline from the basin.

(5) Hyperinflate or hyperoxygenate the client, or do both, before suctioning, using manual resuscitation Ambu-bag connected to the oxygen source on the mechanical ventilator. Some mechanical ventilators have a button that, when pushed, delivers oxygen for a few minutes and then resets to the previous value.

(6) If the client is receiving mechanical ventilation, open swivel the adapter or, if necessary, remove the oxygen or humidity delivery device with your nondominant hand.

(7) Without applying suction, gently but quickly insert the catheter, using your dominant thumb and forefinger, into the artificial airway (it is best to time catheter insertion with inspiration) until resistance is met or the client coughs; then pull back 1 cm.

(8) Apply intermittent suction by placing and releasing your nondominant thumb over the vent of the catheter; slowly withdraw the catheter while rotating it back and forth between your dominant thumb and forefinger. Encourage the client to cough. Watch for respiratory distress.

(9) If the client is receiving mechanical ventilation, close the swivel adapter or replace the oxygen delivery device.

(10) Encourage the client to breathe deeply, if able. Some clients respond well to several manual breaths from the mechanical ventilator or Ambu bag.

(11) Rinse the catheter and connecting tubing with normal saline until clear. Use continuous suction.

(12) Assess the client's cardiopulmonary status. Repeat steps 17C(5) through 17C(11) once or twice more to clear secretions. Allow adequate time (at least 1 full minute) between suction passes for ventilation and reoxygenation. Perform oropharyngeal and nasopharyngeal suctioning (Steps 17A and 17B). After oropharyngeal and nasopharyngeal suction is performed, the catheter is contaminated; do not reinsert it into the endotracheal or tracheostomy tube.

18. Complete the procedure:

A. Disconnect the catheter from the connecting tubing. Roll the catheter around the fingers of your dominant hand. Pull the glove off inside out so that the catheter remains in the glove. Pull off the other glove over the first glove in the same way to contain contaminants. Discard gloves into an appropriate receptacle. Turn off the suction device.

B. Remove the towel or drape, and discard it in an appropriate receptacle.

C. Reposition the client as indicated by the condition. Put on clean gloves for the client's personal care (e.g., oral hygiene).

D. If indicated, readjust oxygen supply to the original level.

E. Discard the remainder of normal saline into an appropriate receptacle. If the basin is disposable, discard into an appropriate receptacle. If the basin is reusable, rinse and place in soiled utility room.

Continued

		S	U	NP	Comments
F.	Remove and discard the face shield, and perform hand hygiene.	___	___	___	_____
G.	Place an unopened suction kit on the suction machine table or at the head of bed, according to institution preference.	___	___	___	_____
19.	Compare the client's vital signs and SpO$_2$ saturation before and after suctioning.	___	___	___	_____
20.	Ask the client whether breathing is easier and whether congestion is decreased.	___	___	___	_____
21.	Observe airway secretions.	___	___	___	_____

STUDENT: _____ DATE: _____

INSTRUCTOR: _____ DATE: _____

Skill 39–2 Care of an Artificial Airway

	S	U	NP	Comments
1. Perform cardiopulmonary assessment:				
A. Auscultate lung sounds.	___	___	___	_____
B. Assess condition and patency of airway and surrounding tissues.	___	___	___	_____
C. Note type and size of tube, movement of tube, and cuff size.	___	___	___	_____
2. Explain the procedure to the client and family.	___	___	___	_____
3. Position the client. Clients usually prefer to be lying down. A client with a long-term, well-established tracheostomy may be seated.	___	___	___	_____
4. Place a towel across the client's chest.	___	___	___	_____
5. Perform hand hygiene.	___	___	___	_____
6. Perform airway care:				
A. Endotracheal (ET) tube care:				
(1) Observe for signs and symptoms of the need to perform care of the artificial airway:				
(a) Soiled or loose tape	___	___	___	_____
(b) Pressure sores on nares, lip, or corner of mouth	___	___	___	_____
(c) Unstable tube	___	___	___	_____
(d) Excessive secretions	___	___	___	_____
(2) Identify factors that increase risk of complications from ET tubes:				
(a) Type and size of tube	___	___	___	_____
(b) Movement of tube up and down trachea	___	___	___	_____
(c) Cuff size	___	___	___	_____
(d) Duration of placement	___	___	___	_____
(3) Suction ET tube:				
(a) Instruct the client not to bite or move the ET tube with the tongue or pull on tubing; removal of tape can be uncomfortable.	___	___	___	_____
(b) Leave the Yankauer suction catheter connected to the suction source.	___	___	___	_____
(4) Prepare method to secure the ET tube (check agency policy):				
(a) *Tape method:* Cut a piece of tape long enough to go completely around the client's head, from naris to naris, plus 15 cm: for an adult, about 30–60 cm. Lay adhesive side up on the bedside table. Cut and lay 8–16 cm of tape, adhesive side down, in the centre of the long strip to prevent the tape from sticking to the client's hair.	___	___	___	_____
(b) *Commercially available endotracheal tube holder:* Open the package per manufacturer's instructions. Set the device aside with the head guard in place and the Velcro strips open.	___	___	___	_____
(5) Put on gloves, and instruct an assistant to put on a pair of gloves and hold the ET tube firmly at the client's lips. Note the number marking on the ET tube at the gum line.	___	___	___	_____
(6) Remove old tape or device:				
(a) *Tape:* Carefully remove tape from the ET tube and the client's face. If the tape is difficult to remove, moisten it with water or adhesive tape remover. Discard tape in an appropriate receptacle if nearby. If not, place soiled tape on the bedside table or on the distant end of the towel.	___	___	___	_____
(b) *Commercially available device:* Remove Velcro strips from the ET tube, and remove the ET tube holder from the client.	___	___	___	_____
(7) Use adhesive remover swab to remove excess secretions or adhesive left on the client's face.	___	___	___	_____
(8) Remove oral airway or bite block, if present.	___	___	___	_____
(9) Clean the mouth, gums, and teeth opposite the ET tube with mouthwash solution and 4 × 4 gauze, sponge-tipped applicators, or saline swabs. Brush teeth as indicated. If necessary, administer oropharyngeal suctioning with a Yankauer catheter.	___	___	___	_____

Continued

	S	U	NP	Comments

(10) Note "cm" ET tube marking at the lips or gums. With the help of the assistant, move the ET tube to the opposite side or centre of the mouth. Do not change tube depth.   ___ ___ ___ _____

(11) Repeat oral cleaning on the opposite side of the mouth.   ___ ___ ___ _____

(12) Clean the face and neck with a soapy washcloth; rinse and dry. Shave a male client as necessary.   ___ ___ ___ _____

(13) Use a small amount of skin protectant or liquid adhesive on a clean 2 × 2 gauze, and dot on the upper lip (with oral ET tube) or across the nose (with nasal ET tube) and from cheeks to ear. Allow tincture to dry completely.   ___ ___ ___ _____

(14) Secure ET tube.
 (a) Tube method:
  (a1) Slip tape under the client's head and neck, adhesive side up. Do not twist the tape or catch hair. Do not allow tape to stick to itself. It helps to stick tape gently to the tongue blade, which serves as a guide as the tape is passed behind the client's head. Centre tape so that double-faced tape extends around the back of the neck from ear to ear.   ___ ___ ___ _____

  (a2) On one side of the client's face, secure tape from ear to naris (with nasal ET tube) or to the edge of the mouth (with oral ET tube). Tear remaining tape in half lengthwise, forming two pieces that are 1–2 cm wide. Secure the bottom half of the tape across the upper lip (with oral ET tube) or across the top of the nose (with nasal ET tube). Wrap the top half of tape around the tube.   ___ ___ ___ _____

  (a3) Gently pull the other side of tape firmly to pick up slack, and secure to the remaining side of the face. Have the assistant release hold when the tube is secure. You may want the assistant to help reinsert the oral airway.   ___ ___ ___ _____

 (b) Commercially available device:
  (b1) Place the ET tube through the opening designed to secure the ET tube. Ensure that the pilot balloon to the ET tube is accessible.   ___ ___ ___ _____

  (b2) Place the Velcro strips of the ET holder under the client at the occipital region of the head.   ___ ___ ___ _____

  (b3) Verify that the ET tube is at the established position, using the lip or gum line as a guide.   ___ ___ ___ _____

  (b4) Secure the Velcro strips at the base of the client's head. Leave 1 cm slack in the strips.   ___ ___ ___ _____

  (b5) Verify that the tube is secure and that it does not move forward from the client's mouth or backward down into the client's throat. Ensure that there are no pressure areas on the oral mucosa or occipital region of the head.   ___ ___ ___ _____

(15) Clean the oral airway in warm, soapy water, and rinse well. Hydrogen peroxide can aid in removal of crusted secretions. Shake excess water from the oral airway.   ___ ___ ___ _____

(16) For an unconscious client, reinsert the oral airway without pushing the tongue into the oropharynx.   ___ ___ ___ _____

B. Tracheostomy care:
 (1) Observe for signs and symptoms of the need to perform tracheostomy care:
  (a) Soiled or loose ties or dressing   ___ ___ ___ _____
  (b) Nonstable tube   ___ ___ ___ _____
  (c) Excessive secretions   ___ ___ ___ _____

 (2) Suction tracheostomy. Before removing gloves, remove soiled tracheostomy dressing and discard in a glove with the coiled catheter.

 (3) While client is replenishing oxygen stores, prepare equipment on bedside table:
  (a) Open sterile tracheostomy kit. Open three 4 × 4 gauze packages, using aseptic technique, and pour normal saline (NS) on one package and hydrogen peroxide on another. Leave the third package dry. Open two packages of cotton-tipped swabs and pour NS on one package and hydrogen peroxide on the other. Do not recap hydrogen peroxide and NS.   ___ ___ ___ _____

Continued

	S	U	NP	Comments
(b) Open the sterile tracheostomy package.	___	___	___	_____
(c) Unwrap the sterile basin and pour approximately 0.5–2 cm of hydrogen peroxide into it.	___	___	___	_____
(d) Open the small sterile brush package and place it aseptically into the sterile basin.	___	___	___	_____
(e) Prepare a length of twill tape long enough to go around the client's neck two times, approximately 60–75 cm for an adult. Cut ends on the diagonal. Lay aside in a dry area.	___	___	___	_____
(f) If using a commercially available tracheostomy tube holder, open the package according to the manufacturer's directions.	___	___	___	_____
(4) Put on gloves. Keep your dominant hand sterile throughout the procedure.	___	___	___	_____
(5) Remove the oxygen source from the kit. Apply the oxygen source loosely over the tracheostomy if the client desaturates during the procedure.	___	___	___	_____
(6) If a nondisposable inner cannula is used:	___	___	___	_____
(a) While touching only the outer aspect of the tube, remove the inner cannula with your nondominant hand. Drop the inner cannula into the hydrogen peroxide basin.	___	___	___	_____
(b) Place the tracheostomy collar or T tube and ventilator oxygen source over or near the outer cannula. (*Note:* T tube and ventilator oxygen devices cannot be attached to all outer cannulas when the inner cannula is removed.)	___	___	___	_____
(c) To prevent oxygen desaturation in affected clients, quickly pick up the inner cannula and use a small brush to remove secretions from inside and outside the cannula.	___	___	___	_____
(d) Hold the inner cannula over the basin and rinse with NS, using your nondominant hand to pour.	___	___	___	_____
(e) Replace the inner cannula and secure the "locking" mechanism. Reapply the ventilator or oxygen sources.	___	___	___	_____
(7) If a disposable inner cannula is used:				
(a) Remove the cannula from the manufacturer's packaging.	___	___	___	_____
(b) While touching only the outer aspect of the tube, withdraw the inner cannula and replace with the new cannula. Lock into position.	___	___	___	_____
(c) Dispose of the contaminated cannula in an appropriate receptacle, and apply oxygen source.	___	___	___	_____
(8) Using hydrogen peroxide–prepared cotton-tipped swabs and 4 × 4 gauze, clean the exposed outer cannula surfaces and stoma under the faceplate, extending 5–10 cm in all directions from the stoma. Clean in a circular motion from the stoma site outward, using your dominant hand to handle sterile supplies.	___	___	___	_____
(9) Using NS-prepared cotton-tipped swabs and 4 × 4 gauze, rinse the hydrogen peroxide from the tracheostomy tube and skin surfaces.	___	___	___	_____
(10) Using dry 4 × 4 gauze, pat lightly at skin and exposed outer cannula surfaces.	___	___	___	_____
(11) Secure tracheostomy.				
(a) *Tracheostomy tie method:*				
(a1) Instruct assistant, if available, to hold the tracheostomy tube securely in place while ties are cut.	___	___	___	_____
(a2) Take the prepared tie and insert one end of the tie through the faceplate eyelet, and pull ends even.	___	___	___	_____
(a3) Slide both ends of the tie behind the client's head and around the neck to the other eyelet, and insert one tie through the second eyelet.	___	___	___	_____
(a4) Pull snugly.	___	___	___	_____
(a5) Tie ends securely in a double square knot, allowing space for only one finger in the tie.	___	___	___	_____
(a6) Insert fresh tracheostomy dressing under the clean ties and faceplate.	___	___	___	_____

Continued

462

	S	U	NP	Comments
(b) *Tracheostomy tube holder method:*				
(b1) While wearing gloves, maintain a secure hold on the tracheostomy tube. This can be done with an assistant or, when an assistant is not available, by leaving the old tracheostomy tube holder in place until the new device is secure.	____	____	____	_____
(b2) Align strap under the client's neck. Ensure that Velcro attachments are positioned on either side of the tracheostomy tube.	____	____	____	_____
(b3) Place the narrow end of ties under and through the faceplate eyelets. Pull the ends even, and secure with Velcro closures.	____	____	____	_____
(b4) Verify that there is space for only one loose or two snug finger widths under the neck strap.	____	____	____	_____
7. Position the client comfortably, and assess respiratory status.	____	____	____	_____
8. Replace any oxygen delivery devices.	____	____	____	_____
9. Remove and discard gloves. Replace the caps on the hydrogen peroxide and normal saline. Perform hand hygiene.	____	____	____	_____
10. Compare respiratory assessments made before and after the procedure.	____	____	____	_____
11. Observe depth and position of tubes.	____	____	____	_____
12. Assess the security of the tape or commercial ET or ET tube holder by tugging at the tube.	____	____	____	_____
13. Assess the skin around the mouth and the oral mucosa (with ET tube) and the tracheostomy stoma for drainage, pressure, and signs of irritation.	____	____	____	_____

STUDENT: _____ DATE: _____

INSTRUCTOR: _____ DATE: _____

Skill 39–3 Care of Clients With Chest Tubes

	S	U	NP	Comments
1. Perform hand hygiene and assess client: for respiratory distress and chest pain, breath sounds over affected lung area, and vital signs.				
A. Pulmonary status: Assess for respiratory distress, chest pain, breath sounds over affected lung area, and stable vital signs. Signs and symptoms of increased respiratory distress or chest pain include decreased breath sounds over the affected and nonaffected lungs, marked cyanosis, asymmetrical chest movements, presence of subcutaneous emphysema around tube insertion site or neck, hypotension, and tachycardia.	___	___	___	_____
B. Measure vital signs and SpO_2.	___	___	___	_____
C. Pain: If possible, ask the client to rate the level of pain on a scale of 0 to 10.	___	___	___	_____
2. Observe the following:				
A. Chest tube dressing and site surrounding tube insertion	___	___	___	_____
B. Tubing, for kinks, dependent loops, or clots	___	___	___	_____
C. Chest drainage system, which should be upright and below level of tube insertion				
3. Provide two shodded hemostats or approved clamps for each chest tube, and attach them to the top of the client's bed with adhesive tape. Chest tubes are clamped only under specific circumstances per physician order or nursing policy and procedure:	___	___	___	_____
A. To assess air leak	___	___	___	_____
B. To quickly empty or change disposable systems; performed by a nurse who has received education in the procedure	___	___	___	_____
C. If the drainage tubing is accidentally disconnected from the drainage collection device or if the device is damaged	___	___	___	_____
D. To assess whether the client is ready to have the chest tube removed (which is done by physician's order); the client is monitored for recurrent pneumothorax	___	___	___	_____
4. Position client in one of the following ways:				
A. Semi-Fowler's position to evacuate air (pneumothorax)	___	___	___	_____
B. High-Fowler's position to drain fluid (hemothorax, effusion)	___	___	___	_____
5. Maintain the tube connection between the chest and drainage tubes; ensure that it is intact and taped.	___	___	___	_____
A. The water-sealed vent must be without occlusion.	___	___	___	_____
B. The suction-control chamber vent must be without occlusion when suction is used.	___	___	___	_____
6. Avoid excess tubing; the tubing should be laid horizontally across the client's bed or chair before dropping vertically into the drainage bottle. If the client is in a chair and the tubing is coiled, lift the tubing every 15 minutes to promote drainage.	___	___	___	_____
7. Adjust the tubing to hang in a straight line from the top of the mattress to the drainage chamber. If the chest tube is draining fluid, indicate time (e.g., 0900 hours) that drainage began on the drainage bottle's adhesive tape or on the write-on surface of the disposable commercial system. Strip or milk chest tube only if indicated.	___	___	___	_____
8. Perform hand hygiene.	___	___	___	_____
9. Evaluate:				
A. Vital signs and pulse oximetry as ordered or if client's condition changes.	___	___	___	_____
B. Chest tube dressing.	___	___	___	_____
C. Tubing: It should be free of kinks and dependent loops.	___	___	___	_____
D. Chest drainage system: It should be upright and below the level of tube insertion. Note the presence of clots or debris in tubing.	___	___	___	_____
E. Water seal for fluctuations with the client's inspiration and expiration.	___	___	___	_____
(1) Waterless system: diagnostic indicator for fluctuations with client's inspirations and expirations	___	___	___	_____
(2) Water-seal system: bubbling in the water-seal chamber	___	___	___	_____
(3) Water-seal system: bubbling in the suction-control chamber (when suction is used)	___	___	___	_____

Continued

	S	U	NP	Comments

F. Waterless system: Bubbling is diagnostic indicator.

G. Type and amount of fluid drainage: Note colour and amount of drainage, client's vital signs, and skin colour. The normal amount of drainage is as follows:

   (1) In the adult: <50–200 mL/hour immediately after surgery in a mediastinal chest tube; approximately 500 mL in the first 24 hours.

   (2) Between 100 and 300 mL of fluid may drain in a pleural chest tube in an adult during the first 3 hour after insertion. This rate will decrease after 2 hours; 500–1000 mL can be expected in the first 24 hours. Drainage is grossly bloody during the first several hours after surgery and then changes to serous. Remember that a sudden gush of drainage may be retained blood and not active bleeding. This increase in drainage can result from client's position changes.

H. Waterless system: The suction control (float ball) indicates the amount of suction that the client's intrapleural space is receiving.

I. Observe the client for decreased respiratory distress and chest pain; auscultate lung sounds over the affected area, and monitor SpO_2.

J. Pain: Ask the client to evaluate pain on a level of 0–10.

STUDENT: _____ DATE: _____

INSTRUCTOR: _____ DATE: _____

Skill 39–4 Applying a Nasal Cannula or Oxygen Mask

	S	U	NP	Comments
1. Inspect the client for signs and symptoms associated with hypoxia and the presence of airway secretions.	___	___	___	_____
2. Obtain the client's most recent SpO_2 or arterial blood gas (ABG) values.	___	___	___	_____
3. Explain to the client and family what the procedure entails and the purpose of oxygen therapy.	___	___	___	_____
4. Perform hand hygiene.	___	___	___	_____
5. Attach the nasal cannula to the oxygen tubing, and attach the tubing to the humidified oxygen source, adjusted to the prescribed flow rate.	___	___	___	_____
6. Place tips of the cannula into the client's nares. Adjust the elastic headband or plastic slide until the cannula fits snugly and comfortably.	___	___	___	_____
7. Maintain sufficient slack on the oxygen tubing, and secure tubing to the client's clothes.	___	___	___	_____
8. Check the cannula every 8 hours. Keep the humidification jar filled at all times.	___	___	___	_____
9. Observe the client's nares and the superior surface of both ears for skin breakdown.	___	___	___	_____
10. Perform hand hygiene.	___	___	___	_____
11. Check the oxygen flow rate and physician's orders every 8 hours.	___	___	___	_____
12. Inspect the client for relief of symptoms.	___	___	___	_____

STUDENT: _____ DATE: _____

INSTRUCTOR: _____ DATE: _____

Skill 39–5 Using Home Oxygen Equipment

	S	U	NP	Comments
1. While the client is in the hospital, determine the client's and family's ability to use oxygen equipment correctly. In the home setting, reassess for appropriate use of equipment.	___	___	___	_____
2. Assess the home environment for adequate electrical service if an oxygen concentrator is used.	___	___	___	_____
3. Assess client's and family's ability to observe for signs and symptoms of hypoxia.	___	___	___	_____
4. Determine appropriate resources in the community for equipment and assistance, including maintenance and repair services and the medical equipment supplier.	___	___	___	_____
5. In case of power failure, determine appropriate backup system when a compressor is used. Have a spare oxygen tank available.	___	___	___	_____
6. Perform hand hygiene.	___	___	___	_____
7. Place the oxygen delivery system in a clutter-free environment that is well ventilated; away from walls, drapes, bedding, and combustible materials; and at least 8 feet (2.5 m) from a heat source.	___	___	___	_____
8. Demonstrate steps for preparation and completion of oxygen therapy.				
A. Compressed oxygen system:				
(1) Turn the cylinder valve counterclockwise two to three turns with the wrench. Store the wrench with the oxygen tank	___	___	___	_____
(2) Check cylinders by reading the amount on the pressure gauge.	___	___	___	_____
B. Oxygen concentrator system:				
(1) Plug the concentrator into an appropriate outlet.	___	___	___	_____
(2) Turn on the power switch.	___	___	___	_____
(3) Alarm will sound for a few seconds.	___	___	___	_____
C. Liquid oxygen system:				
(1) Check liquid system by depressing the button at the lower right corner and reading the dial on the stationary oxygen reservoir or ambulatory tank.	___	___	___	_____
(2) Collaborate with the medical equipment provider to supply instruction on refilling the ambulatory tank.	___	___	___	_____
(3) Refilling the oxygen tank:				
(a) Wipe both filling connectors with a clean, dry, lint-free cloth.	___	___	___	_____
(b) Turn off the flow selector of the ambulatory unit.	___	___	___	_____
(c) Attach the ambulatory unit to the stationary reservoir by inserting the adapter of the ambulatory tank into the adapter of the stationary reservoir.	___	___	___	_____
(d) Open the fill valve on the ambulatory tank, and apply firm pressure to the top of the stationary reservoir. Stay with the unit while it is filling. You will hear a loud hissing noise. The tank fills in about 2 minutes.	___	___	___	_____
(e) Disengage the ambulatory unit from the stationary reservoir when the hissing noise changes and a vapor cloud begins to form from the stationary unit.	___	___	___	_____
(f) Wipe both filling connectors with a clean, dry, lint-free cloth.	___	___	___	_____
9. Connect the oxygen delivery device to the oxygen system.	___	___	___	_____
10. Adjust to the prescribed flow rate (litres per minute).	___	___	___	_____
11. Place the oxygen delivery device on the client.	___	___	___	_____
12. Perform hand hygiene.	___	___	___	_____
13. Instruct the client and family not to change the oxygen flow rate.	___	___	___	_____
14. Guide the client and family as they perform each step. Provide written material for reinforcement and review.	___	___	___	_____
15. Instruct the client or family to notify the physician if signs or symptoms of hypoxia or respiratory tract infection occur.	___	___	___	_____
16. Discuss emergency plans for power loss, natural disaster, and acute respiratory distress. Instruct the client or family to call 911 and notify the physician and home care agency.	___	___	___	_____
17. Instruct the client in safe home oxygen practices, including not allowing smoking in the home, keeping oxygen tanks away from open flames, and storing tanks upright.	___	___	___	_____
18. Monitor rate of oxygen delivery.	___	___	___	_____

STUDENT: _____   DATE: _____

INSTRUCTOR: _____   DATE: _____

Skill 40–1 Initiating a Peripheral Intravenous Infusion

	S	U	NP	Comments
1. Review the physician's order for the type and amount of intravenous (IV) fluid, rate of fluid administration, and purpose of infusion. Follow seven rights for administration of medications.	___	___	___	_____
2. Observe the client for signs and symptoms indicating fluid or electrolyte imbalances that may be affected by IV fluid administration:				
A. Peripheral edema	___	___	___	_____
B. Greater than 20% change in body weight	___	___	___	_____
C. Dry skin and mucous membranes	___	___	___	_____
D. Distended neck veins	___	___	___	_____
E. Blood pressure changes	___	___	___	_____
F. Irregular pulse rhythm; tachycardia	___	___	___	_____
G. Auscultation of abnormal lung sounds	___	___	___	_____
H. Decreased skin turgor	___	___	___	_____
I. Thirst	___	___	___	_____
J. Anorexia, nausea, and vomiting	___	___	___	_____
K. Decreased urine output	___	___	___	_____
L. Behavioural changes	___	___	___	_____
3. Assess the client's prior or perceived experience with IV therapy and arm placement preference.	___	___	___	_____
4. Determine whether the client is to undergo any planned surgeries or is to receive blood infusion later.	___	___	___	_____
5. Assess laboratory data and client's history of allergies.	___	___	___	_____
6. Assess for the following risk factors: child or older adult, presence of heart failure or renal failure, or low platelet count.	___	___	___	_____
7. Prepare the client and family by explaining the procedure, its purpose, and what is expected of the client.	___	___	___	_____
8. Perform hand hygiene.	___	___	___	_____
9. Assist the client to a comfortable sitting or supine position.	___	___	___	_____
10. Organize equipment on a clean, clutter-free bedside stand or overbed table.	___	___	___	_____
11. Change the client's gown to a more easily removable gown with snaps at the shoulder, if available.	___	___	___	_____
12. Open sterile packages, using sterile aseptic technique.	___	___	___	_____
13. Check IV solution, using the rights of drug administration. Make sure prescribed additives (e.g., potassium, vitamins) have been added. Check solution for colour, clarity, and expiration date. Check bag for leaks, which is best if done before reaching the bedside.	___	___	___	_____
14. Open the infusion set, maintaining sterility of both ends of tubing. Many sets allow for priming of tubing without removal of end cap.	___	___	___	_____
15. Place a roller clamp about 2–5 cm below the drip chamber and move the roller clamp to closed position.	___	___	___	_____
16. Remove the protective sheath over the IV tubing port on the plastic IV solution bag. For bottled IV solution, remove the metal cap and the metal and rubber discs beneath the cap. Use caution to avoid touching the exposed opening.	___	___	___	_____
17. Insert the infusion set into the fluid bag or bottle by removing the protector cap from the tubing insertion spike (keeping the spike sterile), and inserting the spike into the opening of the IV bag. Cleanse the rubber stopper on the glass-bottled solution with antiseptic, and insert the spike into the black rubber stopper of the IV bottle. Hang the solution container on the IV pole at a minimum height of 90 cm above the planned insertion site.	___	___	___	_____
18. Compress the drip chamber and release, allowing it to fill one third to one half full. Open the clamp and prime the infusion tubing by filling with IV solution, carefully inverting valves and ports in sequence as the solution moves through the tubing.	___	___	___	_____
19. Remove the tubing protector cap (some tubing can be primed without removal) and slowly release the roller clamp to allow fluid to travel from the drip chamber through the tubing to the needle adapter. Return the roller clamp to the closed position after the tubing is primed (filled with IV fluid).	___	___	___	_____

Continued

470

	S	U	NP	Comments

20. Be certain that the tubing is clear of air and air bubbles. To remove small air bubbles, firmly tap the IV tubing where air bubbles are located. Check the entire length of tubing to ensure that all air bubbles are removed.

21. Replace the tubing cap protector on the end of the tubing.

22. *Optional:* Prepare normal saline lock for infusion. Use a sterile technique to connect the IV plug to the loop or short extension tubing. Inject 1–3 mL of normal saline through the plug and through the loop or short extension tubing.

23. Put on disposable gloves. Eye protection and a mask may be worn if splash or spray of blood is possible. *Note:* Gloves can be left off to locate a vein but must be put on before the site is prepared.

24. Identify an accessible vein for IV placement. Place a tourniquet 10–15 cm above the proposed insertion site. Position the tourniquet so that the ends are away from the site. Check for the presence of the radial pulse. *Option:* Apply a blood pressure (BP) cuff instead of a tourniquet. Inflate the cuff to a level just below the client's normal diastolic pressure. Maintain inflation at that pressure until the venipuncture is completed.

25. Select the vein. Common intravenous sites for the adult include cephalic, basilic, and median cubital veins:
    A. Use the most distal site in the client's nondominant arm, if possible.
    B. Avoid areas that are painful to palpation.
    C. Select a vein large enough for catheter placement.
    D. Choose a site that will not interfere with the client's activities of daily or planned procedures.
    E. Use the fingertips to palpate the vein by pressing downward and noting the resilient, soft, bouncy feeling as the pressure is released.
    F. Promote venous distension by instructing the client to open and close the fist several times, lowering the client's arm in a dependent position, applying warmth to the arm for several minutes, and rubbing or stroking the client's arm from distal to proximal below the proposed site.
    G. Avoid sites distal to the previous venipuncture site, sclerosed or hardened cordlike veins, infiltrated site or phlebitic vessels, bruised areas, and areas of venous valves or bifurcation. Avoid veins in the antecubital fossa and ventral surface of the wrist.
    H. Avoid fragile dorsal veins in older adults and vessels in an extremity with compromised circulation (e.g., in cases of mastectomy, dialysis graft, or paralysis).

26. Release tourniquet temporarily. Clip arm hair with scissors (if necessary). Do not shave the area.

27. (If area of insertion appears to need cleansing, use soap and water first.) Cleanse the insertion site, using a firm, circular motion (centre to outward) in concentric circles 5 to 7.5 cm from the insertion site. Use antiseptic preparation as a single agent or in combination, according to agency policy. Two percent chlorhexidine gluconate is the antiseptic cleansing agent of choice. Povidone-iodine is a topical anti-infective agent that reduces skin surface bacteria; 70% alcohol is another antiseptic cleansing agent. Povidone-iodine must dry to be effective in reducing microbial counts. Avoid touching the cleansed site. Allow the site to dry for at least 2 minutes. If the skin is touched after cleansing, repeat cleansing procedure.

28. Reapply tourniquet or BP cuff.

29. Perform venipuncture. Anchor the vein by placing your thumb over the vein beneath the insertion site and by stretching the skin against the direction of insertion 5–7.5 cm distal to the site. Warn the client of a sharp stick. Puncture skin and vein, holding the catheter at a 10- to 30-degree angle with bevel pointed upward.
    A. *Butterfly needle:* Hold the needle at a 10- to 30-degree angle with bevel up, slightly distal to the actual site of venipuncture.
    B. *Needleless over-the-needle catheter (ONC) safety device:* Insert ONC with bevel up, at a 10- to 30-degree angle, slightly distal to the actual site of venipuncture in the direction of the vein.

Continued

	S	U	NP	Comments

30. Look for blood return through the tubing of the butterfly needle or flashback chamber of the ONC, indicating that the needle has entered the vein. Lower the catheter or needle until almost flush with the skin. Advance the butterfly needle until the hub rests at the venipuncture site. Advance the ONC 0.5 cm into the vein and then loosen the stylet. Advance the catheter off the stylet into the vein until the hub rests at the venipuncture site. Do not reinsert the stylet once it is loosened. (Advance the safety device by using the push-tab to thread the catheter.)

31. Stabilize the catheter. Apply gentle but firm pressure with the index finger of your nondominant hand 3 cm above the insertion site. Release the tourniquet or BP cuff you're your dominant hand, and retract the stylet from ONC. Do not recap the stylet. For a safety device, slide the catheter off the stylet while gliding the protective guard over the stylet. A click indicates that the device is locked over the stylet.

32. Quickly connect the adapter of the primed fluid administration set or saline lock to the hub of the ONC or butterfly tubing. Be sure the connection is secure. Do not touch the point of entry of the adapter.

33. Release the roller clamp slowly to begin infusion at a rate to maintain patency of the IV line.
    A. *Intermittent infusion:* Continue to stabilize the catheter with your nondominant hand, and attach the injection cap of the adapter. Insert prefilled flush solution into the injection cap. Flush slowly. Maintain thumb pressure on the syringe during withdrawal, or close the clamp on the extension tubing of the injection cap while still flushing the last 0.2–0.4 mL of flush solution.

34. Tape or secure the catheter:
    A. *If applying transparent dressing:* Secure the catheter with your nondominant hand while preparing to apply dressing.
    B. *If applying a gauze dressing:*
       (1) Tape the IV catheter. Place a narrow piece (1-cm wide) of sterile tape under the hub of the catheter with adhesive side up, and criss-cross tape over the hub to form a chevron.
       (2) Place tape only on the catheter, never over the insertion site. Secure the site to allow easy visual inspection and early recognition of infiltration and phlebitis. Avoid applying tape around the extremity.
    C. Observe the site for swelling.

35. Apply sterile dressing over the site.
    A. Transparent dressing:
       (1) Carefully remove adherent backing. Apply one edge of dressing and then gently smooth remaining dressing over the site, leaving the end of the catheter hub uncovered. Refer to the manufacturer's directions.
       (2) Take a 2.5-cm piece of tape and place it from the end of the catheter hub to the insertion site, over transparent dressing.
       (3) Apply chevron and place only over the tape, not the transparent dressing.
    B. Sterile gauze dressing:
       (1) Fold $2 \times 3 \times 2$ gauze in half and cover with a 2.5-cm-wide piece of sterile tape extending about 2.5 cm from each side. Place under tubing–catheter hub junction. Place a 2×2 gauze pad over venipuncture site and catheter hub. Secure edges with tape.
       (2) Curl a loop of tubing alongside the arm and place a second piece of tape directly over the 2×2 gauze, securing tubing in two places.

36. Prepare the equipment according to expected frequency of use:
    A. *For IV fluid administration:* Adjust the flow rate to correct drops per minute or connect to electronic infusion device (EID).
    B. *For intermittent use:* Saline lock. Flush with 3 mL of sterile normal saline at prescribed frequency or per agency policy.

Continued

	S	U	NP	Comments
37. Label dressing with date, time, gauge size and length of catheter, placement of IV line and dressing, and your initials.	___	___	___	_____
38. Dispose of used needles in an appropriate sharps container. Discard supplies. Remove gloves and perform hand hygiene.	___	___	___	_____
39. Observe the client every hour to determine whether fluid is infusing correctly:	___	___	___	_____
A. Check whether the correct amount of solution is infused as prescribed by looking at the time tape.	___	___	___	_____
B. Count the flow or check the rate on the infusion pump.	___	___	___	_____
C. Check the patency of the IV catheter or needle.	___	___	___	_____
D. Observe the client for signs of discomfort.	___	___	___	_____
E. Inspect the insertion site for absence of phlebitis, infiltration, or inflammation.	___	___	___	_____
40. Observe the client every hour to determine response to therapy (i.e., measure vital signs, conduct postprocedure assessments).	___	___	___	_____

STUDENT: _____ DATE: _____

INSTRUCTOR: _____ DATE: _____

Skill 40–2 Regulating Intravenous Flow Rates

	S	U	NP	Comments
1. Check the client's medical record for the correct solution, additives, and time of infusion. The usual order includes solution for 24 hours, usually divided into 2 or 3 L. On occasion, an intravenous (IV) order contains only 1 L to keep the vein open (KVO). An order also indicates the time over which each litre is to infuse.	___	___	___	_____
2. Perform hand hygiene. Observe for patency of the IV line and the needle or catheter.	___	___	___	_____
A. Open the drip regulator and observe for rapid flow of fluid from the solution into the drip chamber, and then close the drip regulator to the prescribed rate.	___	___	___	_____
3. Check the client's knowledge of how positioning of the IV site affects flow rate.	___	___	___	_____
4. Verify with the client how the venipuncture site feels (e.g., determine whether the client is experiencing pain or a burning sensation).	___	___	___	_____
5. Have paper and pencil or a calculator to calculate the flow rate.	___	___	___	_____
6. Check calibration (drop factor) in drops per millilitre (gtt/mL) of the infusion set: A. *Microdrip:* 60 gtt/mL B. *Macrodrip:* 15 gtt/mL or 10 gtt/mL, depending on manufacturer (will be stated on package)	___	___	___	_____
7. Calculate flow rate (hourly volume) of the prescribed infusion. Flow rate (mL/hr) = total infusion (volume in millilitres) per hours of infusion (time to be infused).	___	___	___	_____
8. Read the physician's orders and follow seven rights for the correct solution and proper additives.	___	___	___	_____
9. Determine how long each litre of fluid should run. IV fluids are usually ordered by rate, such as 100 mL/hr. On occasion, however, IV fluids are ordered over a period of time, such as 1000 mL D$_5$W with 20 mmol KCl over 8 hr	___	___	___	_____
10. Place adhesive or fluid indicator tape on the IV bottle or bag next to volume markings.	___	___	___	_____
11. Select one of the following formulas to calculate minute rate (drops/min) on the basis of the drop factor of the infusion set: A. mL/hr/60 min = mL/min, and drop factor · mL/min = drops/min B. Alternative: mL/hr · drop factor/60 min = drops/min. Using this formula, calculate minute flow rate for bottle 1:1000 mL with 20 mmol KCl: *Microdrip:* 125 mL/hr · 60 gtt/mL = 7500 gtt/hr 7500 gtt ÷ 60 minutes = 125 gtt/min *Macrodrip:* 125 mL/hr · 15 gtt/mL = 1875 gtt/hr 1875 gtt ÷ 60 minutes = 31 gtt/min	___	___	___	_____
12. Establish flow rate by counting drops in the drip chamber for 1 minute by watch; then adjust the roller clamp to increase or decrease the rate of infusion.	___	___	___	_____
13. Follow this procedure for the infusion controller or pump: A. Place the electronic eye on the drip chamber below the origin of the drop and above the fluid level in the chamber, or consult manufacturer's directions for setup of the infusion. If a controller is used, ensure that the IV bag is 1 m above the IV site. B. Place the IV infusion tubing within the ridges of the control box in the direction of flow (i.e., the portion of tubing nearest the IV bag at the top and the portion of tubing nearest the client at the bottom), or consult manufacturer's directions for use of the pump. Some devices require securing tubing through "air in line" alarm system. Close the control chamber door. Turn on the pump. Select required drops per minute or volume per hour and volume to be infused. Open the rate control clamp, and press the start button.	___	___	___	_____

Continued

474

	S	U	NP	Comments
C. Monitor infusion rates and IV site for complications according to agency policy.	___	___	___	_____
D. Assess patency and integrity of the system when the alarm sounds.	___	___	___	_____
14. Follow this procedure for a volume control device:				
A. Place the volume control device between the IV bag and insertion spike of the infusion set, using sterile technique.	___	___	___	_____
B. Place a 2-hour allotment of fluid into the chamber device.	___	___	___	_____
C. Assess the system at least hourly; add fluid to the volume control device as needed. Regulate flow rate.	___	___	___	_____
15. Observe the client for response to therapy and for signs of overhydration or dehydration.	___	___	___	_____
16. Evaluate infusion site for signs of infiltration, inflammation, clot in catheter, or kink or knot in infusion tubing.	___	___	___	_____

STUDENT: _____ DATE: _____

INSTRUCTOR: _____ DATE: _____

Skill 40–3 Maintenance of Intravenous System

	S	U	NP	Comments

CHANGING INTRAVENOUS SOLUTION

	S	U	NP	Comments
1. Check physician's orders.	___	___	___	_____
2. If the order is written for keep vein open (KVO) or to keep open (TKO), contact the physician for clarification of the rate of the infusion. Note date and time when solution was last changed.	___	___	___	_____
3. Determine the compatibility of all intravenous (IV) fluids and additives by consulting appropriate literature or the pharmacy.	___	___	___	_____
4. Determine the client's understanding of the need for continued IV therapy.	___	___	___	_____
5. Assess patency of the current IV access site.	___	___	___	_____
6. Have the next solution prepared at least 1 hour before needed. Check that the solution is correct and properly labelled. Check the solution expiration date and for the presence of precipitate and discoloration.	___	___	___	_____
7. Prepare to change solution when less than 50 mL of fluid remains in the bottle or bag or when a new type of solution is ordered.	___	___	___	_____
8. Prepare the client and family by explaining the procedure, its purpose, and what is expected of the client.	___	___	___	_____
9. Ensure that the drip chamber is at least half full.	___	___	___	_____
10. Perform hand hygiene.	___	___	___	_____
11. Prepare the new solution for changing. If using a plastic bag, remove the protective cover from the IV tubing port. If using a glass bottle, remove the metal cap and the metal and rubber discs.	___	___	___	_____
12. Move the roller clamp to stop the flow rate.	___	___	___	_____
13. Remove the old IV fluid container from the IV pole.	___	___	___	_____
14. Quickly remove the spike from the old solution bag or bottle and, without touching the tip, insert the spike into the new bag or bottle.	___	___	___	_____
15. Hang the new bag or bottle of solution on the IV pole.	___	___	___	_____
16. Check for air in the tubing. If bubbles form, the can be removed by closing the roller clamp, stretching the tubing downward, and tapping the tubing with your finger (the bubbles rise in the fluid to the drip chamber). For larger amounts of air, swab the injection port below the air with alcohol and allow to dry. Connect a syringe to this port and aspirate the air into the syringe. Reduce air in tubing by priming slowly instead of allowing a wide-open flow.	___	___	___	_____
17. Ensure drip chamber is one-third to half full. If the drip chamber is too full, pinch off tubing below the drip chamber, invert the container, squeeze the drip chamber, hang up the bottle, and release the tubing.	___	___	___	_____
18. Regulate flow to the prescribed rate.	___	___	___	_____
19. Mark the date and time on label, and tape it on bag. Do not use felt-tipped pens or permanent markers on intravenous bags.	___	___	___	_____
20. Observe the client for signs of overhydration or dehydration to determine response to IV fluid therapy.	___	___	___	_____
21. Observe IV system for patency and development of complications (e.g., infiltration or phlebitis).	___	___	___	_____

CHANGING INTRAVENOUS TUBING

	S	U	NP	Comments
22. Determine when a new infusion set is needed:				
A. Agency policy will indicate the frequency of routine change for IV administration sets and saline flush tubing.	___	___	___	_____
B. Puncture of infusion tubing necessitates immediate change.	___	___	___	_____
C. Contamination of tubing necessitates immediate change.	___	___	___	_____
D. Occlusions in existing tubing can occur after infusion of packed red blood cells, whole blood, albumin, or other blood components.	___	___	___	_____
23. Prepare the client and family by explaining the procedure, its purpose, and what is expected of the client.	___	___	___	_____
24. Perform hand hygiene.	___	___	___	_____

Continued

	S	U	NP	Comments

25. Open the new infusion set, keeping protective coverings over the infusion spike and distal adapter. Secure all junctions with Luer-Loks, clasping devices, or threaded devices.   _____ _____ _____ _____
26. Apply nonsterile, disposable gloves.   _____ _____ _____ _____
27. If the needle or catheter hub is not visible, remove IV dressing while maintaining the stability of the catheter. If transparent dressing must be removed, place a small piece of sterile tape across the hub temporarily to anchor the catheter during disconnection. Do not remove tape securing the needle or catheter to the skin with gauze dressing.   _____ _____ _____ _____
28. For IV continuous infusion:
   A. Move the roller clamp on new IV tubing to the closed position.   _____ _____ _____ _____
   B. Slow the rate of infusion by regulating the drip rate on the old tubing. Maintain KVO rate.   _____ _____ _____ _____
   C. Compress and fill the drip chamber.   _____ _____ _____ _____
   D. Remove the IV container from the pole, invert the container, and remove old tubing from the container. Carefully hold the container while hanging or taping the drip chamber on the IV pole 1 m above the IV site.   _____ _____ _____ _____
   E. Place the insertion spike of the new tubing into the old solution bag opening, and hang the solution bag on the IV pole.   _____ _____ _____ _____
   F. Compress and release the drip chamber on the new tubing. Slowly fill the drip chamber one-third to half full.   _____ _____ _____ _____
   G. Slowly open the roller clamp, remove the protective cap from the needle adapter (if necessary), and flush the new tubing with solution. Replace the cap.   _____ _____ _____ _____
   H. Turn the roller clamp on the old tubing to the closed position.   _____ _____ _____ _____
29. For saline lock:
   A. If a loop or short extension tubing is needed because of an awkward IV site placement, use sterile technique to connect the new injection cap to the loop or tubing.   _____ _____ _____ _____
   B. Swab the injection cap with alcohol, povidone-iodine, or chlorhexidine. Insert the syringe with 1–3 mL saline and inject through the injection cap into the loop or short extension tubing.   _____ _____ _____ _____
30. Stabilize the hub of the catheter and apply pressure over the vein just above the catheter tip, at least 3 cm above the insertion site. Gently disconnect old tubing from the catheter hub. Maintain stability of the hub and quickly insert the adapter of new tubing or saline or heparin lock into the hub.   _____ _____ _____ _____
31. Open the roller clamp on new tubing. Allow solution to run rapidly for 30–60 seconds.   _____ _____ _____ _____
32. Regulate the IV drip according to physician's orders and monitor the rate hourly.   _____ _____ _____ _____
33. Apply new dressing, if necessary.   _____ _____ _____ _____
34. Discard old tubing in a proper container.   _____ _____ _____ _____
35. Remove and dispose of gloves. Perform hand hygiene.   _____ _____ _____ _____
36. Evaluate the flow rate and observe the connection site for leakage.   _____ _____ _____ _____

DISCONTINUING PERIPHERAL INTRAVENOUS ACCESS

37. Check physician's order for discontinuing IV therapy.   _____ _____ _____ _____
38. Explain the procedure to the client. Explain that the affected extremity must be held still and how long the procedure will take.   _____ _____ _____ _____
39. Perform hand hygiene, and put on disposable gloves.   _____ _____ _____ _____
40. Turn the IV tubing roller clamp to the closed position. Remove the tape securing the tubing.   _____ _____ _____ _____
41. Remove the IV site dressing and tape while stabilizing the catheter.   _____ _____ _____ _____
42. With dry gauze or an alcohol swab held over the site, apply light pressure and withdraw the catheter, using a slow, steady movement, keeping the hub parallel to the skin.   _____ _____ _____ _____
43. Apply pressure to the site for 2–3 minutes, using the dry, sterile gauze pad. Secure with tape.   _____ _____ _____ _____
44. Inspect the catheter for intactness, noting tip integrity and length.   _____ _____ _____ _____
45. Discard used supplies.   _____ _____ _____ _____
46. Remove and discard gloves, and perform hand hygiene.   _____ _____ _____ _____
47. Instruct the client to report any redness, pain, drainage, or swelling that may occur after catheter removal.   _____ _____ _____ _____

STUDENT: _____ DATE: _____

INSTRUCTOR: _____ DATE: _____

Skill 40–4 Changing a Peripheral Intravenous Dressing

	S	U	NP	Comments
1. Determine when dressing was last changed. Many institutions require that the nurse record the date and time on the dressing when the device is first placed.	___	___	___	_____
2. Perform hand hygiene. Observe the present dressing for moisture and intactness.	___	___	___	_____
3. Observe the intravenous (IV) system for proper functioning. Palpate the catheter site through the intact dressing for inflammation or subjective complaints of pain or burning sensation.	___	___	___	_____
4. Inspect the exposed catheter site for swelling or blanching.	___	___	___	_____
5. Assess the client's understanding of the need for continued IV infusion.	___	___	___	_____
6. Explain procedure and purpose to the client and family. Explain that the affected extremity must be held still and how long the procedure will take.	___	___	___	_____
7. Put on disposable gloves.	___	___	___	_____
8. Remove tape, gauze, or transparent dressing from the old dressing, one layer at a time, leaving tape (if present) that secures the IV needle in place. Be cautious to prevent the catheter tubing from becoming tangled between two layers of dressing. When removing transparent dressing, hold the catheter hub and tubing with your nondominant hand.	___	___	___	_____
9. Observe the insertion site for signs and symptoms of infection (redness, swelling, and exudate). If they are present, remove the catheter and insert a new IV line in another site.	___	___	___	_____
10. If infiltration, phlebitis, or clot occurs, or if otherwise ordered by physician, stop infusion and discontinue IV therapy. Restart new IV line if continued therapy is necessary. Place a moist, warm compress over an area of phlebitis.	___	___	___	_____
11. If IV fluid is infusing properly, gently remove tape securing the catheter. Stabilize the needle or catheter with one hand. Use adhesive remover to cleanse skin and remove adhesive residue, if needed.	___	___	___	_____
12. Stabilize the catheter at all times with one finger over the catheter until tape or dressing is replaced.	___	___	___	_____
13. Use circular motion, cleanse the peripheral IV insertion site with an antiseptic swab, starting at the insertion site and working outward, creating concentric circles. Allow swab solution to air-dry completely.	___	___	___	_____
14. Apply new transparent or gauze dressing.	___	___	___	_____
15. Remove and discard gloves.	___	___	___	_____
16. Anchor IV tubing with additional pieces of tape. When using transparent polyurethane dressing, minimize the tape placed over dressing.	___	___	___	_____
17. Write insertion date, date and time of dressing change, size and gauge of catheter, and your initials directly on dressing. Apply arm board, commercial housing device, or both if the site is affected by joint motion.	___	___	___	_____
18. Discard used equipment, and perform hand hygiene.	___	___	___	_____
19. Observe functioning and patency of the IV system in response to changing dressing.	___	___	___	_____
20. Monitor the client's body temperature.	___	___	___	_____

STUDENT: _____   DATE: _____

INSTRUCTOR: _____   DATE: _____

Skill 43–1 Aspiration Precautions

	S	U	NP	Comments
1. Perform nutritional screening.	___	___	___	_____
2. Assess clients who are at increased risk of aspiration for signs and symptoms of dysphagia (e.g., cough, pharyngeal pooling, change in voice after swallowing).	___	___	___	_____
3. Observe the client during mealtime for signs of dysphagia, and allow the client to attempt to feed himself or herself. Observe the client eat foods of various consistencies and drink liquids. Note at the end of the meal whether the client becomes tired.	___	___	___	_____
4. Ask the client about any difficulties with chewing or swallowing various foods with different textures.	___	___	___	_____
5. Report signs and symptoms of dysphagia to the health care professional.	___	___	___	_____
6. Place identification on the client's chart or Kardex indicating that dysphagia is present.	___	___	___	_____
7. Explain to the client why you are observing him or her while the client eats.	___	___	___	_____
8. Perform hand hygiene.	___	___	___	_____
9. Using a penlight and tongue blade, gently inspect the client's mouth for pockets of food.	___	___	___	_____
10. Elevate the head of the client's bed so that the hips are flexed at a 90-degree angle and the head is flexed slightly forward, or help the client to the same position in a chair.	___	___	___	_____
11. Observe the client consume foods and liquids of various consistencies.	___	___	___	_____
12. Add thickener to thin liquids, to create the consistency of mashed potatoes, or serve the client pureed foods.	___	___	___	_____
13. Place ½ to 1 teaspoon of food on the unaffected side of the mouth, allowing the utensil to touch the mouth or tongue.	___	___	___	_____
14. Place your hand on the client's throat to gently palpate the swallowing event as it occurs.	___	___	___	_____
15. Provide verbal coaching and positive reinforcement while feeding the client:				
A. "Feel the food in your mouth."	___	___	___	_____
B. "Chew and taste the food."	___	___	___	_____
C. "Raise your tongue to the roof of your mouth."	___	___	___	_____
D. "Think about swallowing."	___	___	___	_____
E. "Close your mouth and swallow."	___	___	___	_____
F. "Swallow again."	___	___	___	_____
G. "Cough to clear the airway."	___	___	___	_____
16. Observe for coughing, choking, gagging, and drooling of food; suction the airway as necessary.	___	___	___	_____
17. Provide rest periods as necessary during the meal, to avoid rushed or forced feeding.	___	___	___	_____
18. Ask the client to remain sitting upright for at least 30 minutes after the meal.	___	___	___	_____
19. Help the client perform hand hygiene and mouth care.	___	___	___	_____
20. Return the client's tray to the appropriate place, and perform hand hygiene.	___	___	___	_____
21. Observe the client's ability to ingest foods of various textures and thicknesses.	___	___	___	_____
22. Weigh the client weekly at the same time on the same scale.	___	___	___	_____
23. Observe the client's oral cavity after a meal to detect pockets of food.	___	___	___	_____

STUDENT: _____ DATE: _____

INSTRUCTOR: _____ DATE: _____

Skill 44–1 Collecting a Midstream (Clean-Voided) Urine Specimen

	S	U	NP	Comments
1. Assess the client's voiding status:				
A. When client last voided	___	___	___	_____
B. Level of awareness or developmental stage	___	___	___	_____
C. Mobility, balance, and physical limitations	___	___	___	_____
2. Assess the client's understanding of the purpose of the test and method of collection.	___	___	___	_____
3. Explain the procedure to the client:				
A. Reason why midstream specimen is needed	___	___	___	_____
B. Ways in which the client and family can assist	___	___	___	_____
C. Ways to obtain a specimen free of feces	___	___	___	_____
4. Provide fluids to drink a half-hour before collecting the specimen, unless contraindicated (i.e., fluid restriction), if the client does not feel the urge to void.	___	___	___	_____
5. Provide privacy for the client by closing the door or bed curtain.	___	___	___	_____
6. Give the client or family members soap, a washcloth, and a towel to cleanse the perineal area.	___	___	___	_____
7. Perform hand hygiene and put on nonsterile gloves, and assist nonambulatory clients with perineal care. Assist female client onto bedpan.	___	___	___	_____
8. Change gloves if necessary.	___	___	___	_____
9. Using surgical aseptic technique, open the sterile kit or prepare sterile supplies. Put on sterile gloves after opening the sterile specimen cup, placing the cap with sterile inside surface up; do not touch the inside of the container or cap.	___	___	___	_____
10. Pour antiseptic solution over cotton balls or gauze pads unless kit contains prepared gauze pads in antiseptic solution.	___	___	___	_____
11. Assist or allow the client to cleanse the perineal area and collect the specimen.	___	___	___	_____
A. Female client:				
(1) Spread the client's labia with the thumb and forefinger of your nondominant hand.	___	___	___	_____
(2) Cleanse the area with a cotton ball or gauze, moving from front (above urethral orifice) to back (toward anus).	___	___	___	_____
(3) If agency policy indicates, rinse area with sterile water, and dry with a cotton ball or gauze.	___	___	___	_____
(4) While you continue holding the client's labia apart, the client should initiate urine stream; after stream begins, pass container into stream and collect 30–60 mL of urine.				
B. Male client:				
(1) Hold the client's penis with one hand; using circular motion and antiseptic swab, cleanse the end of the penis, moving from centre to outside. In uncircumcised men, the foreskin should be retracted before cleansing.	___	___	___	_____
(2) If agency policy indicates, rinse the area with sterile water, and dry with a cotton ball or gauze.	___	___	___	_____
(3) After client has initiated urine stream, pass specimen collection container into stream and collect 30–60 mL of urine.	___	___	___	_____
12. Remove specimen container before urine flow stops and before you release labia or penis. The client finishes voiding in the bedpan or toilet. If the foreskin was retracted for specimen collection, it must be replaced over the glans.	___	___	___	_____
13. Replace cap securely on the specimen container (touch only the outside).	___	___	___	_____
14. Cleanse any urine from the exterior surface of the container. Place the container in a plastic specimen bag.	___	___	___	_____
15. Remove the bedpan (if applicable), assist the client to a comfortable position, and provide a handwashing basin, if needed.	___	___	___	_____
16. Label the specimen and attach a laboratory requisition slip.	___	___	___	_____
17. Remove gloves, dispose of them in a proper receptacle, and perform hand hygiene.	___	___	___	_____
18. Transport the specimen to the laboratory within 15 minutes, or refrigerate it immediately.	___	___	___	_____

STUDENT: _____ DATE: _____

INSTRUCTOR: _____ DATE: _____

Skill 44–2 Inserting a Straight or In-Dwelling Catheter

	S	U	NP	Comments
1. Review the client's medical record, including physician's order and nurses' notes.	___	___	___	_____
2. Close bedside curtain or door.	___	___	___	_____
3. Assess the status of the client:				_____
A. Urinary status: Ask the client when he or she last voided, or check intake and output flow sheet, or palpate bladder	___	___	___	_____
B. Level of awareness or developmental stage	___	___	___	_____
C. Mobility and physical limitations of the client	___	___	___	_____
D. The client's gender and age	___	___	___	_____
E. Bladder distension	___	___	___	_____
F. Perineum, for erythema, drainage, and odour: Perform hand hygiene, put on clean gloves, and inspect perineum	___	___	___	_____
G. Any pathological condition that may impair passage of catheter (e.g., enlarged prostate in men)	___	___	___	_____
H. Allergies	___	___	___	_____
4. Assess the client's knowledge of the purpose of catheterization.	___	___	___	_____
5. Explain the procedure to the client.	___	___	___	_____
6. Arrange for extra nursing assistance if necessary.	___	___	___	_____
7. Perform hand hygiene.	___	___	___	_____
8. Raise the bed to an appropriate working height.	___	___	___	_____
9. Facing the client, stand on the left side of the bed if you are right-handed (on the right side if you are left-handed). Clear the bedside table, and arrange equipment.	___	___	___	_____
10. Raise the side rail on the opposite side of the bed, and put the side rail down on the working side.	___	___	___	_____
11. Place a waterproof pad under the client.	___	___	___	_____
12. Position the client.				
A. Female client:				
(1) Assist the client to the dorsal recumbent position. Ask the client to relax her thighs so that the hips can be rotated externally.	___	___	___	_____
(2) Assist the client to a side-lying (Sims') position with the upper leg flexed at the hip if the client is unable to assume the dorsal recumbent position. If this position is used, you must take extra precautions to cover the rectal area with a drape to reduce chance of cross-contamination.	___	___	___	_____
B. Male client:				
(1) Assist the client to a supine position with thighs slightly abducted.	___	___	___	_____
13. Drape client.				
A. Female client:				
(1) Drape with a bath blanket. Place the blanket in a diamond shape over the client, with one corner at the client's midsection, side corners over each thigh and the abdomen, and the last corner over the perineum.	___	___	___	_____
B. Male client:				
(1) Drape the client's upper trunk with a bath blanket and cover the lower extremities with bedsheets so that only genitalia are exposed.	___	___	___	_____
14. Wearing disposable gloves, wash the perineal area with soap and water as needed; dry thoroughly. Remove and discard gloves; perform hand hygiene.	___	___	___	_____
15. Position a lamp to illuminate the perineal area. (If you use a flashlight, have an assistant hold it.)	___	___	___	_____
16. Open the package containing the drainage system. Place the drainage bag over the edge of the bottom bed frame, and bring the drainage tube up between side rail and mattress.	___	___	___	_____
17. Open the catheterization kit according to directions, keeping the bottom of the container sterile.	___	___	___	_____

Continued

	S	U	NP	Comments

18. Place the plastic bag that contained the kit within reach of the work area to use as a waterproof bag in which used supplies can be disposed.

19. Put on sterile gloves.

20. Organize supplies on a sterile field. Open the inner sterile package containing the catheter. Pour sterile antiseptic solution into the correct compartment containing sterile cotton balls. Open the packet containing lubricant. Remove the specimen container (the lid should be placed loosely on top) and the prefilled syringe from the collection compartment of the tray, and set them aside on the sterile field.

21. Before inserting an in-dwelling catheter, test the balloon by injecting fluid from the prefilled syringe into the balloon port.

22. Lubricate 2.5–5 cm of the catheter for female clients and 12.5–17.5 cm for male clients.

23. Apply the sterile drape:
    A. Female client:
       (1) Allow the top edge of the drape to form a cuff over both gloved hands. Place the drape on the bed between the client's thighs. Slip the cuffed edge just under the client's buttocks, taking care not to touch the contaminated surface with gloves.
       (2) Pick up the fenestrated sterile drape and allow it to unfold without touching any unsterile objects. Apply the drape over the client's perineum, exposing labia, taking care not to touch the contaminated surface with gloves.
    B. Male client:
       (1) Two methods are used for draping, depending on preference.
           First method: Apply the drape over the thighs and under the penis without completely opening fenestrated drape.
           Second method: Apply the drape over the thighs just below the penis. Pick up the fenestrated sterile drape, allow it to unfold without touching any unsterile objects, and drape it over the penis, with the fenestrated slit resting over the penis.

24. Place the sterile tray and contents on the sterile drape. Open the specimen container.

25. Cleanse the urethral meatus.
    A. Female client:
       (1) With your nondominant hand, carefully retract the labia to fully expose the urethral meatus. Maintain position of your nondominant hand throughout the procedure.
       (2) Holding forceps in your sterile dominant hand, pick up a cotton ball saturated with antiseptic solution and clean the client's perineal area, wiping from clitoris toward anus (front to back). Using a new cotton ball for each area, wipe along the far labial fold, the near labial fold, and directly over the centre of the urethral meatus.
    B. Male client:
       (1) If the client is not circumcised, retract the foreskin with your nondominant hand. Grasp the penis at the shaft, just below the glans. Retract the urethral meatus between your thumb and forefinger. Maintain your nondominant hand in this position throughout the procedure.
       (2) With your sterile dominant hand, use forceps to pick up a cotton ball saturated with antiseptic solution, and clean the penis. Move the cotton ball in circular motion from the urethral meatus down to the base of the glans. Repeat cleansing three more times, using a clean cotton ball each time.

26. Pick up the catheter with your gloved dominant hand, 7.5–10 cm from the catheter tip. Hold the end of the catheter loosely coiled in the palm of your dominant hand. (Optional: Grasp the catheter with forceps.)

27. Insert the catheter.
    A. Female client:
       (1) Ask the client to bear down gently as if to void urine, and slowly insert the catheter through the urethral meatus.

Continued

	S	U	NP	Comments

(2) Advance the catheter a total of 5–7.5 cm in an adult or until urine flows out the catheter's end. When urine appears, advance the catheter another 2.5–5 cm. Do not use force against resistance.   ____ ____ ____ _____

(3) Release the labia and hold the catheter securely with your nondominant hand. Slowly inflate the balloon if the in-dwelling catheter is being used.   ____ ____ ____ _____

B. Male client:

(1) Lift the client's penis to position perpendicular to the client's body, and apply light traction.   ____ ____ ____ _____

(2) Ask the client to bear down gently as if to void urine, and slowly insert the catheter through the urethral meatus.   ____ ____ ____ _____

(3) Advance the catheter 17–22.5 cm (7–9 inches) in an adult or until urine flows out the catheter's end. If resistance is felt, withdraw the catheter; do not force it through the urethra. When urine appears, advance the catheter another 2.5–5 cm. Do not use force against resistance.   ____ ____ ____ _____

(4) Lower the client's penis and hold the catheter securely in your nondominant hand. Place the end of the catheter in the urine tray. Inflate the balloon if an in-dwelling catheter is being used.   ____ ____ ____ _____

(5) Reduce (or reposition) the foreskin.   ____ ____ ____ _____

28. Collect the urine specimen as needed. Fill the specimen cup or jar to the desired level (20–30 mL) by holding the end of the catheter over the cup with your dominant hand.   ____ ____ ____ _____

29. Allow the client's bladder to empty fully (about 800–1000 mL) unless institution policy restricts the maximal volume of urine to drain with each catheterization. Check institution policy before beginning catheterization.   ____ ____ ____ _____

30. Inflate the balloon fully per manufacturer's recommendation, and then release the catheter with your nondominant hand and pull gently.   ____ ____ ____ _____

31. Attach the end of the in-dwelling catheter to the collecting tube of the drainage system. The drainage bag must be below the level of the bladder. Attach the bag to the bed frame; do not place the bag on the bed's side rails.   ____ ____ ____ _____

32. Anchor the catheter.

A. Female client:

(1) Secure the catheter tubing to the client's inner thigh or abdomen with a strip of nonallergenic tape (or multipurpose tube holders with a Velcro strap). Allow for slack so that movement of the thigh does not create tension on the catheter.   ____ ____ ____ _____

B. Male client:

(1) Secure the catheter tubing to the top of the thigh or lower abdomen (with the penis directed toward the chest). Allow for slack so that movement does not create tension on the catheter.   ____ ____ ____ _____

33. Assist the client to a comfortable position. Wash and dry the perineal area as needed.   ____ ____ ____ _____

34. Remove gloves and dispose of equipment, drapes, and urine in proper receptacles.   ____ ____ ____ _____

35. Perform hand hygiene.   ____ ____ ____ _____

36. Palpate the client's bladder.   ____ ____ ____ _____

37. Ask whether the client is comfortable.   ____ ____ ____ _____

38. Observe the character and amount of urine in the drainage system.   ____ ____ ____ _____

39. Ensure that no urine is leaking from the catheter or tubing connections.   ____ ____ ____ _____

40. Record and report catheterization, characteristics and amount of urine, specimen collection (if performed), and client's response to procedure and teaching concepts.   ____ ____ ____ _____

41. Initiate intake and output records.   ____ ____ ____ _____

STUDENT: _____ DATE: _____

INSTRUCTOR: _____ DATE: _____

Skill 44–3 In-Dwelling Catheter Care

	S	U	NP	Comments
1. Assess for episodes of bowel incontinence or client discomfort, or provide care as per agency routine regarding hygiene measures.	___	___	___	_____
2. Explain the procedure to the client. Offer the able client an opportunity to perform self-care.	___	___	___	_____
3. Close the door or bedside curtain.	___	___	___	_____
4. Perform hand hygiene.				
5. Position client.				
A. Female client:				
(1) Dorsal recumbent position	___	___	___	_____
B. Male client:				
(1) Supine or Fowler's position	___	___	___	_____
6. Place a waterproof pad under the client.	___	___	___	_____
7. Drape a bath blanket over the client so that only the perineal area is exposed.	___	___	___	_____
8. Put on disposable gloves.	___	___	___	_____
9. Remove the anchor device to free the catheter tubing.	___	___	___	_____
10. With your nondominant hand, prepare the client for the procedure.				
A. Female client:				
(1) Gently retract the labia to expose the urethral meatus and the catheter insertion site fully, maintaining the position of your hand throughout the procedure.	___	___	___	_____
B. Male client:				
(1) Retract foreskin if the client is not circumcised, and hold the penis at the shaft just below the glans, maintaining this position throughout the procedure.	___	___	___	_____
11. Assess the urethral meatus and surrounding tissue for inflammation, swelling, and discharge. Note amount, colour, odour, and consistency of discharge. Ask the client whether any burning sensation or discomfort has been experienced.	___	___	___	_____
12. Cleanse the perineal tissue.				
A. Female client:				
(1) Use a clean cloth, soap, and water. Cleanse around the urethral meatus and catheter. Moving from pubis toward anus, clean the labia minora. Use a clean side of the cloth for each wipe. Clean around the anus. Dry each area well.	___	___	___	_____
B. Male client:				
(1) While spreading the urethral meatus, cleanse around the catheter first, and then wipe in circular motion around meatus and glans.	___	___	___	_____
13. Reassess the urethral meatus for discharge.	___	___	___	_____
14. With the towel and perineal cleanser, wipe in a circular motion along the length of the catheter for 10 cm.	___	___	___	_____
15. In a male client, reduce (or reposition) the foreskin.	___	___	___	_____
16. Reanchor the catheter tubing.	___	___	___	_____
17. Place the client in a safe, comfortable position.	___	___	___	_____
18. Dispose of contaminated supplies, remove gloves, and perform hand hygiene.	___	___	___	_____

STUDENT: _____ DATE: _____

INSTRUCTOR: _____ DATE: _____

Skill 44–4 Closed and Open Catheter Irrigation

	S	U	NP	Comments
1. Assess the physician's order for type of irrigation and irrigation solution to use.	___	___	___	_____
2. Assess the colour of urine and the presence of mucus or sediment.	___	___	___	_____
3. Determine the type of catheter in place:				_____
A. Triple-lumen (one lumen to inflate the balloon, one to instill irrigation solution, one to allow outflow of urine)	___	___	___	_____
B. Double-lumen (one lumen to inflate the balloon, one to allow outflow of urine)	___	___	___	_____
4. Determine the patency of the drainage tubing.	___	___	___	_____
5. Assess the amount of urine in the drainage bag (you may want to empty the drainage bag before irrigation).	___	___	___	_____
6. Explain the procedure and purpose to the client.	___	___	___	_____
7. Perform hand hygiene, and put on clean disposable gloves for closed methods.	___	___	___	_____
8. Provide privacy by pulling bed curtains closed. Fold back covers so that the catheter is exposed. Cover the client's upper torso with the bath blanket.				_____
9. Assess the lower abdomen for bladder distension.	___	___	___	_____
10. Position the client in the dorsal recumbent or supine position.	___	___	___	_____
11. Closed intermittent irrigation (with double-lumen catheter):				_____
A. Prepare prescribed solution in a sterile graduated cup.	___	___	___	_____
B. Draw sterile solution into a syringe, using aseptic technique.	___	___	___	_____
C. Clamp in-dwelling catheter just distal to soft injection (specimen) port.	___	___	___	_____
D. Cleanse injection port with antiseptic swab (same port used for specimen collection).	___	___	___	_____
E. Insert the syringe at a 30-degree angle toward the bladder.	___	___	___	_____
F. Slowly inject fluid into the catheter and bladder.	___	___	___	_____
G. Withdraw the syringe, remove the clamp, and allow solution to drain into the drainage bag. If ordered by the physician, keep the bag clamped to allow solution to remain in the bladder for a short time (20–30 minutes).	___	___	___	_____
12. Closed continuous irrigation (with triple-lumen catheter):				
A. Using aseptic technique, insert the tip of the sterile irrigation tubing into the bag of sterile irrigating solution.	___	___	___	_____
B. Close the clamp on the tubing and hang the bag of solution on the intravenous (IV) pole.	___	___	___	_____
C. Open the clamp and allow solution to flow through tubing, keeping the end of tubing sterile. Close the clamp.	___	___	___	_____
D. Wipe off the irrigation port of the triple-lumen catheter, or attach a sterile Y connector to the double-lumen catheter and then attach to irrigation tubing.	___	___	___	_____
E. Be sure that the drainage bag and tubing are securely connected to drainage port of the triple-lumen catheter or other arm of the Y connector.	___	___	___	_____
F. For intermittent flow, clamp the tubing on the drainage system, open the clamp on the irrigation tubing, and allow the prescribed amount of fluid to enter the bladder. Close the irrigation clamp and then open the drainage tubing clamp. (Optional: Leave the clamp closed for 20–30 minutes if ordered.)	___	___	___	_____
G. For continuous drainage, calculate the drip rate and adjust the clamp on the irrigation tubing accordingly. Ensure that the clamp on the drainage tubing is open, and check the volume of drainage in the drainage bag. Ensure that drainage tubing is patent and avoid kinks.	___	___	___	_____
13. Open irrigation (with double-lumen catheter):				
A. Open the sterile irrigation tray, establish a sterile field, pour the required volume of sterile solution into the sterile container, and replace the cap on the large container of solution.	___	___	___	_____
B. Put on sterile gloves.	___	___	___	_____

Continued

	S	U	NP	Comments

C. Position the sterile waterproof drape under the catheter.   ____ ____ ____ _____

D. Aspirate 30 mL of solution into the sterile irrigating syringe.   ____ ____ ____ _____

E. Move the sterile collection close to the client's thighs.   ____ ____ ____ _____

F. Disconnect the catheter from the drainage tubing, allowing urine from the catheter to flow into the collection basin. Allow urine in tubing to flow into the drainage bag. Cover the end of tubing with a sterile protective cap. Position tubing in a safe place.   ____ ____ ____ _____

G. Insert the tip of the syringe into the catheter lumen, and gently instill solution.   ____ ____ ____ _____

H. Withdraw the syringe, lower the catheter, and allow solution to drain into the basin. Repeat instillation until the prescribed solution has been used or until drainage is clear, depending on the purpose of irrigation.   ____ ____ ____ _____

I. If solution does not return, have the client turn onto the side facing you. If changing position does not help, reinsert the syringe and gently aspirate solution.   ____ ____ ____ _____

J. After irrigation is complete, remove the protector cap from the tubing, cleanse the end with an alcohol swab (or the agency's recommended solution), and re-establish the drainage system.   ____ ____ ____ _____

14. Reanchor the catheter to the client with tape or an elastic tube holder.   ____ ____ ____ _____

15. Assist the client to a comfortable position.   ____ ____ ____ _____

16. Lower the bed to the lowest position. Put the side rails up if appropriate.   ____ ____ ____ _____

17. Dispose of contaminated supplies, remove gloves, and perform hand hygiene.   ____ ____ ____ _____

18. Calculate the amount of fluid used to irrigate the bladder, and subtract from total output.   ____ ____ ____ _____

19. Assess characteristics of output: viscosity, colour, and presence of matter (e.g., sediment, clots, blood).   ____ ____ ____ _____

STUDENT: _____ DATE: _____

INSTRUCTOR: _____ DATE: _____

Skill 45–1 Administering a Cleansing Enema

	S	U	NP	Comments
1. Assess the status of the client: last bowel movement, normal bowel patterns, presence of hemorrhoids, mobility, external sphincter control, and abdominal pain.	___	___	___	_____
2. Assess the client for the presence of increased intracranial pressure, glaucoma, or recent rectal or prostate surgery.	___	___	___	_____
3. Check the client's medical record to clarify the rationale for the enema.	___	___	___	_____
4. Review the physician's order for the enema.	___	___	___	_____
5. Determine the client's level of understanding of the purpose of the enema.	___	___	___	_____
6. Perform hand hygiene. Collect appropriate equipment.	___	___	___	_____
7. Correctly identify the client and explain the procedure.	___	___	___	_____
8. Assemble the enema bag with the appropriate solution and rectal tube.	___	___	___	_____
9. Perform hand hygiene and put on gloves.	___	___	___	_____
10. Provide privacy by closing the curtains around the bed or by closing the door.	___	___	___	_____
11. Raise the bed to an appropriate working height; raise the side rail on the client's left side.	___	___	___	_____
12. Assist the client into a position lying on the left side with the right knee flexed (i.e., Sims' position). Children may instead be placed in a dorsal recumbent position.	___	___	___	_____
13. Place a waterproof pad under the hips and buttocks.	___	___	___	_____
14. Cover the client with a bath blanket, exposing only the rectal area, with the anus clearly visible.	___	___	___	_____
15. Place the bedpan or commode in an easily accessible position. If the client will be expelling contents in a toilet, ensure the toilet is available. (If the client will be walking to the bathroom to expel the enema, place the client's slippers and bathrobe in an easily accessible position.)	___	___	___	_____
16. Administer the enema.				
A. Enema bag:				
(1) Add warmed solution to the enema bag: warm the tap water as it flows from the faucet, place the saline container in a basin of hot water before adding saline to the enema bag, and check the temperature of the solution with a bath thermometer or by pouring a small amount of solution over your inner wrist.	___	___	___	_____
(2) Raise the container, release the clamp, and allow the solution to flow long enough to fill the tubing.	___	___	___	_____
(3) Reclamp the tubing.	___	___	___	_____
(4) Lubricate 6–8 cm of the tip of the rectal tube with lubricating jelly.	___	___	___	_____
(5) Gently separate the buttocks and locate the anus. Instruct the client to relax by breathing out slowly through the mouth.	___	___	___	_____
(6) Insert the tip of the rectal tube slowly by pointing the tip in the direction of the client's umbilicus. The length of the insertion varies: Adult: 7.5–10 cm Child: 5–7 cm Infant: 2.5–3.75 cm	___	___	___	_____
(7) Hold the tubing in the rectum constantly until the end of the fluid instillation.	___	___	___	_____
(8) Open the regulating clamp and allow the solution to enter slowly with the enema container at the client's hip level.	___	___	___	_____
(9) Raise the height of the enema container slowly to the appropriate level above the anus: 30–45 cm for a high enema, 30 cm for a regular enema, 7.5 cm for a low enema. Instillation time varies, depending on the volume of solution administered.	___	___	___	_____

Continued

492

	S	U	NP	Comments

(10) Lower the container or clamp tubing if the client complains of cramping or if fluid escapes around the rectal tube.

(11) Clamp the tubing after all solution is instilled.

B. Prepackaged disposable container:

(1) Remove the plastic cap from the rectal tip. The tip is already lubricated, but more jelly can be applied as needed.

(2) Gently separate the buttocks and locate the rectum. Instruct the client to relax by breathing out slowly through the mouth.

(3) Insert the tip of the bottle gently into the rectum:
Adult: 7.5–10 cm
Child: 5–7.5 cm
Infant: 2.5–3.75 cm

(4) Squeeze the bottle until all the solution has entered the rectum and colon. Instruct the client to retain the solution until the urge to defecate occurs, usually within 2–5 minutes.

17. Place layers of toilet tissue around the tube at the anus and gently withdraw the rectal tube.

18. Explain to the client that the feeling of distension is normal. Ask the client to retain the solution for as long as possible while lying quietly in bed. (For an infant or young child, gently hold the buttocks together for a few minutes.)

19. Discard the enema container and tubing in the proper receptacle, or rinse thoroughly with warm soap and water if the container is to be reused.

20. Assist the client to the bathroom or help to position the client on a bedpan.

21. Observe the character of the feces and solution (caution the client against flushing the toilet until you can inspect the feces).

22. Assist the client as needed to wash the anal area with warm soap and water (if providing perineal care, use gloves).

23. Remove and discard gloves and perform hand hygiene.

24. Inspect the colour, consistency, and amount of stool and fluid passed.

25. Assess the condition of the client's abdomen; cramping, rigidity, or distension can indicate a serious problem.

STUDENT: _____ DATE: _____

INSTRUCTOR: _____ DATE: _____

Skill 45–2 Inserting and Maintaining a Nasogastric Tube

	S	U	NP	Comments
1. Perform hand hygiene. Inspect the condition of the client's nasal and oral cavities.	___	___	___	_____
2. Ask whether the client has a history of nasal surgery, and note whether a deviated nasal septum is present.	___	___	___	_____
3. Palpate the client's abdomen for distension, pain, and rigidity. Auscultate for bowel sounds.	___	___	___	_____
4. Assess the client's level of consciousness and ability to follow instructions.	___	___	___	_____
5. Check the medical record for the surgeon's order, the type of nasogastric tube to be placed, and whether the tube is to be attached to suction equipment.	___	___	___	_____
6. Perform hand hygiene. Prepare equipment at the bedside. Cut a piece of tape approximately 10 cm long and split one end in half to form a "V," or have the nasogastric tube fixator device available.	___	___	___	_____
7. Identify the client and explain the procedure.	___	___	___	_____
8. Put on disposable gloves.	___	___	___	_____
9. Position the client in a high Fowler's position with pillows behind the head and shoulders. Raise the bed to a horizontal level that is comfortable for you.	___	___	___	_____
10. Place a bath towel over the client's chest; give facial tissues to the client. Place the emesis basin within reach.	___	___	___	_____
11. Pull the curtain around the bed, or close the room door.	___	___	___	_____
12. Stand on the client's right side if you are right-handed, on the left side if you are left-handed.	___	___	___	_____
13. Instruct the client to relax and breathe normally while you occlude one naris. Repeat this action for the other naris. Select the nostril with the greater airflow.	___	___	___	_____
14. Measure the distance to insert the tube:				
A. Measure the distance from the tip of the client's nose to the earlobe and then to the xiphoid process.	___	___	___	_____
B. Mark the 50-cm point on the tube, then take a traditional measurement. The tube should be inserted to a midway point between 50 cm and the traditional mark.	___	___	___	_____
15. Mark the length of tube to be inserted by using a small piece of tape placed so that it can easily be removed.	___	___	___	_____
16. Curve 10–15 cm of the end of the tube tightly around your index finger, then release.	___	___	___	_____
17. Lubricate 7.5–10 cm of the end of the tube with water-soluble lubricating jelly.	___	___	___	_____
18. Alert the client that the procedure is to begin.	___	___	___	_____
19. Instruct the client to extend the neck back against the pillow; insert the tube gently and slowly through the naris with the curved end pointing downward.	___	___	___	_____
20. Continue to insert the tube along the floor of the nasal passage aiming down toward the client's ear. If resistance is met, apply gentle downward pressure to advance the tube (do not force the tube past the area of resistance).	___	___	___	_____
21. If resistance is met, try to rotate the tube to see whether it advances. If resistance continues, withdraw the tube, allow the client to rest, relubricate the tube, and insert the tube into the other naris.	___	___	___	_____
22. Continue insertion of tube by gently rotating the tube toward the opposite naris. Insert until the tube is just past the nasopharynx.				
A. Stop the tube advancement; allow the client to relax. Provide the client with tissues.	___	___	___	_____
B. Explain to the client that the next step requires that the client swallow. Give the client a glass of water, unless this is contraindicated.	___	___	___	_____

Continued

	S	U	NP	Comments

23. With the tube just above the oropharynx, instruct the client to flex the head forward, while you place your hand at the back of the neck to support it. Have the client take a small sip of water and swallow. Advance the tube 2.5–5 cm with each swallow of water. If client is not allowed fluids, instruct the client to dry swallow or to suck air through a straw.

24. If the client begins to cough, gag, or choke, withdraw the tube slightly (do not completely remove the tube) and stop tube advancement. Instruct the client to breathe easily and take sips of water.

25. If the client continues to gag and cough or if the client complains that the tube feels as though it is coiling in the back of the throat, check the back of the oropharynx using a tongue blade. If the tube has coiled, withdraw it until the tip is back in the oropharynx. Reinsert the tube while the client swallows.

26. Continue to advance the tube with swallowing until the tape or mark on the tube is reached. Temporarily anchor the tube to the client's cheek with a piece of tape until the tube placement is checked.

27. Verify tube placement. Check agency policy for the preferred methods for checking nasogastric tube placement:
    A. Ask the client to talk.
    B. Inspect the posterior pharynx for the presence of coiled tube.
    C. Aspirate gently back on the syringe to obtain gastric contents. Note the colour and other characteristics.
    D. Measure the pH of the aspirate with colour-coded pH paper with a range of whole numbers 1 to 11.
    E. Have an X-ray examination performed of the chest or abdomen.
    F. If the tube is not in the stomach, advance another 2.5–5 cm and repeat steps 27B, C, and D to check the tube position.

28. Anchor the tube:
    A. After the tube is properly inserted and positioned, either clamp the end or connect the end to the drainage bag or a suction machine.
    B. Tape the tube to the nose; avoid putting pressure on both nares.
       (1) Before taping the tube to the nose, apply a small amount of tincture of benzoin to the lower end of the nose and allow it to dry (optional). Ensure the top end of the tape over the nose is secure.
       (2) Carefully wrap the two split ends of tape around the tube.
       (3) Alternative: Apply the tube fixation device by using a shaped adhesive patch.
    C. Fasten the end of the nasogastric tube to the client's gown by looping a rubber band around the tube into a slip knot. Pin the rubber band to the client's gown (to provide slack for movement).
    D. Unless the physician orders otherwise, the head of the bed should be elevated 30 degrees.
    E. Explain to the client that the sensation of the tube will decrease with time.
    F. Remove gloves and perform hand hygiene.

29. Once placement is confirmed:
    A. Place a mark, either a red mark or tape, on the tube to indicate where the tube exits the nose.
    B. Alternatively, measure the length of the tube from the naris to the connector.
    C. Document the tube length in the client's record.

30. Tube irrigation:
    A. Perform hand hygiene, and put on gloves.
    B. Check for tube placement in the stomach (see Step 27). Reconnect the nasogastric tube to the connecting tube.
    C. Draw up 30 mL of normal saline into Asepto or catheter-tipped syringe.
    D. Clamp the nasogastric tube. Disconnect from the connection tubing, and lay the end of the connection tubing on a towel.
    E. Insert the tip of the irrigating syringe into the end of the nasogastric tube. Remove the clamp. Hold the syringe with the tip pointed at the floor and inject the saline slowly and evenly. Do not force the solution.

Continued

	S	U	NP	Comments
F. If resistance occurs, check for kinks in the tubing. Turn the client onto the left side. Repeated resistance should be reported to the physician.	___	___	___	_____
G. After instilling saline, immediately aspirate or pull back slowly on the syringe to withdraw fluid. If the amount aspirated is greater than the amount instilled, record the difference as output. If the amount aspirated is less than the amount instilled, record the difference as intake.	___	___	___	_____
H. Reconnect the nasogastric tube to the drainage bag or suction equipment (if the solution does not return, repeat the irrigation).	___	___	___	_____
I. Remove gloves and perform hand hygiene.	___	___	___	_____
31. Observe the amount and character of the contents draining from the nasogastric tube. Ask whether the client feels nauseated.	___	___	___	_____
32. Palpate the client's abdomen periodically, noting any distension, pain, or rigidity. Turn off the suction, and auscultate for the presence of bowel sounds.	___	___	___	_____
33. Inspect the condition of the nares and the nose.	___	___	___	_____
34. Observe the position of the tubing.	___	___	___	_____
35. Ask whether the client has a sore throat or feels irritation in the pharynx.	___	___	___	_____
36. Discontinuation of a nasogastric tube:				
A. Verify the order to discontinue the nasogastric tube.	___	___	___	_____
B. Explain the procedure to the client and reassure the client that removal is less distressing than insertion.	___	___	___	_____
C. Perform hand hygiene and put on disposable gloves.	___	___	___	_____
D. Turn off the suction and disconnect the nasogastric tube from the drainage bag or suction equipment. Remove tape from the bridge of the client's nose and unpin the tube from the gown.	___	___	___	_____
E. Stand on the client's right side if you are right-handed, on the left side if you are left-handed.	___	___	___	_____
F. Hand the client a facial tissue; place a clean towel across the chest. Instruct the client to take a deep breath and to hold the breath.	___	___	___	_____
G. While the client holds the breath, clamp or kink the tubing securely and then pull the tube out steadily and smoothly into a towel held in your other hand.	___	___	___	_____
H. Measure the amount of drainage, and note the character of the contents. Dispose of the tube and drainage equipment into the proper container.	___	___	___	_____
I. Clean the client's nares and provide mouth care.	___	___	___	_____
J. Position the client comfortably and explain the procedure for drinking fluids, if they are not contraindicated.	___	___	___	_____
37. Clean the equipment and return to their proper place. Place soiled linen in the utility room or the proper receptacle.	___	___	___	_____
38. Remove gloves and perform hand hygiene.	___	___	___	_____
39. Inspect the condition of the client's nares and nose.	___	___	___	_____
40. Ask whether the client has a sore throat or feels irritation in the pharynx.	___	___	___	_____

497

STUDENT: _____ DATE: _____

INSTRUCTOR: _____ DATE: _____

Skill 45–3 Pouching an Ostomy

	S	U	NP	Comments
1. Perform hand hygiene, and auscultate for bowel sounds.	___	___	___	_____
2. Put on gloves. Observe the skin barrier and pouch for leakage and the length of time in place. Depending on the type of pouching system used (e.g., an opaque pouch), you may need to remove the pouch to fully observe the stoma. Clear pouches allow the viewing of the stoma without their removal.	___	___	___	_____
3. Observe the stoma for colour, swelling, trauma, and healing; the stoma should be moist and reddish pink. Assess the type of stoma. Stomas can be flush with the skin or can be a budlike protrusion on the abdomen.	___	___	___	_____
4. Measure the stoma at each pouching change. Follow the pouch manufacturer's directions and measuring guide to determine which pouch to use on the basis of the client's stoma size. The opening around the appliance should be no greater than 2 mm larger than the stoma.	___	___	___	_____
5. Observe the abdominal incision (if present).	___	___	___	_____
6. Observe the effluent from the stoma, and record the intake and output. Ask the client about skin tenderness. Remove gloves and perform hand hygiene.	___	___	___	_____
7. Assess the client's abdomen for the best type of pouching system to use. Consider the following:				
A. Contour and peristomal plane	___	___	___	_____
B. Presence of scars, incisions	___	___	___	_____
C. Location and type of stoma	___	___	___	_____
8. Assess the client's self-care ability, to determine the best type of pouching system to use.	___	___	___	_____
9. After removing the skin barrier and pouch, assess the skin around the stoma, noting scars, folds, skin breakdown, and the peristomal suture line, if present. Keep the pouch loosely attached to the stoma to collect any drainage while the system is being changed.	___	___	___	_____
10. Determine the client's emotional response, knowledge, and understanding of an ostomy and its care.	___	___	___	_____
11. Explain the procedure to the client; encourage the client's interaction and questions.	___	___	___	_____
12. Perform hand hygiene. Assemble the equipment, and close the room curtains or door.	___	___	___	_____
13. Position the client either standing or supine and draped. If the client is seated, position the client either on or in front of the toilet.	___	___	___	_____
14. Perform hand hygiene, and put on disposable gloves.	___	___	___	_____
15. Place the towel or disposable waterproof barrier under the client.	___	___	___	_____
16. Completely remove the used pouch and skin barrier by gently pushing the skin away from the barrier. An adhesive remover may be used to facilitate removal of the skin barrier.	___	___	___	_____
17. Clean the peristomal skin gently with warm tap water, using gauze pads or a clean washcloth; do not scrub the skin. Dry completely by patting the skin with gauze or a towel.	___	___	___	_____
18. Measure the stoma for the correct size of pouching system needed, using the manufacturer's measuring guide.	___	___	___	_____
19. Select the appropriate pouch for the client on the basis of your client assessment. For a custom cut-to-fit pouch, use an ostomy guide to cut an opening on the pouch 2 mm larger than the stoma before removing the backing. Prepare the pouch by removing the backing from the barrier and adhesive. For an ileostomy, apply a thin circle of barrier paste around the opening in the pouch; allow to dry.	___	___	___	_____
20. Apply the skin barrier and pouch. If creases occur next to the stoma, use a barrier paste to fill in; let dry 1–2 minutes.	___	___	___	_____

Continued

Copyright © 2010 Elsevier Canada, a division of Reed Elsevier Canada, Ltd.

		S	U	NP	Comments

A. For a one-piece pouching system:
   (1) Use skin sealant wipes on the skin directly under the adhesive skin barrier or pouch; allow to dry. Press the adhesive backing of the pouch or skin barrier smoothly against the skin, starting from the bottom and working up and around the sides. ____ ____ ____ _____

   (2) Hold the pouch by the barrier, centre it over the stoma, and press down gently on the barrier; the bottom of the pouch should point toward the client's knees. ____ ____ ____ _____

   (3) Maintain gentle finger pressure around the barrier for 1–2 minutes. ____ ____ ____ _____

B. For a two-piece pouching system:
   (1) Apply the flange (the barrier with adhesive) as in the steps above for a one-piece system. Then snap on the pouch and maintain finger pressure. ____ ____ ____ _____

C. For both pouching systems, gently tug on the pouch in a downward direction. ____ ____ ____ _____

21. Apply a nonallergenic paper tape around the pectin skin barrier in a "picture frame" method. Half of the tape should be on the skin barrier and half on the client's skin. Some clients prefer a belt attached to the pouch for extra security in place of the tape. ____ ____ ____ _____

22. Although many ostomy pouches are odour-proof, some nurses and clients like to put a small amount of ostomy deodorant into the pouch. Do not use "home remedies," such as aspirin, to control the ostomy odour. ____ ____ ____ _____

23. Fold the bottom of drainable open-ended pouches up once and close, using a closure device such as a clamp (or follow the manufacturer's instructions for closure). ____ ____ ____ _____

24. Properly dispose of the old pouch and the soiled equipment. Consider spraying deodorant in the room if needed. ____ ____ ____ _____

25. Remove gloves and perform hand hygiene. ____ ____ ____ _____

26. Change a one- or two-piece pouch every 3–7 days unless it is leaking. A pouch can remain in place for a tub bath or shower; after a bath or shower, pat the adhesive dry. ____ ____ ____ _____

27. Ask whether the client feels discomfort around the stoma. ____ ____ ____ _____

28. While the pouch is removed and the skin is being cleaned, note the appearance of the stoma around the skin and the existing incision (if present). Reinspect the condition of the skin barrier and adhesive. ____ ____ ____ _____

29. Auscultate for bowel sounds and observe the characteristics of the stool. ____ ____ ____ _____

30. Observe the client's nonverbal behaviours as the pouch is applied. Ask whether the client has any questions about the pouching. ____ ____ ____ _____

STUDENT: _____   DATE: _____

INSTRUCTOR: _____   DATE: _____

Skill 46–1 Moving and Positioning Clients in Bed

	S	U	NP	Comments
1. Assess the client's body alignment and comfort level while the client is lying down.	___	___	___	_____
2. Assess for risk factors that may contribute to complications of immobility:				
A. Paralysis: Hemiparesis resulting from cerebrovascular accident; decreased sensation	___	___	___	_____
B. Impaired mobility: Traction or arthritis or other contributing disease processes	___	___	___	_____
C. Impaired circulation	___	___	___	_____
D. Age: Very young children, older adults	___	___	___	_____
E. Level of consciousness and mental status	___	___	___	_____
F. Condition of client's skin	___	___	___	_____
3. Assess client's physical ability to help with moving and positioning:				
A. Age	___	___	___	_____
B. Level of consciousness and mental status	___	___	___	_____
C. Disease process	___	___	___	_____
D. Strength, coordination	___	___	___	_____
E. Range of motion	___	___	___	_____
4. Assess physician's orders. Clarify whether any positions are contraindicated because of the client's condition (e.g., spinal cord injury; respiratory difficulties; certain neurological conditions; presence of incisions, drain, or tubing).				
5. Perform hand hygiene.	___	___	___	_____
6. Assess for the presence of tubes, incisions, and equipment (e.g., traction).	___	___	___	_____
7. Assess the ability and motivation of the client, family members, and primary caregiver to participate in moving and positioning the client in bed in anticipation of discharge to home.	___	___	___	_____
8. Raise the level of the bed to a comfortable working height. Get extra help if needed.	___	___	___	_____
9. Perform hand hygiene.	___	___	___	_____
10. Explain the procedure to the client.	___	___	___	_____
11. Position the client flat in bed, if this is tolerated.	___	___	___	_____
12. Position the client in bed:				
A. Assist the client in moving up in bed (one or two nurses). *Note:* Only a young child or a lightweight client requiring minimal assistance can be safely moved by one nurse:	___	___	___	_____
(1) Remove the pillow from under the client's head and shoulders, and place the pillow at the head of the bed. Ask the client to cross arms across the chest.	___	___	___	_____
(2) Face the head of the bed.	___	___	___	_____
(a) Each nurse should have one arm under the client's shoulders and one arm under the client's thighs.	___	___	___	_____
(b) Alternative position: Position one nurse at client's upper body. The nurse's arm nearest the head of the bed should be under the client's head and opposite shoulder; other arm should be under the client's closest arm and shoulder. Position the other nurse at the client's lower torso. The nurse's arms should be under the client's lower back and torso.	___	___	___	_____
(3) Place your feet apart, with the foot nearest head of bed behind the other foot (forward–backward stance).	___	___	___	_____
(4) Ask the client to flex knees with feet flat on the bed.	___	___	___	_____
(5) Instruct the client to flex the neck, tilting the chin toward the chest.	___	___	___	_____
(6) Instruct the client to assist moving by pushing with feet on the bed surface.	___	___	___	_____
(7) Flex your knees and hips, bringing your forearms closer to the level of the bed.	___	___	___	_____

Continued

	S	U	NP	Comments

(8) Instruct the client to push with heels and elevate the trunk while breathing out, thus moving toward the head of the bed, on a count of three.

(9) On a count of three, rock and shift weight from back to front leg. At the same time, client pushes with heels and elevates the trunk.

B. Move immobile client up in bed with drawsheet or friction-reducing device (two nurses are needed):

(1) Adjust the bed to an appropriate height for the caregiver's body mechanics. Place a drawsheet or friction-reducing device under the client by turning the client side to side. Have the sheet extend from shoulders to thighs. Return the client to the supine position.

(2) Position one nurse at each side of client.

(3) Grasp the drawsheet or friction-reducing device firmly near the client, with your palms facing up.

(4) Place your feet apart in forward–backward stance. Flex your knees and hips. Shift weight from front to back leg, and move client and drawsheet or friction-reducing device to the desired position in bed.

(5) Realign the client in correct body alignment.

C. Position the client in supported Fowler's position:

(1) Elevate the head of the bed 45–60 degrees.

(2) Rest the client's head against the mattress or on a small pillow.

(3) Use pillows to support the client's arms and hands if the client does not have voluntary control or use of them.

(4) Position the pillow at the client's lower back.

(5) Place a small pillow or roll under the thigh.

(6) Position the client's heel in heel boots or other heel pressure-relief device.

D. Position a hemiplegic client in supported Fowler's position:

(1) Elevate the head of the bed 45–60 degrees.

(2) Position the client in a sitting position as straight as possible.

(3) Position the client's head on a small pillow with the chin slightly forward. If the client is totally unable to control head movement, hyperextension of the neck must be avoided.

(4) Flex the client's knees and hips by using a pillow or folded blanket under the knees.

(5) Support the client's feet in dorsiflexion with a firm pillow or therapeutic boots or splints.

E. Position the client in the supine position:

(1) Be sure the client is comfortable on the back, with the head of the bed flat.

(2) Place a small rolled towel under the lumbar area of the back.

(3) Place a pillow under the upper shoulders, neck, or head.

(4) Place trochanter rolls or sandbags parallel to the lateral surface of the thighs.

(5) Place a small pillow or roll under the ankles to elevate the heels.

(6) Place firm pillows against the bottom of the client's feet.

(7) Place foot boots on the client's feet, if necessary.

(8) Place pillows under the client's pronated forearms, and keep the client's upper arms parallel to the client's body.

(9) Place hand rolls in client's hands. Consider occupational therapy referral for the use of hand splints, if necessary.

F. Position a hemiplegic client in the supine position:

(1) Place the client on the back, with the head of the bed flat.

(2) Place a folded towel or small pillow under the client's shoulder or affected side.

(3) Keep the affected arm away from the client's body, with the elbow extended and palm up. (An alternative is to place the arm out to the side, with the elbow bent and hand toward the head of the bed.)

(4) Place a folded towel under the hip of the client's involved side.

(5) Flex the client's affected knee 30 degrees by supporting it on a pillow or folded blanket.

Continued

	S	U	NP	Comments

(6) Support the client's feet with soft pillows at a right angle to the leg.

G. Position the client in prone position. Two staff members are required in order to position the client safely:
 (1) With the drawsheet under the client, move the client toward one side of the bed. Ensure that the side rail on the opposite side is up for safety. With the client supine, roll the client over the arm positioned close to the body, with elbow straight, and hand under hip. Position on abdomen in the centre of the bed.
 (2) Turn the client's head to one side, and support the head with a small pillow.
 (3) Place a small pillow under the client's abdomen, below the level of the diaphragm.
 (4) Support the arms in flexed position, level at the shoulders.
 (5) Support the lower legs with pillows to elevate the toes.

H. Position a hemiplegic client in prone position:
 (1) Move the client toward the unaffected side.
 (2) Roll the client onto that side.
 (3) Place a pillow on the client's abdomen.
 (4) Roll the client onto the abdomen by positioning the involved arm close to the client's body, with the elbow straight and hand under hip. Roll the client carefully over the arm.
 (5) Turn the client's head toward the involved side.
 (6) Position the client's involved arm out to the side, with elbow bent, hand toward the head of the bed, and fingers extended (if possible).
 (7) Flex the knees slightly by placing a pillow under the legs from knees to ankles.
 (8) Keep feet at right angles by using a pillow high enough to keep toes off the mattress.

I. Position the client in lateral (side-lying) position:
 (1) Lower the head of bed completely or as low as the client can tolerate.
 (2) Position the client to the side of the bed.
 (3) Prepare to turn the client onto the side. Flex the client's knee that will not be next to the mattress. Place one of your hands on the client's hip and your other hand on the client's shoulder.
 (4) Roll the client onto the side, toward you.
 (5) Place a pillow under the client's head and neck.
 (6) Bring the shoulder blade forward.
 (7) Position both of the client's arms in slightly flexed position. The upper arm is supported by a pillow level with shoulder; other arm, by the mattress.
 (8) Place a tuck-back pillow behind the client's back. (Make it by folding a pillow lengthwise. The smooth area is slightly tucked under the client's back.)
 (9) Place a pillow under the semiflexed upper leg for support.
 (10) Place a sandbag parallel to the plantar surface of the dependent foot.

J. Position the client in Sims' (semiprone) position:
 (1) Lower the head of the bed completely.
 (2) Be sure the client is comfortable in the supine position.
 (3) Position the client in the lateral position, with the dependent arm straight along the client's body and with the client lying partially on the abdomen.
 (4) Carefully lift the client's dependent shoulder and bring the arm back behind the client.
 (5) Place a small pillow under the client's head.
 (6) Place a pillow under the flexed upper arm, supporting the arm level with the shoulder.
 (7) Place pillow under flexed upper leg, supporting the leg level with the hip.
 (8) Place sandbags or pillows parallel to the plantar surface of the foot.

K. Logroll the client (this requires three nurses):
 (1) Place a pillow between the client's knees.

Continued

	S	U	NP	Comments
(2) Cross the client's arms on the chest.	___	___	___	_____
(3) Position two nurses on the side of the bed to which the client will be turned. Position the third nurse on the other side of the bed.	___	___	___	_____
(4) Fan-fold or roll the drawsheet or pull sheet.	___	___	___	_____
(5) Move the client as one unit in a smooth, continuous motion on the count of three.	___	___	___	_____
(6) The nurse on the opposite side of the bed places pillows along the length of the client.	___	___	___	_____
(7) Gently lean the client as a unit back toward the pillows.	___	___	___	_____
13. Perform hand hygiene.	___	___	___	_____
14. Evaluate the client's comfort level and ability to assist in position change.	___	___	___	_____
15. After each position change, evaluate the client's body alignment and the presence of any pressure areas. Observe for areas of erythema or breakdown involving skin.	___	___	___	_____

STUDENT: _____ DATE: _____

INSTRUCTOR: _____ DATE: _____

Skill 46–2 Using Safe and Effective Transfer Techniques

	S	U	NP	Comments
1. Assess the client for the following:				
A. Muscle strength (legs and upper arms)	___	___	___	_____
B. Joint mobility and contracture formation	___	___	___	_____
C. Paralysis or paresis (spastic or flaccid)	___	___	___	_____
D. Orthostatic hypotension	___	___	___	_____
E. Activity tolerance	___	___	___	_____
F. Presence of pain	___	___	___	_____
G. Vital signs	___	___	___	_____
2. Assess the client's sensory status:				
A. Adequacy of central and peripheral vision	___	___	___	_____
B. Adequacy of hearing	___	___	___	_____
C. Loss of sensation	___	___	___	_____
3. Assess the client's cognitive status.	___	___	___	_____
4. Assess the client's level of motivation:				
A. The client's eagerness or unwillingness to be mobile	___	___	___	_____
B. Whether the client avoids activity and offers excuses	___	___	___	_____
5. Assess previous mode of transfer (if applicable).	___	___	___	_____
6. Assess client's specific risk of falling when transferred.	___	___	___	_____
7. Assess special transfer equipment needed for the home setting. Assess the home environment for hazards.	___	___	___	_____
8. Perform hand hygiene.	___	___	___	_____
9. Explain the procedure to the client.	___	___	___	_____
10. Transfer the client:				
A. Assist the client to a sitting position (bed at waist level):				
(1) Place the client in supine position.	___	___	___	_____
(2) Face the head of the bed at a 45-degree angle, and remove pillows.	___	___	___	_____
(3) Place your feet apart, with the foot nearer the bed behind the other foot, continuing at a 45-degree angle to the head of the bed.	___	___	___	_____
(4) Place your hand farther from the client under the client's shoulders, supporting the client's head and cervical vertebrae.	___	___	___	_____
(5) Place your other hand on the bed surface.	___	___	___	_____
(6) Raise the client to a sitting position by shifting weight from your front to your back leg. Pivot your feet as weight is shifted from your front to your back leg so that your upper body does not twist.	___	___	___	_____
(7) Push against the bed, using your arm that is placed on the bed surface.	___	___	___	_____
B. Assist the client to sitting position on the side of the bed with the bed in low position:				
(1) Turn the client to the side, facing you on the side of the bed on which the client will be sitting.	___	___	___	_____
(2) With the client supine, raise the head of the bed 30 degrees.	___	___	___	_____
(3) Stand opposite the client's hips. Turn diagonally so that you face the client and the far corner of the foot of the bed.	___	___	___	_____
(4) Place your feet apart, with the foot closer to the head of the bed in front of the other foot.	___	___	___	_____
(5) Place your arm nearer the head of the bed under the client's shoulder, supporting the client's head and neck.	___	___	___	_____
(6) Place your other arm over the client's thighs.	___	___	___	_____
(7) Move the client's lower legs and feet over the side of the bed. Pivot toward your rear leg, allowing the client's upper legs to swing downward.	___	___	___	_____
(8) At the same time, shift weight to your rear leg and elevate the client. Pivot your feet in the direction of movement to avoid twisting your upper body.	___	___	___	_____
C. Transfer the client from bed to chair with the bed in low position:				
(1) Assist the client to a sitting position on the side of the bed. Position the chair at a 45-degree angle to the bed.	___	___	___	_____

Continued

		S	U	NP	Comments
(2)	Apply a transfer belt or other transfer aids.	___	___	___	_____
(3)	Ensure that the client has stable, nonskid shoes. The client's weight-bearing or unaffected (strong) leg is placed back and the affected (weak) knee is slightly forward or parallel.	___	___	___	_____
(4)	Place your feet shoulder-width apart.	___	___	___	_____
(5)	Flex your hips and knees, supporting the client's weaker knee or leg with your knees.	___	___	___	_____
(6)	Grasp the transfer belt from underneath.	___	___	___	_____
(7)	Rock the client up to a standing position on a count of three while straightening your hips and legs and keeping your knees slightly flexed. Unless it is contraindicated, the client may be instructed to use hands to push up, if applicable.	___	___	___	_____
(8)	Maintain stability of the client's weak or paralyzed leg between your knees.	___	___	___	_____
(9)	Pivot on your foot farther from the chair. Instruct the client to stand straight. Pivot your body in the direction of the chair, instructing the client to take small steps toward the chair. Ask the client to tell you when the chair touches the back of his or her knees.	___	___	___	_____
(10)	Instruct the client to use armrests on the chair for support, and ease the client into the chair.	___	___	___	_____
(11)	Flex your hips and knees while lowering the client into the chair.	___	___	___	_____
(12)	Assess the client for proper alignment for the sitting position. Provide support for paralyzed extremities. Use a lapboard or sling to support a flaccid arm. Stabilize the client's legs with a bath blanket or pillow.	___	___	___	_____
(13)	Praise the client's progress, effort, and performance.	___	___	___	_____

D. Transfer the client from bed to stretcher or another bed, using a drawsheet or friction-reducing device:

		S	U	NP	Comments
(1)	Place the bed flat, and position at the same level as the stretcher. Ensure that bed brakes are locked.	___	___	___	_____
(2)	Lower the side rails. Have two caregivers stand on the side where the stretcher will be, while the third caregiver stands on the other side.	___	___	___	_____
(3)	Two caregivers help the client roll onto the side toward one caregiver.	___	___	___	_____
(4)	Work together to position the friction-reducing device properly under the client's back.	___	___	___	_____
(5)	Roll the stretcher alongside the bed. Lock the wheels of the stretcher once it is in place. Instruct the client to place his or her arms across the chest and not to move.	___	___	___	_____
(6)	All three caregivers place feet widely apart with one foot slightly in front of the other, and grasp the friction-reducing device.	___	___	___	_____
(7)	On the count of three, caregivers pull the client from the bed onto the stretcher, using the friction-reducing device and shifting weight appropriately.	___	___	___	_____
(8)	Put up the side rail of the stretcher on the side where caregivers are, and then roll the stretcher away from the side of the bed and put side rails up on that side.	___	___	___	_____

E. Use mechanical or hydraulic lift to transfer the client from bed to chair. Before using the lift, be thoroughly familiar with its operation. Gather all necessary equipment and caregivers.

		S	U	NP	Comments
(1)	Choose the appropriate-size sling for the client's weight and height. Position lift properly at the bedside.	___	___	___	_____
(2)	Position a chair near the bed and allow adequate space to manoeuvre the lift.	___	___	___	_____
(3)	Raise the bed to a high position, with the mattress flat. Lower the side rail.	___	___	___	_____
(4)	Keep the bed side rail up on the side opposite you.	___	___	___	_____
(5)	Roll the client on the side away from you.	___	___	___	_____
(6)	Place the sling under the client. Place the lower edge under the client's knees (wide piece) and the upper edge under the client's shoulders (narrow piece).	___	___	___	_____
(7)	Roll the client to the opposite side, and pull the sling through.	___	___	___	_____

Continued

	S	U	NP	Comments
(8) Roll the client supine onto the sling.	___	___	___	_____
(9) Remove the client's glasses, if present.	___	___	___	_____
(10) If you are using a transportable Hoyer lift, place the lift's horseshoe bar under the side of the bed (on the side with the chair).	___	___	___	_____
(11) Lower the horizontal bar to sling level by releasing the hydraulic valve. Lock the valve.	___	___	___	_____
(12) Attach hooks on the strap (chain) to holes in the sling. Short straps hook to top holes of the sling; longer straps hook to bottom holes of the sling.	___	___	___	_____
(13) Elevate the head of the bed.	___	___	___	_____
(14) Fold the client's arms over the chest.	___	___	___	_____
(15) Pump hydraulic handle using long, slow, even strokes until client is raised off bed. Use the steering handle to pull the lift from the bed and manoeuvre to the chair.	___	___	___	_____
(16) Position the client and slowly lower into the chair.	___	___	___	_____
(17) Close the check valve as soon as the client is down, and release straps.	___	___	___	_____
(18) Remove straps and mechanical or hydraulic lift.	___	___	___	_____
(19) Check the client's sitting alignment.	___	___	___	_____
11. Perform hand hygiene.	___	___	___	_____
12. With each transfer, evaluate the client's tolerance and level of fatigue and comfort.	___	___	___	_____
13. After each transfer, evaluate the client's body alignment.	___	___	___	_____

STUDENT: _____ DATE: _____

INSTRUCTOR: _____ DATE: _____

Skill 47–1 Assessment for Risk of Pressure Ulcer Development

	S	U	NP	Comments
1. Identify at-risk individuals needing prevention and the specific factors placing them at risk:				
A. Use a validated risk assessment tool (e.g., the Braden Scale).	___	___	___	_____
B. Assess the client on admission to the hospital, long-term care facility, home care program, or other health care facility.	___	___	___	_____
C. Inspect the condition of the client's skin at least once a day and examine all bony prominences, noting skin integrity. (Check agency policy for reassessment, and reassess at periodic intervals.) If redness or discoloration is noted, use your thumb to gently palpate area of redness. The discoloration may vary from pink to deep red.	___	___	___	_____
D. Observe all assistive devices, such as braces or casts, and medical equipment, such as nasogastric and enteral tubes and catheters, for pressure points.	___	___	___	_____
2. Determine the client's ability to respond meaningfully to pressure-related discomfort (sensory perception).	___	___	___	_____
3. Assess the degree to which the client's skin is exposed to moisture.	___	___	___	_____
4. Evaluate the client's activity level:				
A. Determine the client's ability to change and control body position (mobility).	___	___	___	_____
B. Determine client's preferred positions.	___	___	___	_____
5. Assess the client's usual food and fluid intake pattern (nutrition and hydration):				
A. Review weight pattern and nutritional laboratory values.	___	___	___	_____
B. Complete a fluid intake assessment.	___	___	___	_____
6. Evaluate the presence of friction and shear.	___	___	___	_____
7. Document the risk assessment on admission, on a regular basis according to institutional policy, and if any change in status occurs.	___	___	___	_____
A. Observe the Braden Scale scores: As they become lower, predicted risk becomes higher.	___	___	___	_____
B. Link the risk assessment to preventive protocols.	___	___	___	_____
C. Institute mild-risk interventions (score of 15–16). Plan of care should include frequent turning; maximum remobilization; off-load heel pressure; use of pressure-reducing support surface; management of moisture, nutrition, and friction and shear.	___	___	___	_____
D. Institute moderate-risk interventions (score of 13–14). Plan of care should include interventions for mild risk, as well as use of foam wedges to position the client in the 30-degree lateral position.	___	___	___	_____
E. Institute high-risk interventions (score of 10–12). Plan of care should include interventions for moderate risk, as well as instructions to turn the client with small shifts in weight.	___	___	___	_____
F. Institute very high-risk interventions (score <10). Plan of care should include interventions for high risk, as well as use of a pressure-relieving surface if the client has uncontrolled pain or severe pain exacerbated by turning.	___	___	___	_____
8. Provide education to the client and family regarding pressure ulcer risk and prevention.	___	___	___	_____
9. Evaluate measures to reduce pressure ulcer development:				
A. Observe the client's skin for areas at risk.	___	___	___	_____
B. Observe the client's tolerance for positioning.	___	___	___	_____
C. Monitor the success of a toileting program or other measures to reduce the frequency of incontinence of urine or stool.	___	___	___	_____
D. Evaluate laboratory nutrition values.	___	___	___	_____

STUDENT: _____ DATE: _____

INSTRUCTOR: _____ DATE: _____

Skill 47–2 Treating Pressure Ulcers

	S	U	NP	Comments
1. Assess the client's level of comfort, using a scale of 1–10 and the need for pain medication.	___	___	___	_____
2. Determine whether the client has allergies to topical agents.	___	___	___	_____
3. Review physician's order for topical agent or dressing.	___	___	___	_____
4. Close the room door or bedside curtains. Position the client to allow dressing removal.	___	___	___	_____
5. Perform hand hygiene, and put on clean gloves. Remove dressing and place it in a plastic bag.	___	___	___	_____
6. Assess pressure ulcer(s). All pressure ulcers need individual assessments:				
A. Note colour, type, and percentage of tissue present in the wound base.	___	___	___	_____
B. Measure width and length of the ulcer(s). Determine width by measuring the dimension from left to right and the length from top to bottom.	___	___	___	_____
C. Measure depth of pressure ulcer by using a sterile cotton-tipped applicator or other device that will allow measurement of wound depth.	___	___	___	_____
D. Measure depth of undermining, using a cotton-tipped applicator to gently probe under skin edges.	___	___	___	_____
7. Assess the periwound skin; check for maceration, redness, and denuded areas.	___	___	___	_____
8. Change to sterile gloves (check agency policy).	___	___	___	_____
9. Cleanse ulcer thoroughly with normal saline or a cleansing agent. Use an irrigating syringe for deep ulcers.	___	___	___	_____
10. Apply topical agents, as prescribed:				
A. Enzymes (where available):				
(1) Apply a thin, even layer of ointment over only necrotic areas of the ulcer. Do not apply enzyme to surrounding skin.	___	___	___	_____
(2) Apply secondary nonadherent gauze dressing directly over the ulcer.	___	___	___	_____
(3) Tape securely in place.	___	___	___	_____
B. Hydrogel:				
(1) Cover the surface of the ulcer with a thin layer of hydrogel, using the applicator or your gloved hand.	___	___	___	_____
(2) Apply secondary nonadherent gauze dressing or transparent dressing over the wound, and make it adhere to intact skin.	___	___	___	_____
C. Calcium alginate:				
(1) Lightly pack wound with alginate, using an applicator or your gloved fingers.	___	___	___	_____
(2) Apply secondary dressing of nonadherent gauze, absorbent pad, or foam over alginate. Tape in place.	___	___	___	_____
11. Remove gloves, and dispose of soiled supplies. Perform hand hygiene.	___	___	___	_____
12. Assess the pressure ulcer at each dressing change or sooner if the wound or client's condition deteriorates. Utilize the agency's tool for wound assessment.	___	___	___	_____
13. Compare wound assessment to the identified plan of care. If the wound is not progressing toward healing, as indicated by an increase in size, increased presence of pain, foul-smelling drainage, or an increase in devitalized tissue, discuss findings with the health care team.	___	___	___	_____
14. Complete wound documentation required for one of the wound assessment instruments per agency's protocol.	___	___	___	_____

STUDENT: _____ DATE: _____

INSTRUCTOR: _____ DATE: _____

Skill 47–3 Applying Dry and Moist Dressings

	S	U	NP	Comments
1. Perform hand hygiene. Obtain information about size and location of the wound.	___	___	___	_____
2. Assess the client's level of comfort.	___	___	___	_____
3. Review orders for dressing change procedure.	___	___	___	_____
4. Explain procedure to the client, and instruct the client not to touch the wound area or sterile supplies.	___	___	___	_____
5. Close the room or cubicle curtains and windows.	___	___	___	_____
6. Position the client comfortably, and drape with a bath blanket to expose only the wound site.	___	___	___	_____
7. Place a disposable bag within reach of the work area. Fold the top of bag to make a cuff.	___	___	___	_____
8. Put on a face mask and protective eyewear, if splashing occurs.	___	___	___	_____
9. Put on clean, disposable gloves, and remove tape, bandage, or ties.	___	___	___	_____
10. Remove tape: Pull parallel to skin toward dressing; remove remaining adhesive from skin.	___	___	___	_____
11. With your gloved hand, carefully remove gauze dressings one layer at a time, taking care not to dislodge drains or tubes.	___	___	___	_____
A. If dressing sticks on a wet-to-dry dressing, do not moisten it; instead, gently free the dressing, and alert the client to potential discomfort.	___	___	___	_____
12. Observe the character and amount of drainage on the dressing and the appearance of wound.	___	___	___	_____
13. Fold dressings with drainage contained inside, and remove gloves inside out. With small dressings, remove gloves inside out over the dressing. Dispose of gloves and soiled dressings in disposable bag. Perform hand hygiene.	___	___	___	_____
14. Open the sterile dressing tray or individually wrapped sterile supplies. Place on the bedside table.	___	___	___	_____
15. If ordered, cleanse or irrigate the wound:				
A. Pour the ordered solution into the sterile irrigation container.	___	___	___	_____
B. Using a syringe, gently allow the solution to flow over the wound.	___	___	___	_____
C. Continue until the irrigation flow is clear.	___	___	___	_____
D. Dry the surrounding skin.	___	___	___	_____
16. Apply dressing.				
A. Dry dressing:				
(1) Put on sterile gloves.	___	___	___	_____
(2) Inspect the wound for appearance, drains, drainage, and integrity.	___	___	___	_____
(3) Cleanse the wound with solution:				
(a) Clean from the least contaminated area to the most contaminated area.	___	___	___	_____
(4) Dry the area.	___	___	___	_____
(5) Apply sterile, dry dressing to cover the wound.	___	___	___	_____
(6) Apply topper dressing if indicated.	___	___	___	_____
B. Moist dressing:				
(1) Put on clean gloves.	___	___	___	_____
(2) Remove and discard old dressings.	___	___	___	_____
(3) Assess the surrounding skin. Discard gloves.	___	___	___	_____
(4) Put on sterile gloves.	___	___	___	_____
(5) Cleanse the wound base with normal saline or commercially prepared wound cleanser. Assess the wound base.	___	___	___	_____
(6) Moisten gauze with the prescribed solution. Gently wring out excess solution. Unfold gauze.	___	___	___	_____

Continued

512

	S	U	NP	Comments

(7) Apply gauze as a single layer directly onto the wound surface. If the wound is deep, gently pack dressing into the wound base by hand or with forceps until all wound surfaces are in contact with the gauze. If tunnelling is present, use a cotton-tipped applicator to place gauze into the tunnelled area. Be sure gauze does not touch the surrounding skin.

(8) Cover with sterile dry gauze and topper dressing.

17. Secure dressing:

A. Tape: Apply nonallergenic tape to secure dressing in place.

B. Montgomery ties.

(1) Expose adhesive surface of tape on the end of each tie.

(2) Place ties on opposite sides of the dressing.

(3) Place adhesive directly on the skin, or use a skin barrier.

C. For dressings on an extremity, secure dressing with rolled gauze or an elastic net.

18. Remove gloves, and dispose of them in the bag. Remove any mask or eyewear.

19. Dispose of supplies, and perform hand hygiene.

20. Assist the client to a comfortable position.

STUDENT: _____ DATE: _____

INSTRUCTOR: _____ DATE: _____

Skill 47–4 Performing Wound Irrigation

	S	U	NP	Comments
1. Assess the client's level of pain. Administer prescribed analgesic 30–45 minutes before starting wound irrigation procedure.	___	___	___	_____
2. Review the medical record for physician's prescription for irrigation of open wound and type of solution to be used.	___	___	___	_____
3. Assess recent recording of signs and symptoms related to client's open wound:				
A. Condition of skin and wound	___	___	___	_____
B. Elevation of body temperature	___	___	___	_____
C. Drainage from wound (amount, colour)	___	___	___	_____
D. Odour	___	___	___	_____
E. Consistency of drainage	___	___	___	_____
F. Size of wound, including depth, length, and width	___	___	___	_____
4. Explain the procedure of wound irrigation and cleansing to the client.	___	___	___	_____
5. Perform hand hygiene.	___	___	___	_____
6. Position the client comfortably to permit gravitational flow of irrigating solution through the wound and into the collection receptacle. Position the client so that the wound is vertical to the collection basin.	___	___	___	_____
7. Warm irrigation solution to approximately body temperature.	___	___	___	_____
8. Form a cuff on the waterproof bag, and place the bag near the bed.	___	___	___	_____
9. Close the room door or bed curtains.	___	___	___	_____
10. Put on gown and goggles, if needed.	___	___	___	_____
11. Put on disposable gloves, remove soiled dressing, and discard in waterproof bag. Discard gloves.	___	___	___	_____
12. Prepare equipment; open sterile supplies.	___	___	___	_____
13. Put on sterile gloves (check agency policy).	___	___	___	_____
14. Irrigating a wound with a wide opening:				
A. Fill a 35-mL syringe with irrigation solution.	___	___	___	_____
B. Attach a 19-gauge needle or angiocatheter.	___	___	___	_____
C. Hold the syringe tip 2.5 cm above the upper end of the wound and over the area being cleansed.	___	___	___	_____
D. Using continuous pressure, flush the wound; repeat Steps 14A, B, and C until the solution draining into the basin is clear.	___	___	___	_____
15. Irrigating a deep wound with a very small opening:				
A. Attach a soft angiocatheter to the filled irrigating syringe.	___	___	___	_____
B. Lubricate the tip of the catheter with irrigating solution; then gently insert the tip of the catheter and pull out about 1 cm.	___	___	___	_____
C. Using slow, continuous pressure, flush wound.	___	___	___	_____
D. Pinch off the catheter just below the syringe while keeping the catheter in place.	___	___	___	_____
E. Remove and refill the syringe. Reconnect it to the catheter, and repeat Steps 15A to D until solution draining into basin is clear.	___	___	___	_____
16. Cleanse the wound with a hand-held shower:				
A. With the client seated comfortably in the shower chair, adjust the spray to gentle flow; water temperature should be warm.	___	___	___	_____
B. Cover the showerhead with a clean washcloth, if needed.	___	___	___	_____
C. Have the client shower for 5–10 minutes with the showerhead 30 cm from the wound.	___	___	___	_____
17. Obtain cultures, if needed, after cleansing with nonbacteriostatic saline.	___	___	___	_____
18. Dry the wound edges with gauze; dry the client, if a shower or whirlpool is used.	___	___	___	_____
19. Apply appropriate dressing.	___	___	___	_____
20. Remove gloves and, if worn, mask, goggles, and gown.	___	___	___	_____
21. Dispose of equipment and soiled supplies. Perform hand hygiene.	___	___	___	_____
22. Assist the client to a comfortable position.	___	___	___	_____
23. Assess the type of tissue in the wound bed.	___	___	___	_____
24. Inspect the dressing periodically.	___	___	___	_____
25. Evaluate skin integrity.	___	___	___	_____
26. Observe the client for signs of discomfort.	___	___	___	_____
27. Observe for presence of retained irrigant.	___	___	___	_____

STUDENT: _____ DATE: _____

INSTRUCTOR: _____ DATE: _____

Skill 47–5 Applying an Abdominal or Breast Binder

	S	U	NP	Comments
1. Observe the client with a need for support of the thorax or abdomen. Observe ability to breathe deeply and cough effectively.	___	___	___	_____
2. Review the medical record for whether a medical prescription for a particular binder is required and reasons for application.	___	___	___	_____
3. Inspect the skin for actual or potential alterations in integrity. Observe for irritation, abrasion, skin surfaces that rub against each other or allergic response to adhesive tape used to secure dressing.	___	___	___	_____
4. Inspect any surgical dressing.				
5. Assess the client's comfort level, using an analogue scale of 0–10, noting any objective signs and symptoms of pain.	___	___	___	_____
6. Gather necessary data regarding the size of client and appropriate binder.	___	___	___	_____
7. Explain the procedure to the client.	___	___	___	_____
8. Teach the skill to the client or significant other.	___	___	___	_____
9. Perform hand hygiene and put on gloves (if you are likely to contact wound drainage).	___	___	___	_____
10. Close the curtains or room door.	___	___	___	_____
11. Apply the binder.				
A. Abdominal binder:				
(1) Position the client in the supine position with the head slightly elevated and knees slightly flexed.	___	___	___	_____
(2) Fanfold the far side of the binder toward the midline of the binder.	___	___	___	_____
(3) Instruct and help the client to roll away from you toward the raised side rail while firmly supporting the abdominal incision and dressing with hands.	___	___	___	_____
(4) Place the fan-folded ends of the binder under the client.	___	___	___	_____
(5) Instruct or assist client to roll over the folded ends.	___	___	___	_____
(6) Unfold and stretch the ends out smoothly on the far side of the bed.	___	___	___	_____
(7) Instruct the client to roll back into the supine position.	___	___	___	_____
(8) Adjust the binder so that the supine client is centred over the binder; use the symphysis pubis and costal margins as lower and upper landmarks.	___	___	___	_____
(9) Close the binder. Pull one end of the binder over the centre of the client's abdomen. While maintaining tension on that end of the binder, pull the opposite end of binder over the centre and secure with Velcro closure tabs, metal fasteners, or horizontally placed safety pins.	___	___	___	_____
B. Breast binder:				
(1) Assist the client in placing arms through the binder's armholes.	___	___	___	_____
(2) Assist the client to the supine position in bed.	___	___	___	_____
(3) Pad the area under the breasts, if necessary.	___	___	___	_____
(4) Using Velcro closure tabs or horizontally placed safety pins, secure the binder at nipple level first. Continue closure process above and then below the nipple line until the entire binder is closed.	___	___	___	_____
(5) Make appropriate adjustments, including individualizing fit of shoulder straps and pinning waistline darts to reduce binder size.	___	___	___	_____
(6) Instruct the client in self-care related to reapplying breast binder, and observe skill development.	___	___	___	_____
12. Remove gloves, and perform hand hygiene.	___	___	___	_____
13. Assess the client's comfort level, using an analogue scale of 0–10, noting any objective signs and symptoms.	___	___	___	_____
14. Adjust the binder, as necessary.	___	___	___	_____
15. Observe the site for skin integrity, circulation, and characteristics of the wound. (Periodically remove binder and surgical dressing to assess wound characteristics.)	___	___	___	_____
16. Assess the client's ability to ventilate properly.				
17. Identify the client's need for assistance with activities such as hair combing.	___	___	___	_____

STUDENT: _____ DATE: _____

INSTRUCTOR: _____ DATE: _____

Skill 47–6 Applying an Elastic Bandage

	S	U	NP	Comments
1. Perform hand hygiene and put on gloves, if needed. Inspect the client's skin for alterations in integrity as indicated by abrasions, discoloration, chafing, or edema. (Look carefully at bony prominences.)	___	___	___	_____
2. Inspect surgical dressing. Remove gloves and perform hand hygiene.	___	___	___	_____
3. Observe adequacy of circulation (distal to bandage) by noting surface temperature, skin colour, and sensation of body parts to be wrapped.	___	___	___	_____
4. Review the medical record for specific orders related to application of elastic bandage. Note the area to be covered, the type of bandage required, the frequency of change, and previous response to treatment.	___	___	___	_____
5. Identify client's and primary caregiver's current knowledge level of skill, if bandaging will be continued at home.	___	___	___	_____
6. Explain the procedure to the client.				
7. Teach the skill to the client or primary caregiver.	___	___	___	_____
8. Perform hand hygiene and put on gloves if drainage is present.	___	___	___	_____
9. Close the room door or curtains.	___	___	___	_____
10. Help the client assume a comfortable, anatomically correct position.	___	___	___	_____
11. Hold a roll of elastic bandage in your dominant hand, and use your other hand to lightly hold beginning of bandage at the distal body part. Continue transferring roll to dominant hand as bandage is wrapped.	___	___	___	_____
12. Apply bandage from the distal point toward the proximal boundary, using a variety of turns to cover various shapes of body parts.	___	___	___	_____
13. Unroll and very slightly stretch bandage.	___	___	___	_____
14. Overlap turns by one-half to two-thirds' width of the bandage roll.	___	___	___	_____
15. Secure the first bandage with a clip or tape before applying additional rolls.	___	___	___	_____
16. Apply additional rolls without leaving any skin surface uncovered. Secure the last bandage applied.	___	___	___	_____
17. Remove gloves, if worn, and perform hand hygiene.	___	___	___	_____
A. Assess distal circulation when the bandage application is complete and at least twice during the next 8-hour period.	___	___	___	_____
B. Observe skin colour for pallor or cyanosis.	___	___	___	_____
C. Palpate skin for warmth.	___	___	___	_____
D. Palpate pulses and compare bilaterally.	___	___	___	_____
E. Ask whether the client is aware of pain, numbness, tingling, or other discomfort.	___	___	___	_____
F. Observe mobility of the extremity.	___	___	___	_____
18. Have the client demonstrate bandage application.	___	___	___	_____

STUDENT: _____   DATE: _____

INSTRUCTOR: _____   DATE: _____

Skill 49–1 Demonstrating Postoperative Exercises

	S	U	NP	Comments
1. Assess the client for risk of postoperative respiratory complications. Review the medical history to identify the presence of chronic pulmonary conditions (e.g., emphysema, chronic bronchitis, asthma), any condition that affects chest wall movement, history of smoking, and presence of reduced hemoglobin.	___	___	___	_____
2. Assess the client's ability to cough and breathe deeply by having the client take a deep breath and observing movement of shoulders and chest wall. Measure chest excursion during deep breath. Ask the client to cough after taking a deep breath.	___	___	___	_____
3. Assess risk for postoperative thrombus formation. (Older clients, those with active cancer, and those immobilized for more than 3 days are most at risk.) Observe for localized tenderness along the distribution of the venous system, swollen calf or thigh, calf swelling more than 3 cm in comparison with asymptomatic leg, pitting edema in symptomatic leg, and collateral superficial veins. If any of these signs are present, notify the physician.	___	___	___	_____
4. Assess the client's ability to move independently while in bed.	___	___	___	_____
5. Explain postoperative exercises to the client, including their importance to recovery and physiological benefits.	___	___	___	_____
6. Demonstrate exercises:				
A. Diaphragmatic breathing:				
(1) Assist the client to a comfortable sitting position on the side of the bed or in a chair or to standing position.	___	___	___	_____
(2) Stand or sit facing the client.	___	___	___	_____
(3) Instruct the client to place the palms of the hands across from each other, down and along the lower borders of the anterior rib cage. Place the tips of the third fingers lightly together. Demonstrate for the client.	___	___	___	_____
(4) Have the client take slow, deep breaths, inhaling through the nose and pushing the abdomen against the hands. Tell the client to feel the middle fingers separate during inhalation. Demonstrate.	___	___	___	_____
(5) Explain that the client will feel normal downward movement of the diaphragm during inspiration. Explain that abdominal organs descend and the chest wall expands.	___	___	___	_____
(6) Avoid using auxiliary chest and shoulder muscles while inhaling, and instruct client in the same manner.	___	___	___	_____
(7) Have the client hold a slow, deep breath for count of three and then slowly exhale through the mouth as if blowing out a candle (with pursed lips). Tell the client that the middle fingertips will touch as the chest wall contracts.	___	___	___	_____
(8) Repeat breathing exercise three to five times.	___	___	___	_____
(9) Have the client practise the exercise. Instruct the client to take 10 slow, deep breaths every hour while awake during postoperative period until mobile.	___	___	___	_____
B. Incentive spirometry:				
(1) Perform hand hygiene.	___	___	___	_____
(2) Instruct the client to assume semi-Fowler's or high-Fowler's position.	___	___	___	_____
(3) Either set or indicate to the client on the device scale the volume level to be attained with each breath.	___	___	___	_____
(4) Demonstrate to the client how to place the mouthpiece of the spirometer so that the lips completely cover it.	___	___	___	_____
(5) Instruct client to inhale slowly and maintain constant flow through the unit, attempting to reach goal volume. When maximal inspiration is reached, the client should hold breath for 2–3 seconds and then exhale slowly. Number of breaths should not exceed 10–12 per minute in each session.	___	___	___	_____
(6) Instruct the client to breathe normally for short period.	___	___	___	_____

Continued

	S	U	NP	Comments

(7) Have the client repeat the manoeuvre until goals are achieved.

(8) Perform hand hygiene.

C. Positive expiratory pressure (PEP) therapy and "huff" coughing:

(1) Perform hand hygiene.

(2) Set PEP device to the setting ordered.

(3) Instruct the client to assume semi-Fowler's or high-Fowler's position, and place nose clip on the client's nose.

(4) Have the client place lips around the mouthpiece. The client should take a full breath and then exhale two to three times longer than inhalation. This pattern should be repeated for 10–20 breaths.

(5) Remove device from the client's mouth and have the client take a slow, deep breath and hold for 3 seconds.

(6) Instruct the client to exhale in quick, short, forced inhalations, or "huffs."

D. Controlled coughing:

(1) Explain the importance of maintaining an upright position.

(2) Demonstrate coughing. Take two slow, deep breaths, inhaling through the nose and exhaling through the mouth.

(3) Inhale deeply a third time and hold breath to a count of three. Cough fully for two or three consecutive coughs without inhaling between coughs. (Tell the client to push all air out of lungs.)

(4) Caution the client against simply clearing the throat instead of coughing. Explain that coughing will not cause injury to the incision when done correctly.

(5) If the surgical incision will be abdominal or thoracic, teach the client to place one hand over the incisional area and the other hand on top of it. During breathing and coughing exercises, the client presses gently against incisional area to splint or support it. A pillow over the incision is optional.

(6) The client continues to practise coughing exercises, splinting the imaginary incision. Instruct the client to cough two to three times every 2 hours while awake.

(7) Instruct the client to examine any sputum for consistency, odour, amount, and colour changes.

E. Turning:

(1) Instruct the client to assume the supine position and move to the side of the bed if permitted by surgery. Have the client move by bending knees and pressing heels against the mattress to raise and move buttocks. Top side rails on both sides of the bed should be raised.

(2) Instruct the client to place the right hand over the incisional area to splint it.

(3) Instruct the client to keep the right leg straight and flex the left knee up. If back or vascular surgery is being performed, the client will need to logroll or will require assistance with turning.

(4) Have the client grab the right side rail with the left hand, pull toward the right, and roll onto the right side.

(5) Instruct the client to turn every 2 hours while awake.

F. Leg exercises:

(1) Have the client assume the supine position in bed. Demonstrate leg exercises by performing passive range-of-motion exercises and simultaneously explaining exercise.

(2) Rotate each ankle in a complete circle. Instruct the client to draw imaginary circles with the big toe. Repeat five times.

(3) Alternate dorsiflexion and plantar flexion of both feet. Direct the client to feel calf muscles contract and relax alternately. Repeat five times.

(4) Perform quadriceps setting by tightening thigh muscles and bringing the knee down toward the mattress, then relaxing. Repeat five times.

Continued

	S	U	NP	Comments
(5) Have the client alternately raise each leg straight up from the bed surface, keeping legs straight, and then have the client bend the leg at the hip and knee. Repeat five times.	___	___	___	_____
7. Have the client practise exercises at least every 2 hours while awake. Instruct the client to coordinate turning and leg exercises with diaphragmatic breathing, incentive spirometry, and coughing exercises.	___	___	___	_____
8. Observe the client's ability to perform all five exercises independently.	___	___	___	_____

Answer Key for Study Guide Review Questions

Chapter 1

1. The correct answer is d.
2. The correct answer is a.
3. The correct answer is a.
4. The correct answer is b.
5. The correct answer is c.
6. The correct answer is b.
7. The correct answer is c.
8. The correct answer is b.
9. The correct answer is d.
10. The correct answer is c.

Chapter 2

1. The correct answer is a.
2. The correct answer is c.
3. The correct answer is a.
4. The correct answer is b.
5. The correct answer is b.

Chapter 3

1. The correct answer is a.
2. The correct answer is d.
3. The correct answer is b.
4. The correct answer is b.
5. The correct answer is a.

Chapter 4

1. The correct answer is c.
2. The correct answer is a.
3. The correct answer is a.
4. The correct answer is d.
5. The correct answer is c.

Chapter 5

1. The correct answer is b.
2. The correct answer is d.
3. The correct answer is b.

Chapter 6

1. The correct answer is a.
2. The correct answer is a.
3. The correct answer is d.
4. The correct answer is c.
5. The correct answer is c.

Chapter 7

1. The correct answer is a.
2. The correct answer is d.
3. The correct answer is c.
4. The correct answer is b.
5. The correct answer is c.

Chapter 8

1. The correct answer is a.
2. The correct answer is c.
3. The correct answer is c.
4. The correct answer is b.
5. The correct answer is a.

Chapter 9

1. The correct answer is a.
2. The correct answer is d.
3. The correct answer is b.
4. The correct answer is d.
5. The correct answer is d.
6. The correct answer is d.
7. The correct answer is a.
8. The correct answer is b.
9. The correct answer is b.
10. The correct answer is d.

Chapter 10

1. The correct answer is b.
2. The correct answer is b.
3. The correct answer is a.
4. The correct answer is b.
5. The correct answer is c.

Chapter 11

1. The correct answer is c.
2. The correct answer is c.
3. The correct answer is d.
4. The correct answer is c.
5. The correct answer is c.

Chapter 12

1. The correct answer is b.
2. The correct answer is c.
3. The correct answer is a.
4. The correct answer is b.

Chapter 13

1. The correct answer is c.
2. The correct answer is d.

3. The correct answer is b.
4. The correct answer is d.

Chapter 14

1. The correct answer is d.
2. The correct answer is c.
3. The correct answer is d.
4. The correct answer is c.

Chapter 15

1. The correct answer is c.
2. The correct answer is c.

Chapter 16

1. The correct answer is b.
2. The correct answer is c.
3. The correct answer is c.
4. The correct answer is c.
5. The correct answer is d.

Chapter 17

1. The correct answer is b.
2. The correct answer is d.
3. The correct answer is a.
4. The correct answer is a.
5. The correct answer is c.
6. The correct answer is d.

Chapter 18

1. The correct answer is a.
2. The correct answer is b.
3. The correct answer is b.
4. The correct answer is b.
5. The correct answer is a.

Chapter 19

1. The correct answer is c.
2. The correct answer is c.
3. The correct answer is d.
4. The correct answer is a.
5. The correct answer is c.
6. The correct answer is d.

Chapter 20

1. The correct answer is a.
2. The correct answer is c.

3. The correct answer is a.
4. The correct answer is c.
5. The correct answer is d.
6. The correct answer is c.

Chapter 21

1. The correct answer is b.
2. The correct answer is c.
3. The correct answer is d.
4. The correct answer is c.
5. The correct answer is b.

Chapter 22

1. The correct answer is b.
2. The correct answer is d.
3. The correct answer is a.
4. The correct answer is c.
5. The correct answer is d.

Chapter 23

1. The correct answer is c.
2. The correct answer is d.
3. The correct answer is d.
4. The correct answer is d.
5. The correct answer is d.
6. The correct answer is d.

Chapter 24

1. The correct answer is b.
2. The correct answer is b.
3. The correct answer is c.
4. The correct answer is a.
5. The correct answer is a.

Chapter 25

1. The correct answer is b.
2. The correct answer is a.
3. The correct answer is c.
4. The correct answer is b.

Chapter 26

1. The correct answer is b.
2. The correct answer is c.
3. The correct answer is a.
4. The correct answer is c.
5. The correct answer is d.

Chapter 27

1. The correct answer is b.
2. The correct answer is d.
3. The correct answer is c.
4. The correct answer is a.
5. The correct answer is d.

Chapter 28

1. The correct answer is a.
2. The correct answer is a.
3. The correct answer is b.
4. The correct answer is c.
5. The correct answer is a.

Chapter 29

1. The correct answer is b.
2. The correct answer is b.
3. The correct answer is c.
4. The correct answer is b.

Chapter 30

1. The correct answer is d.
2. The correct answer is a.
3. The correct answer is a.
4. The correct answer is a.
5. The correct answer is d.

Chapter 31

1. The correct answer is d.
2. The correct answer is d.
3. The correct answer is b.
4. The correct answer is c.
5. The correct answer is c.

Chapter 32

1. The correct answer is d.
2. The correct answer is a.
3. The correct answer is c.
4. The correct answer is c.
5. The correct answer is c.
6. The correct answer is d.

Chapter 33

1. The correct answer is d.
2. The correct answer is b.

3. The correct answer is d.
4. The correct answer is a.
5. The correct answer is b.
6. The correct answer is b.

Chapter 34

1. The correct answer is b.
2. The correct answer is a.
3. The correct answer is a.
4. The correct answer is a.
5. The correct answer is b.
6. The correct answer is a.

Chapter 35

1. The correct answer is c.
2. The correct answer is b.
3. The correct answer is d.
4. The correct answer is a.

Chapter 36

1. The correct answer is c.
2. The correct answer is b.
3. The correct answer is a.
4. The correct answer is d.

Chapter 37

1. The correct answer is d.
2. The correct answer is d.
3. The correct answer is c.
4. The correct answer is d.
5. The correct answer is a.

Chapter 38

1. The correct answer is b.
2. The correct answer is a.
3. The correct answer is c.
4. The correct answer is b.
5. The correct answer is c.

Chapter 39

1. The correct answer is a.
2. The correct answer is c.
3. The correct answer is b.
4. The correct answer is b.
5. The correct answer is d.
6. The correct answer is b.

526

Chapter 40

1. The correct answer is b.
2. The correct answer is c.
3. The correct answer is a.
4. The correct answer is c.
5. The correct answer is b.

Chapter 41

1. The correct answer is a.
2. The correct answer is a.
3. The correct answer is c.
4. The correct answer is d.
5. The correct answer is b.

Chapter 42

1. The correct answer is b.
2. The correct answer is d.
3. The correct answer is a.
4. The correct answer is b.
5. The correct answer is c.

Chapter 43

1. The correct answer is c.
2. The correct answer is d.
3. The correct answer is c.
4. The correct answer is c.
5. The correct answer is d
6. The correct answer is c.

Chapter 44

1. The correct answer is a.
2. The correct answer is b.
3. The correct answer is c.
4. The correct answer is a.
5. The correct answer is d.

Chapter 45

1. The correct answer is b.
2. The correct answer is a.
3. The correct answer is c.
4. The correct answer is b.
5. The correct answer is c.

Chapter 46

1. The correct answer is a.
2. The correct answer is d.
3. The correct answer is d.
4. The correct answer is a.

5. The correct answer is b.
6. The correct answer is d.

Chapter 47

1. The correct answer is b.
2. The correct answer is b.
3. The correct answer is a.
4. The correct answer is c.
5. The correct answer is b.
6. The correct answer is d.

Chapter 48

1. The correct answer is c.
2. The correct answer is a.
3. The correct answer is b.
4. The correct answer is c.
5. The correct answer is a.

Chapter 49

1. The correct answer is d.
2. The correct answer is c.
3. The correct answer is b.
4. The correct answer is a.
5. The correct answer is b.

Answers to Critical Thinking Models

528

KNOWLEDGE

- Components of self-concept (identity, body image, self-esteem, role performance)
- Self-concept stressors related to identity, body image, self-esteem, and role
- Therapeutic communication principles, nonverbal indicators of distress
- Cultural factors that influence self-concept
- Growth and development (middle-aged adult)
- Pharmacological effects of medicine (pain medication)

EXPERIENCE

- Caring for a client who had an alteration in body image, self-esteem, role, or identity
- Personal experience of threat to self-concept

Assessment

- Observe Ms. Johnson's behaviours that suggest an alteration in self-concept
- Assess Ms. Johnson's cultural background
- Assess Ms. Johnson's coping skills and resources
- Converse with Ms. Johnson to determine her feelings and perceptions about changes in body image
- Assess the quality of Ms. Johnson's relationships

STANDARDS

- Support Ms. Johnson's autonomy to make choices and express values that support positive self-concept
- Apply intellectual standards of relevance and plausibility for care to be acceptable to Ms. Johnson
- Safeguard Ms. Johnson's right to privacy by judiciously protecting information of a confidential nature

QUALITIES

- Display curiosity in considering why Ms. Johnson might be behaving or responding in this manner
- Display integrity when beliefs and values differ from Ms. Johnson's; admit to any inconsistencies in own values or in the client's
- Risk-taking may be necessary in developing a trusting relationship with Ms. Johnson

CHAPTER 26   Critical Thinking Model for Nursing Care Plan for *Disturbed Body Image* (page 121).

KNOWLEDGE

- A basic understanding of sexual development, sexual orientation, sociocultural dimensions, the impact of self-concept, sexually transmitted infections, safer sex practices
- Ways to phrase questions regarding sexuality and functioning
- Disease conditions that affect sexual functioning
- How interpersonal relationship factors may affect sexual functioning

EXPERIENCE

- Explore your discomfort with discussing topics related to sexuality and develop a plan for addressing these discomforts
- Reflect on your personal sexual experiences and how you have responded

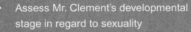

Assessment

- Assess Mr. Clement's developmental stage in regard to sexuality
- Consider self-concept as a factor that will influence sexual satisfaction and functioning
- Perform physical assessment of urogenital area
- Determine Mr. Clement's sexual concerns
- Assess safer sex practices and the use of contraception
- Assess the medical conditions and medications that may be affecting his sexual functioning
- Assess the impact of high-risk behaviours on sexual health

STANDARDS

- Apply intellectual standards of relevance and plausibility for care to be acceptable to Mr. Clement
- Safeguard Mr. Clement's right to privacy by judiciously protecting information of a confidential nature
- Apply the principles of ethic of care

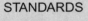

QUALITIES

- Display curiosity, consider why Mr. Clement might behave or respond in a particular manner
- Display integrity; your beliefs and values may differ from Mr. Clement's
- Admit to any inconsistencies in your and Mr. Clement's values
- Risk-taking: Be willing to explore both your and Mr. Clement's sexual issues and concerns

CHAPTER 27 Critical Thinking Model for Nursing Care Plan for *Sexual Dysfunction* (page 128).

KNOWLEDGE

- The concepts of faith, hope, spiritual well-being, and religion
- Caring practices in the individual approach to a client
- Available services in the community (health care professionals and agencies)

EXPERIENCE

- Your past experience in selecting interventions that support a client's spiritual well-being

Planning

- Collaborate with James and his family on choice of interventions
- Consult with pastoral care or other clergy or spiritual leaders as appropriate
- Incorporate religious rituals specific to James
- Ask if the client's expectations have been met

STANDARDS

- Standards of autonomy and self-determination to support James's decisions about the plan

QUALITIES

- Exhibit confidence in your skills and know how to develop a trusting relationship with James
- Be open to any possible conflict between the client's opinion and yours; decide how to reach mutually beneficial outcomes

CHAPTER 28   Critical Thinking Model for Nursing Care Plan for *Spiritual Distress*
(page 133).

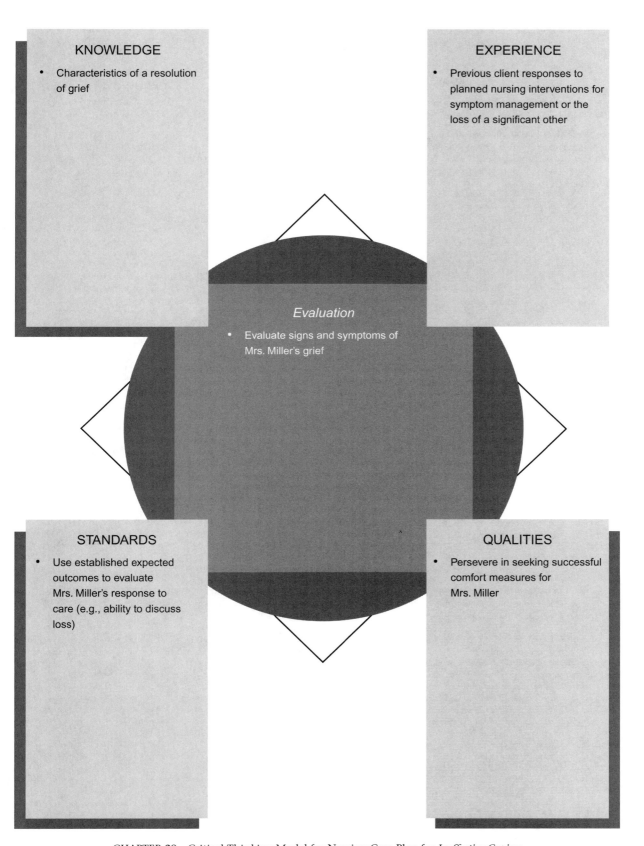

KNOWLEDGE
- Characteristics of a resolution of grief

EXPERIENCE
- Previous client responses to planned nursing interventions for symptom management or the loss of a significant other

Evaluation
- Evaluate signs and symptoms of Mrs. Miller's grief

STANDARDS
- Use established expected outcomes to evaluate Mrs. Miller's response to care (e.g., ability to discuss loss)

QUALITIES
- Persevere in seeking successful comfort measures for Mrs. Miller

CHAPTER 29   Critical Thinking Model for Nursing Care Plan for *Ineffective Coping*
(page 139).

KNOWLEDGE

- Characteristics of adaptive behaviours
- Characteristics of continuing stress response
- Differentiation of stress and trauma

EXPERIENCE

- Previous client responses to planned nursing interventions

Evaluation

- Reassess Carl for the presence of new or recurring stress-related problems or symptoms (fatigue, changes in energy level, weight, or eating habits)
- Determine if change in care promoted Carl's adaptation to stress
- Evaluate if Carl's expectations have been achieved

STANDARDS

- Use established expected outcomes to evaluate Carl's plan of care (rest and relaxation, stable weight, positive feelings about wife and their relationship)
- Apply the intellectual standard of relevance; be sure that Carl achieves his goals relevant to his needs

QUALITIES

- Demonstrate perseverance in redesigning interventions to promote Carl's adaptation to stress
- Display integrity in accurately evaluating nursing interventions

CHAPTER 30   Critical Thinking Model for Nursing Care Plan for *Caregiver Role Strain*
(page 145).

KNOWLEDGE

- Understand the role of physiotherapists and exercise trainers in improving Mrs. Wertenberger's level of activity and exercise pattern
- Determine Mrs. Wertenberger's ability to increase her level of activity
- Assess the impact of medication on Mrs. Wertenberger's activity tolerance

EXPERIENCE

- Eric needs to consider previous client and personal experiences with therapies designed to improve exercise and activity tolerance
- Eric's personal experience with exercise regimens

Planning

- Eric needs to consult and collaborate with members of the health care team to increase Mrs. Wertenberger's activity
- Involve Mrs. Wertenberger and her family in designing an activity and exercise plan
- Eric needs to consider Mrs. Wertenberger's ability to increase her activity level and follow an exercise program

STANDARDS

- Therapies need to be individualized to Mrs. Wertenberger's activity tolerance
- Eric needs to apply the goals of the Health Canada Physical Activity Unit

QUALITIES

- Eric needs to be responsible and creative in designing interventions to improve Mrs. Wertenberger's activity tolerance

CHAPTER 36   Critical Thinking Model for Nursing Care Plan for *Activity Intolerance*
(page 204).

534

KNOWLEDGE

- Basic human needs
- The potential risks to a client's safety from physical and environmental hazards
- The influence of developmental stage on safety needs (older adult)
- The influence of illness and medications on Ms. Cohen's safety (consider the factors of immobilization and visual impairment)

EXPERIENCE

- Mr. Key's past experiences of caring for clients with mobility or sensory impairments that threaten safety
- Personal experiences in caring for older adults

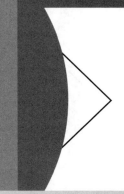

Assessment

- Identification of actual and potential threats to Ms. Cohen's safety
- Determine the impact of Ms. Cohen's underlying disease on her safety
- Identify the presence of risks for Ms. Cohen's developmental stage

STANDARDS

- Mr. Key needs to apply intellectual standards of accuracy, significance, completeness, and fairness when assessing for threats to Ms. Cohen's safety
- Apply all prevention or restraint protocols

QUALITIES

- Perseverance is needed when identifying all threats to Ms. Cohen's safety
- Responsibility for collecting unbiased accurate data regarding threats to Ms. Cohen's safety
- Fairness is appropriate to objectively evaluate the risk to Ms. Cohen's safety within the home and the community

CHAPTER 37   Critical Thinking Model for Nursing Care Plan for *Risk for Injury* (page 210).

KNOWLEDGE

- Theoretical knowledge about the structure of the feet
- Etiology of diabetic foot ulcers
- Collection of subjective and objective data regarding the feet and foot care
- Principles of comfort and safety
- Adult learning principles when teaching the client and his family about foot care
- Resources and services available through community agencies

EXPERIENCE

- Assessment skills
- Communication skills
- Care of previous clients with diabetes mellitus
- Care of previous client with diabetic foot ulcers

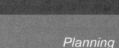

Planning

- Involve Mr. James and his family in planning, evaluating, and follow-up of foot care
- Know community services and resources that would assist Mr. James in regaining optimal health of his feet

STANDARDS

- Individualize the foot care to include Mr. James's preferences
- Apply standards of safety and promotion of client dignity
- Practice standards as set out by the educational institution and CARN (Canadian Association of Registered Nurses)
- Apply foot care guidelines from the Canadian Diabetes Association regarding prevention and management of diabetic foot ulcers

QUALITIES

- Use inquiry and critical and creative thinking when developing a self-care plan for the client
- Take responsibility for following standards of good hygiene practice
- Employ a caring, empathetic attitude

CHAPTER 38   Critical Thinking Model for Nursing Care Plan for *Ineffective Tissue Perfusion, Improper Foot Care and Hygiene*
(page 218).

KNOWLEDGE

- Cardiac and respiratory anatomy and physiology
- Cardiopulmonary pathophysiology
- Clinical signs and symptoms of altered oxygenation
- Developmental factors affecting oxygenation
- Impact on lifestyle
- Environmental impact

EXPERIENCE

- Caring for clients with impaired oxygenation, activity intolerance, and respiratory infections
- Observations of changes in client respiratory patterns made during poor air quality days
- Personal experience with how a change in altitude or physical conditioning affects respiratory patterns
- Personal experience with respiratory infections or cardiopulmonary alterations

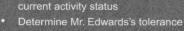

Assessment

- Identify recurring and present signs and symptoms associated with Mr. Edwards's impaired oxygenation
- Determine the presence of risk factors that apply to Mr. Edwards
- Ask Mr. Edwards about his use of medication
- Determine Mr. Edwards's normal and current activity status
- Determine Mr. Edwards's tolerance to activity

STANDARDS

- Apply intellectual standards of clarity, precision, specificity, and accuracy when obtaining a health history from Mr. Edwards

QUALITIES

- Carry out the responsibility of obtaining correct information about Mr. Edwards
- Display confidence while assessing the extent of Mr. Edwards's respiratory alterations

CHAPTER 39   Critical Thinking Model for the Nursing Care Plan for *Ineffective Airway Clearance/Retained Secretions* (page 230).

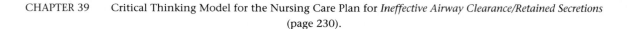

KNOWLEDGE

Consider the following:
- The role of the other health care professionals caring for Mrs. Topping
- The impact of specific fluid regimens on Mrs. Topping's fluid balance
- The effects of new medications on Mrs. Topping's fluid balance

EXPERIENCE

- Consider the previous clinical assignments you have had and how those clients responded to nursing therapies (what worked and what did not)

Planning

- Select nursing interventions to promote fluid, electrolyte, and acid–base balance
- Consult with pharmacists, nutritionists, and intravenous therapy specialists
- Involve Mrs. Topping and her family in designing the interventions

STANDARDS

- Therapies need to be individualized to Mrs. Topping's fluid balance and acid–base requirements
- Apply agency and professional standards for prevention of intravascular infections

QUALITIES

- Use creativity to plan interventions that will achieve fluid balance and integrate those into Mrs. Topping's activities of daily living
- Be responsible in planning nursing interventions consistent with the client's fluid balance and acid–base requirements and with standards of practice

CHAPTER 40　Critical Thinking Model for Nursing Care Plan for *Fluid, Electrolyte, and Acid–Base Balances* (page 243).

KNOWLEDGE

- The characteristics of a desirable sleep pattern
- Behaviours reflecting adequate sleep

EXPERIENCE

- Previous client's responses to planned nursing interventions for promoting sleep
- Previous experience in adapting sleep therapies to personal needs

Evaluation

- Evaluate signs and symptoms of Julie's sleep disturbance
- Review Julie's sleep pattern
- Ask Julie's sleep partner to report her response to sleep therapies
- Ask Julie if her expectations of care are being met

STANDARDS

- Use of established expected outcomes to evaluate Julie's responses to care (e.g., improved duration of sleep, fewer awakenings)

QUALITIES

- Demonstrate humility if an intervention is unsuccessful; rethink your approach
- In the case of chronic sleep problems, display perseverance in staying with the plan of care or in trying new approaches

CHAPTER 41   Critical Thinking Model for Nursing Care Plan for *Disturbed Sleep Pattern* (page 252).

KNOWLEDGE

- Physiology of pain
- Factors that potentially increase or decrease responses to pain
- Pathophysiology of conditions causing pain
- Awareness of biases affecting pain assessment and treatment
- Cultural variations in how pain is expressed
- Knowledge of nonverbal communication

EXPERIENCE

- Caring for clients with acute, chronic, and cancer pain
- Caring for clients who experienced pain as a result of a health care therapy
- Personal experience with pain

Assessment

- Determine Mrs. Mays's perspective of pain, including history of pain, its meaning, and physical, emotional, and social effects
- Measure objectively the characteristics of Mrs. Mays's pain
- Review potential factors affecting Mrs. Mays's pain

STANDARDS

- Refer to AHCPR and RNAO guidelines for acute pain assessment and management
- Apply intellectual standards (e.g., clarity, specificity, accuracy, and completeness) when performing the pain assessment

QUALITIES

- Persevere in exploring causes and possible solutions for chronic pain
- Display confidence when assessing pain to relieve Mrs. Mays's anxiety
- Display integrity and fairness to prevent prejudice from affecting assessment

CHAPTER 42 Critical Thinking Model for Nursing Care Plan for *Acute Pain*
(page 260).

KNOWLEDGE

- Roles of dietitians and nutritionists in caring for clients with altered nutrition
- Impact of community support groups and other resources in assisting clients to manage nutrition
- Impact of inappropriate diets on clients' overall nutritional status

EXPERIENCE

- Previous client responses to nursing interventions for altered nutrition
- Personal experiences with dietary change strategies (what worked and what did not)

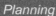

Planning

- Select nursing interventions to promote optimal nutrition
- Select nursing interventions consistent with therapeutic diets
- Consult with other health care professionals (dietitians, nutritionists, physicians, pharmacists, physiotherapists, and occupational therapists) to adopt interventions that reflect Mrs. Cooper's needs
- Involve Mrs. Cooper's family when designing interventions
- Plan regular follow-up and revise interventions to respond to Mrs. Cooper's changing nutritional status

STANDARDS

- Individualize therapy according to client needs
- Select therapies consistent with professional standards of nutrition
- Select therapies consistent with established standards for therapeutic diets

QUALITIES

- Display confidence when selecting interventions
- Creatively adapt interventions for the client's physical limitations, culture, personal preferences, budget, and home care needs

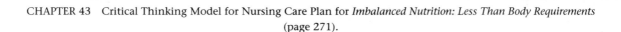

CHAPTER 43 Critical Thinking Model for Nursing Care Plan for *Imbalanced Nutrition: Less Than Body Requirements* (page 271).

KNOWLEDGE

- Physiology of fluid balance
- Anatomy and physiology of normal urine production and urination
- Pathophysiology of selected urinary alterations
- Factors affecting urination
- Principles of communication used to address issues related to self-concept and sexuality

EXPERIENCE

- Caring for clients with alterations in urinary elimination
- Caring for clients at risk for urinary infection
- Personal experience with changes in urinary elimination

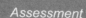

Assessment

- Gather health history of the urination pattern, symptoms, and factors affecting urination
- Conduct a physical assessment of body systems potentially affected by urinary change
- Assess the characteristics of urine
- Assess Mrs. Grayson's perception of urinary problems as it affects her self-concept

STANDARDS

- Maintain Mrs. Grayson's privacy and dignity
- Apply intellectual standards to ensure history and assessment are complete and in depth
- Apply agency and professional standards of care from professional organizations such as the CNA and the Canadian Continence Foundation

QUALITIES

- Display humility in recognizing limitations in knowledge
- Establish trust with Mrs. Grayson to encourage her to reveal the full picture of this potentially sensitive topic

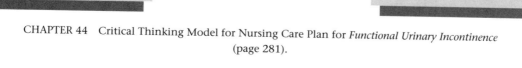

CHAPTER 44 Critical Thinking Model for Nursing Care Plan for *Functional Urinary Incontinence* (page 281).

KNOWLEDGE

- Role of the other health care professionals in returning the client's bowel elimination pattern to normal
- Impact of specific therapeutic diets and medication on bowel elimination patterns
- Expected results of cathartics, laxatives, and enemas on bowel elimination

EXPERIENCE

- Previous client response to planned nursing therapies for improving bowel elimination (what worked and what did not)

Planning

- Javier needs to select nursing interventions to promote normal bowel elimination
- Consult with nutritionists
- Involve Larry and his family in designing nursing interventions

STANDARDS

- Individualize therapies to Larry's bowel elimination needs
- Select therapies that comply with wound and ostomy professional practice standards

QUALITIES

- Javier needs to be creative when planning interventions for Larry to achieve normal bowel elimination patterns
- He should display independence when integrating interventions from other disciplines in Larry's plan of care
- He must act responsibly by ensuring that interventions are consistent within standards

CHAPTER 45   Critical Thinking Model for Nursing Care Plan for *Constipation*
(page 290).

KNOWLEDGE

- Effects of improved mobility status on all physiological systems and the client's psychosocial and developmental status

EXPERIENCE

- Previous client responses to planned mobility interventions
- Level of weakness may not permit active transfer

Evaluation

- Reassess Ms. Adams for signs and symptoms of improved or decreased mobility status
- Ask for Ms. Adams's perceptions of her mobility status after the intervention
- Ask if Ms. Adams's expectations of care have been met
- Ask for Ms. Adams's suggestions for increasing mobility

STANDARDS

- Use established expected outcomes for Ms. Adams's plan of care (e.g., lung fields remain clear) to evaluate her response to care

QUALITIES

- Display humility when identifying those interventions that were not successful
- Use creativity when redesigning new interventions to improve Ms. Adams's mobility status
- Display confidence with early interventions

CHAPTER 46   Critical Thinking Model for Nursing Care Plan for *Impaired Physical Mobility*
(page 298).

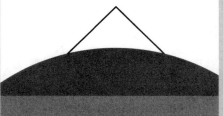

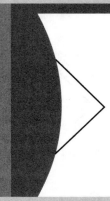

KNOWLEDGE

- Pathogenesis of pressure ulcers
- Factors contributing to pressure ulcer formation or poor wound healing
- Factors contributing to wound healing
- Impact of underlying disease process on skin integrity
- Impact of medication on skin integrity and wound healing

EXPERIENCE

- Caring for clients with wounds or impaired skin integrity
- Observation of normal wound healing

Assessment

- Identify Mrs. Stein's risk for developing impaired skin integrity
- Identify signs and symptoms associated with impaired skin integrity or poor wound healing
- Examine Mrs. Stein's skin for actual impairment in skin integrity

STANDARDS

- Apply intellectual standards of accuracy, relevance, completeness, and precision when obtaining the health history regarding skin integrity and wound management
- Apply agency and professional standards for prevention and management of pressure ulcers (e.g., AHCPR, RNAO)

QUALITIES

- Use discipline to obtain complete and correct assessment data regarding Mrs. Stein's skin or wound integrity
- Demonstrate responsibility for collecting appropriate specimens for diagnostic and laboratory tests related to wound management

CHAPTER 47   Critical Thinking Model for *Impaired Skin Integrity*
(page 306).

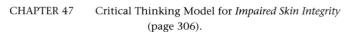

KNOWLEDGE

- Understand how a sensory deficit can affect Judy's functional status
- Understand the role other health professionals might have in sensory function management
- Services of community resources
- Adult learning principles to apply when educating Judy and her family

EXPERIENCE

- Previous client responses to planned nursing interventions to promote sensory function

Planning

- Select strategies that assist Judy to remain functional in her home
- Adapt therapies based on whether the sensory deficit is short or long term
- Involve the family in helping Judy adjust to her limitations
- Refer Judy to an appropriate health care professional and/or community agency

STANDARDS

- Individualize therapies that allow Judy to adapt to sensory loss in any setting
- Apply standards of safety

QUALITIES

- Use creativity to find interventions that help Judy adapt to home environment

CHAPTER 48   Critical Thinking Model for Nursing Care Plan for *Disturbed Sensory Perception* (page 312).

KNOWLEDGE

- Behaviours that demonstrate learning
- Characteristics of anxiety and/or fear
- Signs and symptoms or conditions that contraindicate surgery

EXPERIENCE

- Previous client responses to planned preoperative care
- Any personal experience Joe has had with surgery

Evaluation

- Evaluate Mrs. Campana's knowledge of the surgical procedure and planned postoperative care
- Have Mrs. Campana demonstrate postoperative exercises
- Observe behaviours or nonverbal expressions for anxiety or fear
- Ask if Mrs. Campana's expectation are being met

STANDARDS

- Use established expected outcomes to evaluate Mrs. Campana's response to care (e.g., the ability to perform postoperative exercises)

QUALITIES

- Demonstrate perseverance if Mrs. Campana has difficulty performing postoperative exercises

CHAPTER 49   Critical Thinking Model for Nursing Care Plan for *Deficient Knowledge Regarding Preoperative and Postoperative Care Requirements*
(page 321).